The Environmental, Public Health, and Human Rights Impacts on Enhancing the Quality of Life of People with Intellectual Disability

The Environmental, Public Health, and Human Rights Impacts on Enhancing the Quality of Life of People with Intellectual Disability

Editor

Laura Elisabet Gomez Sanchez

MDPI • Basel • Beijing • Wuhan • Barcelona • Belgrade • Manchester • Tokyo • Cluj • Tianjin

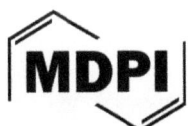

Editor
Laura Elisabet Gomez Sanchez
Psychology
Universidad de Oviedo
Oviedo
Spain

Editorial Office
MDPI
St. Alban-Anlage 66
4052 Basel, Switzerland

This is a reprint of articles from the Special Issue published online in the open access journal *International Journal of Environmental Research and Public Health* (ISSN 1660-4601) (available at: www.mdpi.com/journal/ijerph/special_issues/health_disability).

For citation purposes, cite each article independently as indicated on the article page online and as indicated below:

LastName, A.A.; LastName, B.B.; LastName, C.C. Article Title. *Journal Name* **Year**, *Volume Number*, Page Range.

ISBN 978-3-0365-1316-4 (Hbk)
ISBN 978-3-0365-1315-7 (PDF)

© 2021 by the authors. Articles in this book are Open Access and distributed under the Creative Commons Attribution (CC BY) license, which allows users to download, copy and build upon published articles, as long as the author and publisher are properly credited, which ensures maximum dissemination and a wider impact of our publications.

The book as a whole is distributed by MDPI under the terms and conditions of the Creative Commons license CC BY-NC-ND.

Contents

About the Editor vii

Robert L. Schalock, Ruth Luckasson and Karrie A. Shogren
Going beyond Environment to Context: Leveraging the Power of Context to Produce Change
Reprinted from: *International Journal of Environmental Research and Public Health* **2020**, *17*, 1885, doi:10.3390/ijerph17061885 1

Laura E. Gómez, Asunción Monsalve, Mª Lucía Morán, Mª Ángeles Alcedo, Marco Lombardi and Robert L. Schalock
Measurable Indicators of CRPD for People with Intellectual and Developmental Disabilities within the Quality of Life Framework
Reprinted from: *International Journal of Environmental Research and Public Health* **2020**, *17*, 5123, doi:10.3390/ijerph17145123 15

Michael L. Wehmeyer
The Importance of Self-Determination to the Quality of Life of People with Intellectual Disability: A Perspective
Reprinted from: *International Journal of Environmental Research and Public Health* **2020**, *17*, 7121, doi:10.3390/ijerph17197121 41

Eva Vicente, Cristina Mumbardó-Adam, Verónica M. Guillén, Teresa Coma-Roselló, María-Ángeles Bravo-Álvarez and Sergio Sánchez
Self-Determination in People with Intellectual Disability: The Mediating Role of Opportunities
Reprinted from: *International Journal of Environmental Research and Public Health* **2020**, *17*, 6201, doi:10.3390/ijerph17176201 49

Laura García-Domínguez, Patricia Navas, Miguel Ángel Verdugo and Víctor B. Arias
Chronic Health Conditions in Aging Individuals with Intellectual Disabilities
Reprinted from: *International Journal of Environmental Research and Public Health* **2020**, *17*, 3126, doi:10.3390/ijerph17093126 63

Kristel Vlot-van Anrooij, Thessa I.M. Hilgenkamp, Geraline L. Leusink, Anneke van der Cruijsen, Henk Jansen, Jenneken Naaldenberg and Koos van der Velden
Improving Environmental Capacities for Health Promotion in Support Settings for People with Intellectual Disabilities: Inclusive Design of the DIHASID Tool
Reprinted from: *International Journal of Environmental Research and Public Health* **2020**, *17*, 794, doi:10.3390/ijerph17030794 75

Laura Arcangeli, Alice Bacherini, Cristina Gaggioli, Moira Sannipoli and Giulia Balboni
Attitudes of Mainstream and Special-Education Teachers toward Intellectual Disability in Italy: The Relevance of Being Teachers
Reprinted from: *International Journal of Environmental Research and Public Health* **2020**, *17*, 7325, doi:10.3390/ijerph17197325 89

Juan Carlos García, Emiliano Díez, Dominika Z. Wojcik and Mónica Santamaría
Communication Support Needs in Adults with Intellectual Disabilities and Its Relation to Quality of Life
Reprinted from: *International Journal of Environmental Research and Public Health* **2020**, *17*, 7370, doi:10.3390/ijerph17207370 111

Víctor B. Arias, Antonio M. Amor, Miguel A. Verdugo, María Fernández, Benito Arias and Alba Aza
Toward a Better "Person–Environment Fit" through Items Calibration of the SIS-C
Reprinted from: *International Journal of Environmental Research and Public Health* **2020**, *17*, 3471, doi:10.3390/ijerph17103471 . . . . **127**

Carmen Francisco Mora, Alba Ibáñez and Anna Balcells-Balcells
State of the Art of Family Quality of Life in Early Care and Disability: A Systematic Review
Reprinted from: *International Journal of Environmental Research and Public Health* **2020**, *17*, 7220, doi:10.3390/ijerph17197220 . . . . **145**

Anna Balcells-Balcells, Joana M. Mas, Natasha Baqués, Cecilia Simón and Simón García-Ventura
The Spanish Family Quality of Life Scales under and over 18 Years Old: Psychometric Properties and Families' Perceptions
Reprinted from: *International Journal of Environmental Research and Public Health* **2020**, *17*, 7808, doi:10.3390/ijerph17217808 . . . . **161**

About the Editor

Laura Elisabet Gomez Sanchez

Laura E. Gómez, PhD, is an Associate Professor of Psychology at University of Oviedo (Spain) and a member of the Institute on Community Integration (INICO). She has received awards such as "Infanta Cristina"National and Iberoamerican Research Award, "Young Researcher Award on Ageing in Intellectual Disabilities"and "Saphiro Award"by IASSIDD, and International award by AAIDD. She is an AAIDD Fellow. She is Associate Editor of "Psicothema", editorial board member of "Siglo Cero"and "Clinica y Salud". Her research is mainly focused on quality of life scales of people with intellectual and developmental disabilities. She is a co-author of several instruments to assess quality of life-related personal outcomes for adults with intellectual disabilities (KidsLife Scale, Gencat Scale, INICO-FEAPS Scale, Fumat Scale, San Martin Scale, CAVIDACE Scale).

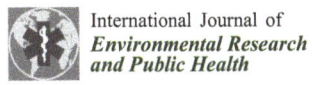

Article

Going beyond Environment to Context: Leveraging the Power of Context to Produce Change

Robert L. Schalock [1,*], Ruth Luckasson [2] and Karrie A. Shogren [3]

[1] Hastings College, Hastings, NE 68901, USA
[2] Department of Special Education, University of New Mexico, Albuquerque, NM 87106, USA; ruthl@unm.edu
[3] Kansas University Center on Developmental Disabilities, University of Kansas, Lawrence, KS 69703, USA; shogren@ku.edu
* Correspondence: rschalock@ultraplix.com

Received: 31 January 2020; Accepted: 11 March 2020; Published: 13 March 2020

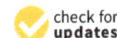

Abstract: This article discusses the processes and implications of going beyond environment to context. The article (a) provides an operational definition of context; (b) describes a multidimensional model of context that views context as being multilevel, multifactorial, and interactive; (c) describes how conceptual models of quality of life, human rights, and human functioning can be used in conjunction with the multidimensional model of context to identify opportunities and develop context-based change strategies that improve quality of life, human rights, and human functioning outcomes; and (d) describes a four-step approach to leveraging an understanding of context to produce change. The article concludes with a discussion of the advantages of and barriers to moving beyond environment to context.

Keywords: context; change strategies; conceptual models; human functioning; human rights; person–environment fit; quality of life; valued outcomes

---

1. Introduction and Overview

The functioning of individuals is highly influenced by their current situations. Historically, these situations were labeled as their "environments," and an individual's functioning was often described as the "person–environmental fit." The concept of person–environmental fit has been very instrumental in conceptualizing disability as resulting from the interaction between a person and their environment, and implementing the supports paradigm that focuses on reducing the discrepancy between an individual's capabilities and environmental requirements.

Despite this contribution, the concept of "person–environmental fit" is not sufficient to capture the totality of the circumstances that influence human functioning and valued outcomes. This is especially true given the significant international trends and developments impacting the disability field. These trends include (a) a commitment to the human and legal rights of persons with disabilities as reflected in the United Nations Convention on the Rights of Persons with Disabilities—UNCRPD [1–3]; (b) the influence of the social-ecological model of disability that emphasizes the interaction between individuals and the multiple factors at the micro-, meso-, and macrosystem that affect human functioning and personal outcomes [4]; (c) the transformative effects of the supports paradigm [5]; (d) the use of the quality of life concept as a framework for program and policy development and evaluation [6,7]; (e) the capacities approach to disability that emphasizes the core values of freedom and human dignity and the obligation of society to improve peoples' lives [8–11]; (f) the impact of positive psychology that shifts the emphasis in disability from defectology to optimum human functioning and well-being [12]; and (g) the use of outcomes evaluation to develop outcome indicators associated with quality of life, human rights, and human functioning [13–16].

Because of these significant trends and developments, it has become necessary to move beyond the "person–environment fit paradigm" to the "context paradigm" that focuses on the interrelated conditions that surround the phenomenon being examined. Once these contextual factors and influencing conditions are understood, individuals, organizations, systems, and policy makers are in a better position to use this understanding to pursue the many opportunities that multiple stakeholders have to unfreeze the status quo and drive change through policies and practices that build contexts to enhance quality of life, human rights, and human functioning outcomes [17–20].

The purpose of this article is to discuss the processes and implications of going beyond environment to context in reference to quality of life, human rights, and human functioning. In the article, we (a) provide an operational definition of context; (b) describe a multidimensional model of context that views context as being multilevel, multifactorial, and interactive; (c) describe how conceptual models of quality of life, human rights, and human functioning can be used in conjunction with a multidimensional conceptual model of context to guide the identification of opportunities and the development of context-based change strategies that enhance personal/valued outcomes; (d) describe a four-step approach to leveraging an understanding of context to produce change; and (e) discuss the advantages of and barriers to moving beyond environment to context.

2. Operational Definition of Context

The concept of context allows one to capture more of the complexity in the lives and functions of individuals by incorporating the micro-, meso-, and macrosystems, as well as multiple factors and interactions that influence outcomes. We define context as *"a concept that integrates the totality of circumstances that comprise the milieu of human life and human functioning"* [21] and propose that context can be viewed as an independent variable, an intervening variable, and an integrative construct.

- As an *independent variable*, context includes personal and environmental characteristics that are not usually manipulated, such as age, language, culture and ethnicity, gender, and family.
- As an *intervening variable*, context includes organizations, systems, and societal policies and practices that can be manipulated to enhance human functioning and personal outcomes.
- As an *integrative concept*, context provides a framework for (a) describing and analyzing aspects of human functioning such as personal and environmental factors, planning systems of supports, and developing disability policy; and (b) delineating the factors that affect, both positively and negatively, human functioning.

3. A Multidimensional Model of Context

Based on our most recent work [22] we have developed a multidimensional model of context that is shown in Figure 1. This multidimensional model conceptualizes context as being multilevel, multifactorial, and interactive. Each of these components is described next.

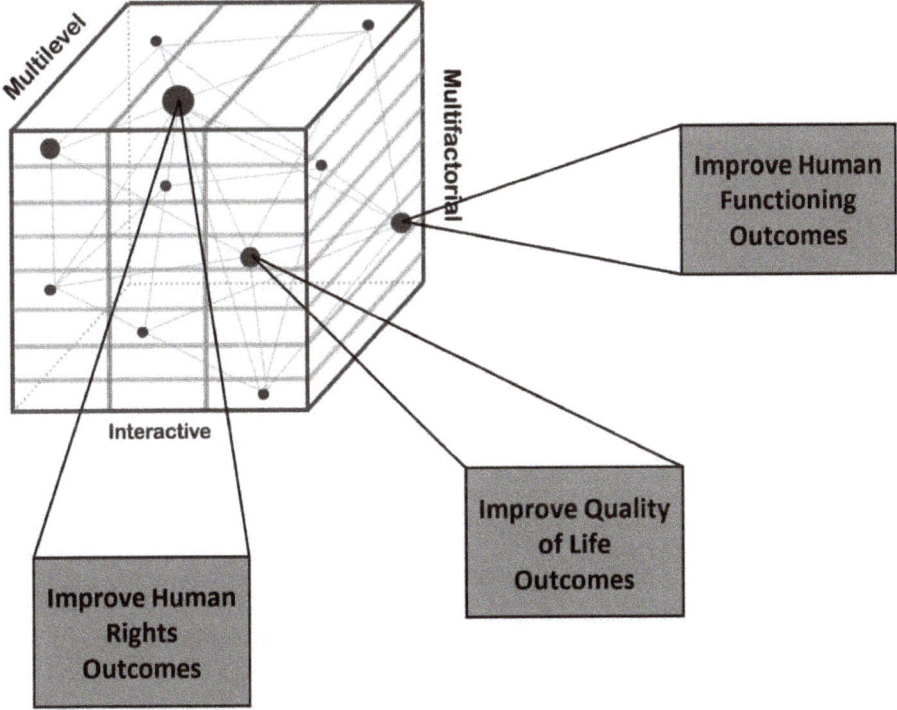

Figure 1. A Multidimensional Model of Context.

3.1. Multilevel

This component of the multidimensional model identifies and describes the ecological systems within which people live, are educated, work, and recreate. The person and these environments interact over time and thereby influence personal outcomes differentially over time. The *micro level* typically includes immediate social settings, such as the person's family, close friends, and advocates. The *meso level* typically includes one's neighborhood and community, and the organizations providing services and supports. The *macro level* typically includes the larger policy context and supports delivery system, and the overarching pattern of culture, society, country, or social-political influences [23].

3.2. Multifactorial

This component of the model identifies and describes the potentially influential factors within the ecological systems within which people live, are educated, work, and recreate. Some of these factors (e.g., age, language, culture and ethnicity, and family structure) are not typically manipulated or changed to enhance outcomes, but need to be understood in order to identify opportunities and develop context-based change strategies. Other contextually based influencing factors can be manipulated or changed to achieve policy goals and enhance personal outcomes. Based on the authors' work to date, Table 1 lists a number of these contextually-based factors that influence outcomes related to quality of life, human rights, and and/or human functioning.

Table 1. Factors that influence quality of life, human rights, and/or human functioning outcomes.

Microsystem Level	Mesosystem Level	Macrosystem Level
-Personal strengths/assets -Health condition -Limitations in intellectual functioning and/or adaptive behavior -Social networks -Family involvement -Choices/opportunities -Decision making supports -Self-advocacy -Augmentative communication systems -Information and assistive technology devices -Natural supports	-Alignment of services and supports to personal goals and assessed support needs -Person-centered planning -User-friendly personal support plans -Environmental accommodation -Organization policies that emphasize improved quality of life, human rights, and/or human functioning.	-Opportunities for increased interdependence, productivity, and community integration -Community access and participation -Community-based alternatives -Living and employment supports -Justice and fairness in the legal system -Legal rights and protections -Transportation availability -Societal attitudes, public policies, and system practices

3.3. Interactive

This component of the multidimensional model of context identifies and describes the variety of ways in which levels and factors interact to influence personal outcomes. *An interaction is a reciprocal action or influence that occurs between multilevel and multifactor contextual variables.* These interactions are denoted by dots in Figure 1, and vary in size depending on their relevance and importance to an individual. The dots also represent a *connection point* between the three elements of the multidimensional model of context (multilevel, multifactor, and interaction) with parallel elements of quality of life, human rights, and human functioning conceptual models (to be described in the following section). *These connection points allow service/supports providers and consumers to successfully leverage an understanding of context to identify opportunities and develop change strategies to improve quality of life, human rights, and/or human functioning outcomes* [24].

In the following section, we describe the elements of conceptual models related to quality of life, human rights, and human functioning, and align these elements to the elements of the multidimensional model of context presented in Figure 1. Based on this alignment and an understanding of context, policy makers, service/support providers, and consumers can identify opportunities and develop context-based change strategies to improve quality of life, human rights, and human functioning outcomes. In Section 6 we explain a four-step approach that facilitates this process.

4. Conceptual Models That Facilitate the Identification of Opportunities and the Development of Context-Based Change Strategies

Identifying opportunities and selecting context-based change strategies to improve quality of life, human rights, and human functioning outcomes is facilitated by using a conceptual model of each of these three targeted areas. A conceptual model is a representation of a phenomenon, such as quality of life, human rights, or human functioning, and incorporates context-based concepts that are used to help people understand the phenomenon and use that understanding to bring about change. As used in this article, the major purposes of a conceptual model are to (a) organize and synthesize information about quality of life, human rights, and human functioning that will facilitate identifying opportunities to improve personal outcomes; and (b) guide the selection of context-based change strategies to enhance this goal. The use of a clearly articulated conceptual model also facilitates integrating theoretical perspectives on intellectual disability that include biomedical, psychoeducational, sociocultural, and justice [25], selecting relevant evidence-based strategies [26,27] and defining operational disability-related constructs and associated outcome measures [22].

A conceptual model can be research based (as in the case of the quality of life and human functioning models) or a consensus document (such as the *United Nations Convention on the Rights of Persons with Disabilities*; UNCRPD). Examples of each, including their key features, are presented next.

4.1. Quality of Life Conceptual Model

The concept of quality of life (QOL) has emerged internationally as a value-based framework for opportunity development, supports provision, and outcomes evaluation [28]. Although QOL is defined and conceptualized in multiple ways, two conceptual models are frequently referenced. The first is that proposed by the World Health Organization that conceptualizes quality of life as a multidimensional phenomenon encompassing physical, mental, and social functioning and well-being [7]. The six core QOL dimensions operationalizing this conceptual model are physical health, psychological state, level of independence, social relationships, environment (e.g., financial resources and opportunities), and spirituality or religion or personal beliefs. The second commonly referenced QOL conceptual model is that proposed by Schalock, Verdugo, Gomez, and Renders [29]. These authors/investigators conceptualize QOL as a multidimensional phenomenon that is composed of domains that reflect one's personal well-being. These domains include personal development, self-determination, interpersonal relations, social inclusion, rights, emotional well-being, physical well-being, and material well-being. These domains are influenced by systems of supports (i.e., choice and personal autonomy, inclusive environments, generic supports, and specialized supports) that can act as moderators or mediators in influencing QOL outcomes [30].

Quality of life dimensions/domains and supports interact due to the reciprocal action or influence that occurs between multilevel and multifactorial contextual variables. Specifically:

- *Multilevel factors* influence QOL outcomes at the micro-level through factors such as personal and family attitudes and expectations about the person's disability, strengths, and limitations, and the availability of resources, services, and supports. At the meso level, QOL outcomes are affected by legislative and statutory opportunities and systems of supports provided at the community level. At the macro level, QOL outcomes are influenced by societal and cultural concepts of disability, with associated stereotypes and attitudes, and the resources a society devotes to quality of life enhancement.
- *Multifactors* influence QOL outcomes through the influencing factors listed in Table 1 and the provision of systems of supports. As summarized in Table 1, these contextually based influencing factors can occur at the micro-, meso-, and/or macrosystem level.
- *Interactions* occur between multilevels and multifactors and affect QOL outcomes through (a) *quality of life* facilitating conditions, such as participation in the community, promoting a sense of belonging, maximizing capabilities, freedom to engage in major life activities, commitment to goals that are important to the person or family, and respect for and enhancement of differences; and (b) *support facilitating conditions*, such as the availability and accessibility of supports, safe and secure environments, information about systems of support, competent support providers, consistency of supports provision, coordination and management of supports, and collaboration among professionals and support providers.

The alignment of the quality of life conceptual model with the multilevel, multifactor, and interactive elements of the multidimensional model of context depicted in Figure 1 can be used to (a) identify opportunities related to enhancing quality of life by understanding the multiple systems that affects one's quality of life, the multiple factors that impact one's QOL, and how multiple-levels and multiple factors interact in terms of quality of life and support facilitating conditions; and (b) to develop context-based change strategies to enhance one's quality of life. Specific details about this process are discussed in Section 6.

4.2. Human Rights Model

A human rights conceptual model based on the *United Nations Convention of the Rights of Persons with Disabilities* provides the framework to identify opportunities and develop context-based strategies to maximize peoples' human rights [2,3,31,32]. The convention calls for a fundamental reappraisal of policy and practice by society, governments, members of professional and voluntary organizations, service and support providers, and individuals regarding peoples' human and legal rights. The parameters of the UNCRPD can be aligned with the multiple elements of the multidimensional model of context presented in Figure 1. Specifically:

- *Multilevels* are reflected in the obligations that signatories are committed to. These obligations involve modification or repeal of laws, customs, and practices that discriminate directly or indirectly against people with disabilities; inclusion of disability in all relevant policies; reframing any practice inconsistent with the UNCRPD; consulting with people with disabilities and their organizations in implementing the UNCRPD; and making "reasonable accommodation" to all relevant aspects of the environment so as to enable people with disabilities to exercise their rights.
- *Multifactors* are reflected in the convention's General Principles that encompass respect for inherent dignity and individual autonomy; equality and nondiscrimination; full and active participation and inclusion in society; respect for differences and acceptance of persons with disabilities as part of humanity; accountability; equality between men and women; and respect for the evolving capabilities of children with disabilities and the right to preserve their identities.
- *Interactions* that occur between these multilevels and multifactors have been selected and mandated by the international community to promote the articles identified in the UNCRPD. These convention articles/outcomes relate to equality and non-discrimination (Article 5), accessibility (Article 9), right to life (Article 10), equal recognition before the law (Article 12), liberty and security of person (Article 14), freedom from exploitation, violence, and abuse (Article 16), liberty of movement and nationality (Article 18), living independently and being included in the community (Article 19), personal mobility (Article 20), freedom of expression and opinion and access to information (Article 21), respect for privacy (Article 22), education (Article 24), health (Article 25), habilitation and rehabilitation (Article 26), work and employment (Article 27), adequate standards of living and social protection (Article 28), and participation in political and public life (Article 29).

Parallel with the quality of life conceptual model, the human rights conceptual model described above aligns elements of the UNCRPD with the element of the multidimensional model of context depicted in Figure 1. This alignment can be used to identify opportunities and develop context-based change strategies to maximize peoples' human rights. As described in Section 6, this involves targeting the signatories' obligations, the UNCRPD general principles, and the convention's articles.

4.3. Human Functioning Conceptual Model

The human functioning conceptual model described in this article has it origin in the *International Classification of Functioning, Disability, and Health* [33]. That model, which is based on a definition of health as a state of complete physical, mental, and social well-being, conceived human functioning as an interactive person–environmental process, and disability as problems in functioning. Furthermore, the ICF model viewed human functioning as resulting from the complex interactions among health conditions (disease and disorder), body structures and functions (impairments), activities (activity limitations), participation (participation restrictions), environmental factors (barriers, hindrances), and personal factors. In the model, personal and environmental factors were referred to as "contextual factors" [34].

The human functioning model presented below is a logical extension of the ICF model and incorporates recent work in (a) operationalizing health in terms of human functioning, and (b) applying a human functioning approach to disability. In reference to operationalizing health in terms of human functioning, Stucki and Bickenbach advocate using the concept of human functioning as a measureable indicator of health [16]. Such use, according to the authors, clarifies, conceptually and quantitatively, the link between health and well-being. Building on the ICF model, the authors explain (p. 1790) how functioning is understood biochemically and in terms of the functions and structures of the body and the intrinsic health capacity of a person to perform simple and complex activities, as well as the actual performance of those activities in interaction with features of the person's physical and social environments [16].

In reference to applying a human functioning approach to disability, Luckasson and Schalock defined such an approach as involving "a systems perspective towards understanding human functioning that includes human functioning dimensions, interactive systems of supports, and human functioning outcomes" [35]. From a systems or logic model perspective, the human functioning conceptual model is operationalized through its *input component*, which includes the human functioning dimensions of intellectual functioning, adaptive behavior, health, participation, and context; its *throughput component* that incorporates systems of supports; and its *output component* that encompasses human functioning outcomes related to socio-economic status, health status, and subjective well-being. These outcome categories encompass both the six dimensions of the WHO-QOL Scales (WHO, 1997), and the eight domains of the Schalock et al. QOL model discussed earlier [29]. The human functioning conceptual model presented in this article (a) is consistent with the model incorporated into the 10th and 11th editions of the American Association on Intellectual and Developmental Disabilities Terminology and Classification Manuals [36,37]; and (b) reflects our increased understanding of the multidimensionality of human functioning and the significant progress in our understanding of support strategies and outcomes evaluation [4,28].

As with the QOL and human rights conceptual models described previously, components of the human functioning model described above can be aligned with the three elements of the multidimensional model of context depicted in Figure 1. Specifically:

- *Multilevels* encompass the individual, community and service/support organizations, and governments and society.
- *Multifactors* relate to the individual's status vis-à-vis intellectual functioning, adaptive behavior, health, participation, and context, and the level and type of supports available to the individual [32,34].
- *Interactions* occur between the multiple levels and multiple factors listed above. Human functioning is improved when interactions are targeted and supported across levels and factors.

5. Using the Multidimensional Model of Context to Identify Opportunities and Developi Context-Based Change Strategies

In this section of the article we describe in more detail how an understanding of elements of a multidimensional model of context and analogous elements of a conceptual model of quality of life, human rights, or human functioning can be used to identify opportunities and develop context-based change strategies. As depicted in Figure 1 and described in Table 1, opportunities result from the interaction of the *ecological systems* within which people live, learn, work, and recreate, and the *context-based influencing factors* within these ecological systems. The better one understands these systems, factors and conceptual models, the more able one is to identify opportunities and develop context-based strategies to improve peoples' quality of life, human rights, and human functioning outcomes.

5.1. Identifying Opportunities

The interactive property of context was depicted in Figure 1 as "dots" of various sizes, which reflect the potential relevance to a proposed change, and the importance of the specific interaction to an individual. Each dot also represents a *connection point* between the elements of the multidimensional model of context and respective elements of a quality of life, human rights, or human functioning conceptual model. These interactions create the opportunities for intervention and change. Examples include increasing one's social inclusion in school, increasing opportunities to live independently in the community, or improving one's health status.

Once these opportunities for change are identified, they need to be evaluated as to whether (a) they reflect the person's values, personal goals, and personal desires; (b) are examined as to their cultural relevance and technical feasibility; and (c) consistent with policy goals that have a high priority for a society or organization. As described next, once these opportunities are identified, specific context-based support strategies can be developed to produce change.

5.2. Developing Context-Based Change Strategies

A specific interaction (i.e., "opportunity") can be systematically influenced and changed by manipulating one or more contextually-based influencing factors. Context-based change strategies may involve multiple change mechanisms, such as adding systems of supports elements, advocating for policy changes, or changing personal circumstances and skills. Examples include (a) legislative changes over the last two decades that have strengthened the relation between supported employment initiatives (factor at the macro level) and organizations implementing supported employment opportunities (factor at the mesosystem); (b) the introduction of decision making supports legislation (factor at the macro-level) with the implementation of a new research-based program for supported decision making (meso-level), which has increased decisions being made by the individual with a disability rather than decisions being made for the person (factor at the micro level); and (c) living in a country where the UNCRPD has been adopted and where there is a commitment to the inherent dignity and human rights of people with disabilities through rights-centered policies and practices, community-based services and supports, high quality health services, and the provision of individualized systems of supports. The context-based change strategy or strategies selected should be based on:

- A contextual analysis that identifies factors that hinder change and forces that facilitate change, and a context-based change model that approaches changes from the perspective of a quality improvement loop that involves analysis, planning, doing, and evaluation [24,38,39].
- An understanding of the contextually-based factors that influence personal outcomes (see Table 1 for examples).
- The multilevel/multifactor parameters of the previously discussed multidimensional model of context and the quality of life, human rights, and human functioning conceptual models.

The following section describes a four-step systematic approach that can be used to develop context-based change strategies that leverage an understanding of context to produce change. The approach involves identifying a needed change, identifying interactions, identifying the levels and factors influencing the opportunity for change, and developing a context-based strategy.

6. A Four-Step Approach to Leveraging an Understanding of Context to Produce Change

6.1. Step 1: Identify a Desired and Needed Change

This first step involves identifying, in collaboration with the person, a needed change (which represents "an opportunity") in the person's life, an organization or community's ability to support people, or a government's desire to provide supports. Using a conceptual model such as that described previously on context, quality of life, human rights, or human functioning facilitates this first step. Specifically, and as described previously in reference to each conceptual model, the alignment of elements of the respective conceptual model with the multilevel, multifactor, and interactive elements of the multidimensional model of context (see Figure 1) allows one to identify interactions (see Step 2) and potential contextual factors influencing the opportunity for change (see Step 3)

6.2. Step 2: Identify Interactions That Potentially Influence Desired or Needed Change

This step focuses on "opportunity development" and requires the analysis of the reciprocal action or influence that occur between multilevel and multifactor contextual variables. Conceptual models, such as those for quality of life, human rights, and human functioning, are also useful in this step both to help individuals, service/ support providers, and policy makers develop context-based change strategies and to select outcome indicators to evaluate the current attainment level of the identified needed/desired change [14,40].

Interactions are denoted by dots in Figure 1, and vary in size depending on their relevance to the proposed change and importance to the individual, organization, community, or society. The dots also represent a connection point between the three elements of the multidimensional model of context with parallel elements of the quality of life, human rights, and human functioning conceptual models described previously. As part of the identification process, potential targeted interactions should be examined as to their cultural relevance and technical feasibility and their consistency with policy goals that have a high priority for an organization or society. The interactions identified for needed change should also be based on "the voice of the person" and reflect the individual's values, personal goals, and personal desires.

6.3. Step 3: Identify the Levels and Factors Influencing the Opportunity for Change

Levels and factors influencing an opportunity/desired change can be identified either by using Table 1 that summarizes literature-based systems-level contextual factors that influence personal outcomes, or by analyzing the multilevel and multifactor elements described previously that are associated with a quality of life, human rights, or human functioning conceptual model. The identified levels and factors are considered as intervening variables that can be manipulated to produce change [21], and act as moderator or mediator variables in the production of change [29]. Examples include (a) micro-system level factors, such as personal strengths/assets, choices/opportunities, and the availability of systems of supports; (b) meso-system level factors, such as organization policies and practices; and (c) macro-system level factors, such as community access and participation, community-based alternatives, living and employment supports, justice and fairness in the legal system, and societal attitudes, public policies, and system practices.

6.4. Step 4: Develop a Context-Based Change Strategy

Selecting a context-based change strategy follows the identification of the levels and factors influencing the opportunity for desired change. Context-based change strategies are used to bring about change in the desired interaction/needed change area. Potential change strategies are also selected based on their potential to promote adoption and increase stakeholder participation. These strategies typically involve disability policy changes, organization transformation strategies, and/or providing systems of supports.

- *Disability policy changes* involve *an integrated approach* to disability policy development, implementation, and evaluation [41], and *a cross-cultural approach* that uses a contextual analysis, emphasizes a value-based approach, aligns the service delivery system both horizontally and vertically, and engages in a partnership in policy implementation [42].
- *Organization transformation* involves *transformation pillars* that include values, self-evaluation, critical thinking skills, and innovation, and *transformation strategies* that include analyzing environments, aligning organization practices, incorporating a balanced approach to performance management, integrating ecological systems, and employing strategic execution [39].
- *Systems of supports* emphasize the provision of supports that involve choice and personal autonomy, inclusive environments, generic supports, and specialized supports [4].

Table 2 shows how the four steps just described can be aligned to bring about desired change in quality of life, human rights, and human functioning outcomes.

Table 2. The four-step approach to bring about change.

Identified Needed Change (Step 1)	Identified Multilevel and Multifactor Interactions and Influencing Factors (Steps 2 and 3)	Selected Context-Based Change Strategies (Step 4)
Increase social inclusion in school (quality of life)	-Micro level: attitudes of peers without disabilities (interpersonal level) -Meso level: degree to which the school's leadership prioritizes social inclusion (organization level)	-Implement a program that promotes social inclusion of students with disabilities at multiple levels using a school-wide approach
Increased opportunity to live independently and being included in the community (UNCRPD Article 19)	-Macro level: restrictive laws and customs regarding persons with disabilities -Meso level: lack of community-based residential options and living supports	-Modify housing codes -Work with professionals and self-advocates to demonstrate strengths and capacities -Implement community living options -Provide systems of supports (e.g., "supported living")
Improve health status (human functioning)	-Meso level: poor access to health care system -Micro level: lifestyle and health related beliefs that are incompatible with proper nutrition	-Interface person with the health care system (e.g., community clinic) -Provide information and monitoring about proper nutrition -Establish a productive interaction between the person and the community clinic to monitor nutrition and lifestyle changes

7. The Advantages of and Barriers to Going beyond Environment to Context

7.1. Advantages

Thus far in this article, we have (a) described how a multidimensional model of context can be used to identify opportunities for needed change and implement context-based change strategies; (b) applied this heuristic to the areas of quality of life, human rights, and human functioning; and (c) outlined a four-step approach to leveraging an understanding of context to produce desired change. Although each of these activities is potentially complex since they involve new concepts and terminology that require both changing one's thinking and understanding the multidimensional properties of context, going beyond environment to context has definite advantages to the field. Chief among these are that the approach to context described in this article provides:

- A broader and more complete picture of the complexities of the lives of people with disability.
- A challenge to the field to systematically explore contextually-based levels and factors that influence human functioning and valued personal outcomes.
- An understanding of the power and importance of the interaction (i.e., reciprocal action or influence) that occurs between multilevel and multifactor contextual variables.
- An analytic framework for identifying and prioritizing opportunities for desired or needed change, and context-based change strategies that honor and reflect the complexities of people's lives.
- A systematic approach that is transparent to all parties and facilitates replication and application.

7.2. Barriers

Barriers will be encountered by those advocates, policy makers, practitioners, or researchers who either want to apply the approach to context described in this article, or to extend the systematic approach described to areas other than quality of life, human rights, and human functioning. These barriers potentially relate to (a) the requirement that people who "are committed to" the person–environment model will need to broaden their perspective; (b) the complexity of the contextual analyses used to identify and understand reciprocal interactions; (c) the required participation of more individuals who can contribute to the more complex analyses; (d) the need to understand international trends and developments, such as the UNCRPD, social-ecological model of disability, support paradigm and systems of supports, QOL concept and its application, capacities approach, and outcomes evaluation; (e) the potential exposure of decision making processes that were previously more private; and (f) the need to prepare and support people so that they can effectively participate in the four-step approach to leveraging an understanding of context to produce change.

As stressed by one of the Reviewers, a significant challenge of going beyond environment to context is to overcome the "operationalization hurdle" faced by previous approaches, such as the person–environmental fit concept, the capacities approach, or the social-ecological model of disability. The advantage and contribution of the multidimensional model of context presented in Figure 1 and discussed in this article is that an understanding of the multilevel, multifactor, and interactive properties of context provides an *operationalization framework* to describe and analyze the impact of personal and environmental factors on valued outcomes, including those related to quality of life, human rights, and human functioning. As discussed more fully in Gomez et al., Schalock, Gomez et al., and Schalock, Verdugo et al., five steps are involved in developing and implementing an operationalization framework [26,27,29]. First, define the practices in question. Exemplary practices were identified in Table 1 in reference to contextually based factors that influence quality of life, human rights, and human functioning outcomes. Second, select outcome areas and outcome indicators. This step involves incorporating commonly used outcome areas, such as quality of life domains, human rights areas, and human functioning dimensions, and relating the specific outcome areas to measurable outcome indicators that can be assessed in reliable and valid ways. Third, gather evidence. Evidence gathering involves (a) employing an evidence-gathering strategy that is consistent with the question(s) asked, the practices being evaluated, statutory/regulatory parameters, the constituents involved, and the available expertise; (b) defining operationally the strategies; and (c) demonstrating implementation fidelity. Fourth, establish the credibility of the evidence, which involves evaluating the obtained evidence in terms of its quality, robustness, and relevance. Fifth, evaluate the relation between practice(s) and outcome(s). This final step requires determining if there is substantial evidence that the outcome was caused by the practice; it has been demonstrated that the intervention clearly leads to the outcome, and/or the intervention has a plausible rationale to explain why it should work and with whom.

Although these barriers may be seen as daunting and pose significant challenges, they also represent opportunities to use an understanding of context to unfreeze the status quo and drive change to enhance valued quality of life, human rights, and human functioning outcomes for people with disabilities. Overcoming these barriers is also a primary responsibility of disability organizations and systems as they continue their efforts to provide services and supports that enhance valued outcomes for people with disabilities and their families. To these ends, we offer the following guidelines. First, clearly identify the targeted area (i.e., "the phenomenon under consideration"). Second, integrate the elements or components of a valid conceptual model of the phenomenon under consideration with the multilevel, multifactor, and interactive elements of the multidimensional model of context presented in Figure 1. This will allow one to identify multilevel, multifactor, and interactive elements that can be used to select opportunities for desired change, and the factors influencing the effectiveness of the context-based change strategies selected and implemented. Third, use a systematic approach, such as the previously described four-step process, to leverage an understanding of context to produce change. Fourth, evaluate the change produced. The evaluation should focus on the status of the identified needed change (see Table 2 for examples), and incorporate the five-steps involved in the operationalization framework described above.

8. Conclusions

In conclusion, the field of disability in general, and the field of intellectual and developmental disability specifically, has gone beyond the person–environment paradigm to a multidimensional contextual paradigm with its related terminology and application. This shift is in line with current international trends and developments and the ongoing realities of the lives of people with a disability that involve multiple levels, factors, and interactions that either facilitate or hinder change in their lives. The multidimensional aspects of context need to be understood in order to unfreeze the status quo and drive valued change through policies and practices that build contexts to improve quality of life, human rights, and human functioning outcomes. As reflected in this article, "it is not just about environment anymore".

Author Contributions: Conceptualization, R.L.S., R.L. and K.A.S.; methodology, R.L.S., R.L. and K.A.S.; writing—original draft preparation, R.L.S.; writing—review and editing, R.L. and K.A.S. All authors have read and agreed to the published version of the manuscript.

Funding: This research received no external funding.

Conflicts of Interest: The authors declare no conflict of interest.

References

1. Karr, V.L. A life of quality: Informing the UN Convention on the Rights of Persons with Disabilities. *J. Disabil. Policy Stud.* **2011**, *22*, 67–82. [CrossRef]
2. Mittler, P. The UN Convention on the Rights of Persons with Disabilities: Implementing a paradigm shift. *J. Policy Pract. Intellect. Disabil.* **2015**, *12*, 79–89. [CrossRef]
3. United Nations. Convention on the Rights of Persons with Disabilities. 2006. Available online: http://www.un.org/disabilities/convention/conventionfull.shtmc (accessed on 23 October 2019).
4. Schalock, R.L.; Luckasson, R.; Tasse, M.J. The contemporary view of intellectual and developmental disabilities; Implications for psychologists. *Psicothema* **2019**, *31*, 223–228. [PubMed]
5. Thompson, J.R.; Schalock, R.L.; Agosta, J.; Tenintry, J.; Fortune, J. How the supports paradigm is transforming service systems for persons with intellectual disability and related developmental disabilities. *Inclusion* **2014**, *2*, 86–99. [CrossRef]
6. Schalock, R.L.; Keith, K.D. *Cross-Cultural Quality of Life: Enhancing the Lives of Persons with Intellectual Disability*, 2nd ed.; American Association on Intellectual and Developmental Disabilities: Washington, DC, USA, 2016.
7. World Health Organization. *Measuring Quality of Life: The WHO Quality of Life Instruments*; World Health Organization: Geneva, Switzerland, 1997.
8. Nussbaum, M.C. *Creating Capabilities: The Human Development Approach*; Belknap Press of Harvard University: Cambridge, MA, USA, 2011.
9. Sen, A. *Development as Freedom*; Oxford University Press: New York, NY, USA, 1999.
10. Sen, A. Why health equity? *Health Econ.* **2002**, *11*, 659–666. [CrossRef] [PubMed]
11. Venkatapuram, S. *Health Justice: An Argument from the Capacities Approach*; John Wiley and Sons: Hoboken, NJ, USA, 2013.
12. Wehmeyer, M.L.; Shogren, K.A. Positive psychology and a quality of life agenda. In *Cross-Cultural Quality of Life: Enhancing the Lives of People with Intellectual Disability*; Schalock, R.L., Keith, K.D., Eds.; American Association on Intellectual and Developmental Disabilities: Washington, DC, USA, 2016; pp. 143–148.
13. Claes, C.; Vandebussche, H.; Lombardi, M. Human rights and quality of life domains: Identifying cross-cultural indicators. In *Cross-Cultural Quality of Life: Enhancing the Lives of People with Intellectual Disability*; Schalock, R.L., Keith, K.D., Eds.; American Association on Intellectual and Developmental Disabilities: Washington, DC, USA, 2016; pp. 167–174.
14. Gomez, L.E.; Verdugo, M.A. Outcomes evaluation. In *Cross-Cultural Quality of Life: Enhancing the Lives of People with Intellectual Disability*, 2nd ed.; Schalock, R.L., Keith, K.D., Eds.; American Association on Intellectual and Developmental Disabilities: Washington, DC, USA, 2016; pp. 71–80.
15. Organization for Economic Cooperation and Development. Better Life Initiative: Compendium of OECD Well-Being Indicators. Available online: http://www.oecd.org/sdd/47917288.pdf (accessed on 28 February 2020).
16. Stucki, G.; Bickenbach, J. Health, functioning, and well-being: Individual and societal. *Arch. Phys. Med. Rehabil.* **2019**, *100*, 1788–1792. [CrossRef]
17. Shogren, K.A.; Luckasson, R.; Schalock, R.L. Using context as an integrative framework to align policy goals, supports, and outcomes in intellectual disability. *Intellect. Dev. Disabil.* **2015**, *53*, 367–376. [CrossRef]

18. Shogren, K.A.; Schalock, R.L.; Luckasson, R. The use of a context-based change model to unfreeze the status quo and drive change to enhance personal outcomes of people with intellectual and developmental disabilities. *J. Policy Pract. Intellect. Disabil.* **2018**, *15*, 101–109. [CrossRef]
19. Simplican, S.C.; Leader, G.; Kosciulek, J.; Leahy, M. Defining social inclusion of people with intellectual and developmental disabilities: An ecological model of social networks and community participation. *Res. Dev. Disabil.* **2015**, *38*, 18–29. [CrossRef]
20. Siperstein, G.N.; McDowell, E.D.; Jacobs, H.E.; Stokes, J.E.; Cahn, A.L. Unified extracurricular activities as a pathway to social inclusion in high schools. *Am. J. Intellect. Dev. Disabil.* **2019**, *124*, 568–582. [CrossRef]
21. Shogren, K.A.; Luckasson, R.; Schalock, R.L. The definition of context and its application in the field of intellectual disability. *J. Policy Pract. Intellect. Disabil.* **2014**, *11*, 109–116. [CrossRef]
22. Schalock, R.L.; Luckasson, R. Intellectual disability, developmental disabilities, and the field of intellectual and developmental disabilities. In *Handbook of Intellectual and Developmental Disabilities*; Glidden, L.M., Abbeduto, L.J., McIntyre, L.L., Tasse, M.J., Eds.; American Psychological Association: Washington, DC, USA, 2007.
23. Bronfenbrenner, U. *The Ecology of Human Development: Experiments by Nature and Design*; Harvard University Press: Cambridge, MA, USA, 1999.
24. Shogren, K.A.; Luckasson, R.; Schalock, R.L. Using a multidimensional model to analyze context and enhance personal outcomes. *Intellect. Dev. Disabil.*. stage of publication.
25. Schalock, R.L.; Luckasson, R.; Tasse, M.J.; Verdugo, M.A. A holistic theoretical approach to intellectual disability: Going beyond the four current perspectives. *Intellect. Dev. Disabil.* **2018**, *56*, 79–89. [CrossRef] [PubMed]
26. Schalock, R.L.; Gomez, L.E.; Verdugo, M.A. Evidence-based practices in the field of intellectual and developmental disabilities: An international consensus approach. *Eval. Program Plan.* **2011**, *34*, 79–89. [CrossRef] [PubMed]
27. Schalock, R.L.; Gomez, L.E.; Verdugo, M.A.; Claes, C. Evidence and evidence-based practices: Are we there yet? *Intellect. Dev. Disabil.* **2017**, *55*, 112–119. [CrossRef]
28. Schalock, R.L.; Verdugo, M.A. International developments influencing the field of intellectual and developmental disabilities. In *Cross-Cultural Psychology: Contemporary Themes and Perspectives*; Keith, K.D., Ed.; Wiley Blackwell: Hoboken, NJ, USA, 2019; pp. 309–323.
29. Schalock, R.L.; Verdugo, M.A.; Gomez, L.E.; Reinders, H.S. Moving us toward a theory of individual quality of life. *Am. J. Intellect. Dev. Disabil.* **2016**, *121*, 1–12. [CrossRef] [PubMed]
30. Gomez, L.E.; Schalock, R.L.; Verdugo, M.A. The role of moderators and mediators in implementing and evaluating intellectual and developmental disabilities-related policies and practices. *J. Dev. Phys. Disabil.* **2019**. [CrossRef]
31. Lombardi, M.; Vandenbussche, H.; Claes, C.; Schalock, R.L.; De Maeyer, J. The concept of quality of life as a framework for implementing the UNCRPD. *J. Policy Pract. Intellect. Disabil.* **2019**. [CrossRef]
32. Verdugo, M.A.; Navas, P.; Gomez, L.E.; Schalock, R.L. The concept of quality of life and its role in enhancing human rights in the field of intellectual disability. *J. Intellect. Disabil. Res.* **2012**, *56*, 1036–1045. [CrossRef]
33. World Health Organization. *International Classification of Functioning, Disability, and Health (ICF)*; World Health Organization: Geneva, Switzerland, 2001.
34. Buntinx, W.H.E. The relationship between WHO-ICF and the AAMR-2002 system. In *What Is Mental Retardation? Ideas for an Evolving Disability in the 21st Century*; Switzky, H., Greenspan, G., Eds.; American Association on Mental Retardation: Washington, DC, USA, 2006; pp. 303–323.
35. Luckasson, R.; Schalock, R.L. Defining and applying a functionality approach to intellectual disability. *J. Intellect. Disabil. Res.* **2013**, *57*, 657–668. [CrossRef]
36. Luckasson, R.; Borthwick-Duffy, S.A.; Buntinx, W.; Coulter, D.; Craig, P.; Reeves, A.; Tasse, M.J. *Mental Retardation: Definition, Classification, and Systems of Supports*, 9th ed.; American Association on Mental Retardation: Washington, DC, USA, 2002.
37. Schalock, R.L.; Borthwick-Duffy, S.A.; Bradley, V.J.; Buntinx, W.H.E.; Coulter, D.L.; Craig, E.M.; Yaeger, M. *Intellectual Disability: Diagnosis, Classification, and Systems of Supports*, 11th ed.; American Association on Intellectual and Developmental Disabilities: Washington, DC, USA, 2010.

38. Shogren, K.A.; Luckasson, R.; Schalock, R.L. The responsibility to build contexts that enhance human functioning and promote valued outcomes for people with intellectual disability: Strengthening system responsiveness. *Intellect. Dev. Disabil.* **2018**, *56*, 287–300. [CrossRef] [PubMed]
39. Schalock, R.L.; Verdugo, M.A.; van Loon, J. Understanding organization transformation in evaluation and program planning. *Eval. Prog. Plan.* **2018**, *67*, 53–60. [CrossRef] [PubMed]
40. Claes, C.; Ferket, N.; Vandevelde, S.; Verlet, D.; De Maeyer, J. Disability policy evaluation: Combining logic models and systems thinking. *Intellect. Dev. Disabil.* **2017**, *55*, 247–257. [CrossRef] [PubMed]
41. Shogren, K.A.; Luckasson, R.; Schalock, R.L. An integrated approach to disability policy development, implementation, and evaluation. *Intellect. Dev. Disabil.* **2017**, *55*, 258–268. [CrossRef] [PubMed]
42. Verdugo, M.A.; Jenaro, C.; Calvo, I.; Navas, P. Disability policy implementation from a cross-cultural perspective. *Intellect. Dev. Disabil.* **2017**, *55*, 234–246. [CrossRef]

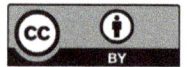

© 2020 by the authors. Licensee MDPI, Basel, Switzerland. This article is an open access article distributed under the terms and conditions of the Creative Commons Attribution (CC BY) license (http://creativecommons.org/licenses/by/4.0/).

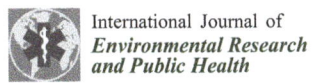

International Journal of
Environmental Research and Public Health

Article

Measurable Indicators of CRPD for People with Intellectual and Developmental Disabilities within the Quality of Life Framework

Laura E. Gómez [1,*], Asunción Monsalve [1], Mª Lucía Morán [1], Mª Ángeles Alcedo [1], Marco Lombardi [2] and Robert L. Schalock [3]

1. Department of Psychology, Universidad de Oviedo, 33003 Oviedo, Spain; monsalve@uniovi.es (A.M.); moranlucia@uniovi.es (M.L.M.); malcedo@uniovi.es (M.Á.A.)
2. E-QUAL, University College Ghent, 9000 Gent, Belgium; marco.lombardi@hogent.be
3. Department of Psychology, Hastings College, Hastings, NE 68901, USA; rschalock@ultraplix.com
* Correspondence: gomezlaura@uniovi.es; Tel.: +34-985-10-3372

Received: 14 June 2020; Accepted: 10 July 2020; Published: 15 July 2020

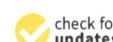

Abstract: This article proposes the quality of life (QOL) construct as a framework from which to develop useful indicators to operationalize, measure, and implement the Articles of the Convention on the Rights of Persons with Disabilities (CRPD). A systematic review of the scientific literature on people with intellectual and developmental disabilities (IDD) was carried out, with the aim of identifying personal outcomes that can be translated into specific and measurable items for each of the CRPD Articles aligned to the eight QOL domains. Following Preferred Reporting Items for Systematic Reviews and Meta-Analyses (PRISMA) guidelines, the systematic review was conducted across the Web of Science Core Collection, Current Contents Connect (CCC), MEDLINE, KCI-Korean Journal Database, Russian Science Citation Index and SciELO Citation Index, for articles published between 2008 and 2020. A total of 65 articles focusing on people with IDD were selected. The results were grouped into four broad categories: conceptual frameworks used to monitor the CRPD; instruments used to assess the rights set out in the CRPD; recommendations on the use of inclusive research; and indicators or personal outcomes associated with specific rights contained in the CRPD.

Keywords: rights; CRPD; intellectual disability; assessment; indicators; quality of life; convention; developmental disabilities; personal outcomes; PRISMA

1. Introduction

Changes in how people with intellectual disabilities and developmental disabilities (IDD) are perceived, and prevailing attitudes toward them, are increasingly reflected not only in national laws and regulations, but also in specific international conventions currently being used worldwide to develop, implement, and monitor social policies and professional practices aimed at promoting the inclusion and independence of people with ID in society [1–3].

More than a decade ago, in an effort to focus attention on the dignity of people with disabilities and their right to participate fully in community life in the same way as any other citizen, the United Nations Convention on the Rights of Persons with Disabilities (CRPD) was approved and ratified by 180 countries [4]. The CRPD was an international milestone recognizing the change in attitudes toward people with disabilities, based on the premise that people with disabilities, including those with ID, should have an active role in making decisions about their own lives, carry out productive activities, be included in society, and receive appropriate supports to allow them to live as full citizens, on an equal basis with others. Thus, the CRPD sets out rights that go far beyond what is strictly required by law, emphasizing economic, social, and cultural rights [3,5]. In its ambition to be more than a mere declaration of principles, the CRPD also underlines the importance of collecting data to assess the extent to which people with disabilities perceive that their rights are being respected and implemented [6].

The CRPD contains 50 Articles. Articles 1 to 4 set out the purpose of the Convention (Art. 1), define the concepts used (Art. 2), and outline the principles on which the CRPD is based (Art. 3) and the general obligations of States Parties (Art. 4). Articles 5 to 30 (i.e., a total of 26) then detail specific obligations for States. These 26 Articles defend the right of persons with disabilities (including those with ID) to enjoy legal capacity in all aspects of life and on an equal basis with others (Art. 12: equal recognition before the law); to have the opportunity to choose their place of residence, where and with whom they live, without being obliged to live in a particular living arrangement (Art. 19: right to live independently and to be included in the community); to access, on an equal basis with others, the physical environment, transportation, information and communications (Art. 9: accessibility); to access information in accessible formats and with technologies appropriate to different types of disability in a timely manner and without additional cost (Art. 21: freedom of expression and opinion, and access to information); to marry and found a family on the basis of free and full consent (Art. 23: respect for the home and the family); not to be excluded from the general education system, ensuring the reasonable accommodation of the individual's requirements, as well as the provision of the necessary individualized support measures to facilitate their effective education within the general education system (Art. 24: education); to access the same range, quality and standard of free or affordable health services as provided to other persons, as close as possible to their communities, including in rural areas (Art. 25: health); to have at their disposal comprehensive habilitation and rehabilitation services and programs in the fields of health, employment, education and social services, available from the earliest possible stage, based on their needs and strengths, and provided by suitably trained professionals (Art. 26: habilitation and rehabilitation); to have the opportunity to earn a living through work freely chosen or accepted in a labor market or work environment that is open, inclusive, and accessible (Art. 27: work and employment); and to participate fully and effectively in political and public life on an equal basis with others, directly or through freely elected representatives (Art. 29: participation in political and public life). Following these 26 Articles containing specific rights, the next 10 (Arts 31–40) deal with data collection and statistics (Art. 31); international cooperation (Art. 32); national implementation and monitoring of the CRPD (Art. 33); the establishment and functioning of the Committee (Art. 34); reports (Arts 35, 36 and 39); the relationship between the Committee, States and other bodies (Arts 37 and 38) and the regular conference with States Parties (Art. 40). Finally, the last 10 Articles (Arts 41–50) are reserved for signature, depositary, entry into force and other similar issues.

Implementing the CRPD is not without its difficulties. The abstract nature of rights and their context-based expression pose a challenge for evaluation and implementation [1,2,7,8], making it essential to define specific targets and objective indicators that can be used to assess progress [9,10]. Because of the significant conceptual and measurement work done in the field of quality of life (QOL) several authors have suggested that the QOL construct provides a valid framework from which to develop useful indicators to operationalize, measure, and implement the CRPD Articles (1,2,11), and to ultimately assist organization and systems transformation. The QOL construct provides an ideal conceptual framework for evaluating rights-related personal outcomes [11–13] and for translating abstract political concepts —such as self-determination, equity, accessibility, or inclusion [1,2,11,14]—into evidence-based practices [15–17].

This article proposes the QOL conceptual framework as a means of evaluating and implementing the CRPD Articles with respect to people with intellectual and developmental disabilities (IDD). The ultimate aim of the purpose of using the QOL framework is not to provide precise statistics on rights violations for the reports submitted to the United Nations Committee, but rather to: (a) give a voice to people with ID regarding everyday situations in their daily lives that are frequently not measured using conventional evaluation methods; (b) serve as a tool that professionals and relatives can use to detect any breach, abuse or denial of rights, thereby helping them enhance the supports they provide to people with ID; and (c) provide guidance to organizations on the strengths and greatest needs of people with ID in relation to rights that are encompassed in the CRPD. In this way, the approach to the evaluation of rights set out in this article focuses more on the microsystem (i.e., improving the lives of people with ID) and on the mesosystem (i.e., improving the provision of generic and professional supports offered by organizations) than on the macrosystem (i.e., lawmaking or production of official national statistics).

Several conceptual models of the QOL construct exist in the field of ID [18–20], although all of them highlight four basic principles in their definition [16]: (a) QOL is composed of several dimensions (i.e., multidimensional) that are the same for all people (i.e., universality); (b) it is influenced by personal and environmental factors; (c) it has both objective and subjective components; and (d) it is enhanced by individualized, person-centered supports. In this article, we focus on the QOL model proposed by Schalock and Verdugo [20]. It is the most widely accepted and cross-culturally validated model of QOL, and is used widely internationally by ID support organizations and systems in support provision, organization transformation, and systems change. [21–27]. According to Schalock and Verdugo's conceptual framework, QOL encompasses eight core domains that interact with each other. These domains include rights, self-determination, social inclusion, interpersonal relationships, personal development, emotional wellbeing, material wellbeing, and physical wellbeing. The eight domains can serve as a basis to evaluate the implementation of the 26 CRPD Articles on specific rights, through the measurement of core indicators and personal outcomes associated with QOL.

Two pioneering studies have sought to operationalize the CRPD through the QOL conceptual framework. The first demonstrated the theoretical foundations of the close relationship between the 26 CRPD Articles and the eight QOL domains, and put forward an initial proposal to organize the Articles by QOL domain [1]. The second article reported on the international consensus on the relationship between the core QOL indicators and the CRPD Articles [2]. To this end, a Delphi study was conducted with 153 experts (comprising people with ID, family members, professionals, researchers, and law experts) from 10 countries (Brazil, Canada, the Czech Republic, Germany, Israel, Italy, Portugal, Spain, Taiwan, and the United States). Consensus was reached on over 80 cross-culturally agreed and validated QOL indicators, which were aligned to the eight QOL domains.

Results from both of these studies are summarized in Table 1. They represent the framework for the systematic review presented in this article. The overall aim of this review is to take the next logical step in the operationalization of the CRPD: to review the scientific literature on people with IDD, in order to identify indicators and personal outcomes that can be translated into specific and measurable items for each of the CRPD Articles that are aligned to the eight QOL domains. In particular, the present systematic review sought to answer the following questions:

- What is discussed in the publications about the CRPD and people with IDD?
- In the literature, what theoretical frameworks and assessment instruments are proposed to monitor the implementation of the CRPD for people with IDD?
- What indicators or personal outcomes are mentioned in the scientific literature discussing the CRPD Articles that protect specific rights for people with IDD?

Table 1. Relationship between QOL domains, QOL indicators, and CRPD Articles [adapted from [1,2]].

Domain.	CRPD Articles Based on Verdugo et al. [1]	QOL Indicators Based on Lombardi et al. [2]
Personal development	24 (education)	– Educational setting – Personal skills – Lifelong learning
Self-determination	14 (liberty and security of person)	– Freedom of movement – Freedom of choice – Personal autonomy – Safe environment – Personal control – Realizing personal goals – Secure environment
Interpersonal relationships	21 (freedom of expression and opinion, access to information)	– Level of understanding the information – Using information – Opportunities to express opinion – Access to information
	23 (respect for home and the family)	– Right to set up their own family – Right to be a parent – Dating and intimate with persons of choice
Social inclusion	8 (awareness-raising)	– Acts of awareness (e.g., projects, campaigns) to increase social inclusion
	9 (accessibility)	– Presence in cultural events – Presence in recreational or leisure events
	18 (liberty of movement and nationality)	– Physical access on community streets – Physical access to public transportation – Physical access in community buildings
	19 (living independently and being included in the community)	– Living in a home with minimum intrusion from others – Home ownership – Rental agreement
	20 (personal mobility)	– A way to be personally mobile (e.g., by walking, using a wheelchair, or using crutches) – A way to transport across environments (e.g., a car, a bike, and public transportation)
	29 (participation in political and public life)	– Membership on boards – Running for public office
	30 (participation in cultural life, recreation, leisure and sport)	– Participation and presence in cultural events (e.g., concerts, movies, theaters, and museums) – Participation in recreational or leisure events (e.g., hobbies and community activity clubs) – Opportunity to travel

Table 1. *Cont.*

Domain	CRPD Articles Based on Verdugo et al. [1]	QOL Indicators Based on Lombardi et al. [2]
Rights	5 (equality and non-discrimination)	– Presence in the community – Engagement in open employment – Participation in community activities – Dating with persons of choice
	6 (women with disabilities)	– Personalized supports – Participation in community life – Adequate financial resources
	7 (children with disabilities)	– Receiving post-natal care – Supports to enhance personal growth and development – Involved in educational program – Provision of adequate medical care – Inclusion in their family – Inclusion in the community
	10 (right to life)	– Making choices about contraception – Making choices about end-of-life decisions
	11 (situations of risk and humanitarian emergencies)	– Supplying immigrants with a disability with sufficient legal, financial, and social supports – Access to health care
	12 (equal recognition before the law)	– Access to legal services – Receiving due process – Being considered legally competent
	13 (access to justice)	– Having a defense attorney – Participation in one's defense – Being adjudicated by a magistrate, a judge, or a jury – If guilty, receiving a fair sentence – Understanding the charge
	15 (freedom from torture or cruel, inhuman or degrading treatment or punishment)	– Personal injuries caused by others (e.g., torture and maiming) – If guilty, the punishment received is commensurate to that received by others
	22 (respect for privacy)	– Control over personal areas (e.g., bedroom, bathroom, home, or dwelling) – Personal access to communication (e.g., letters, e-mails, and phone)

Table 1. Cont.

Domain.	CRPD Articles Based on Verdugo et al. [1]	QOL Indicators Based on Lombardi et al. [2]
Emotional wellbeing	16 (freedom from exploitation, violence and abuse)	– Living in a safe environment – Not being exploited by others (e.g., sexually, financially, socially) – Not being abused by others (e.g., physical and emotional)
	17 (protecting the integrity of the person)	– Experiencing respect – Experiencing dignity – Experiencing equality
Physical wellbeing	25 (health)	– Physical status – Nutritional status – Chronic conditions
	26 (habilitation and rehabilitation)	– Medical intervention if needed – Emotional intervention if needed – Therapy (e.g., physical, occupational, speech)
Material wellbeing	27 (work and employment)	– Full-time paid employment – Part-time paid employment – Job training programs
	28 (adequate standard of living and social protection)	– Annual income covers basic living expenses – Annual income allows for discretionary spending – Adequate housing – Unemployment insurance – Public assistance if necessary

2. Materials and Methods

2.1. Inclusion and Exclusion Criteria

The following inclusion criteria were applied for this systematic review of the scientific literature. First, publications had to be peer-reviewed articles published since 2008, when the CRPD came into force. Thus, articles published between 2008 and January 15, 2020 were included. Second, studies had to refer to the CRPD and to people with IDD. Third, articles had to be published in English or in Spanish.

Given that one of the aims of this research was to locate as many indicators and personal outcomes as possible, added to the fact that the specific nature of the search was unlikely to return a large volume of results, few exclusion criteria were predefined. Following an examination of the complete references, results that had initially met the inclusion criteria set out above were subsequently excluded if they: (a) did not focus on the CRPD; (b) did not include people with IDD; (c) were letters, editorials, books, book chapters, indexes, and proceedings; or (d) were legal texts (i.e., documents limited to describing or analyzing regulations, laws, and conventions).

Articles that met this initial screening were retrieved and read in full, and were subsequently excluded if they: (a) were not related to the CRPD; or (b) did not refer to indicators or personal outcomes associated with any of the 26 Articles pertaining to specific rights (Table 1) for people with IDD.

2.2. Search Procedures

Two separate searches were conducted in parallel: a search of the scientific literature in English and another of the scientific literature in Spanish. The search terms were chosen based on the individual English-language and Spanish-language contexts. In other words, no attempt was made to produce a literal translation of the search terms from English into Spanish or vice versa, but the aim was rather to reproduce the meaning of the search terms and expressions taking into consideration possible cultural differences. For example, the term "learning disabilities" in Spanish is not used as in other countries to refer to people with "intellectual disabilities", but instead refers to people with specific learning disorders, for example, in reading, writing, or solving mathematical problems.

In order to identify studies on the CRPD and people with ID published in English, a systematic review was carried out on Web of Science (WOS). The databases included in the search were Web of Science Core Collection, Current Contents Connect (CCC), MEDLINE, KCI-Korean Journal Database, Russian Science Citation Index and SciELO Citation Index, incorporating the publication timespan 2008–2020 as an inclusion criterion. The search terms used in the TOPIC field were: "Convention" OR "CRPD" OR "UNCRPD", combined with AND "intellectual disability *" OR "developmental disability *" OR "intellectual developmental disorder *" OR "learning disability *". Table 2 summarizes the exact WOS search, which returned a total of 200 publications.

For the search in Spanish, the two platforms of Scopus and ProQuest were used, covering nine databases: Bibliografía de la Literatura Española, EconLit, Literature Online, Philosopher's Index, PsycARTICLES, PsycINFO, PsycTESTS, PTSDpubs and Publicly Available Content Database. In both platforms, the search criteria were set to include papers published in Spanish between the years 2008 and 2020. Furthermore, the search in ProQuest was limited to "peer-reviewed" documents. In both databases, the Spanish-language search terms were "Convención" OR "CDPD" OR "CDPCD", combined with AND "discapacidad intelectual" OR "discapacidad * del desarrollo" OR "trastorno * del desarrollo" in any field in ProQuest and in the "Article title, Abstract, Keywords" fields in Scopus. The Spanish search yielded a total of 53 results (Table 2), giving a combined search total of 253 publications across the two languages.

2.3. Article Selection

Data from the 253 articles identified across the three search platforms were incorporated into one Excel database. After four duplicates were removed—leaving a total of 249 articles—references (title, abstract, publication title, and pages) were screened by the first author of this paper for alignment with the inclusion and the exclusion criteria outlined above. This reference screening phase reduced the initial pool of documents to 136. Articles were removed at this stage primarily because they were not related to the CRPD (44.2%), they were not articles (18.6%), or they were limited to legal aspects (21.2%). A further 12.4% were not written in English or Spanish, and 3.5% did not refer to or include people with IDD. Next, 30% ($n = 75$) of the results were randomly selected and reviewed by the third author in order to examine the reliability of the decisions about inclusion or exclusion. The level of agreement between the two researchers was 89.3% in the first round and was 100% with regard to the reason for excluding a document. The first four authors of this article discussed the eight papers for which there initially had been disagreement and reached a consensus for all of them.

The next step was to retrieve the full-text versions of the 136 selected documents and to assess them for eligibility. After reviewing the full texts, 71 results were excluded because they were not related to the CRPD (11.3%) or because they did not refer to explicit indicators or personal outcomes related to specific rights set out in the CRPD (88.7%). Replicating the process described above, 30% ($n = 41$) of the full-text documents were randomly selected and reviewed, this time by both the first and the third authors of this paper. In the first round, the decision to exclude an article or not on the basis of the two reasons outlined above obtained an inter-rater agreement of 80.5%. The first four authors then discussed the eight papers for which there had been disagreement, and a consensus was ultimately reached. As a result, 65 articles were considered to have met the inclusion criteria (marked with * in References) and form the pool of documents upon which the results of this review are based. The entire process is illustrated in Figure 1.

Table 2. Search procedures for English and Spanish publications.

Platform	Set	Results	Search	Language
WOS	#1	39,949	TOPIC: (Convention) OR TOPIC: (CRPD) OR TOPIC: (UNCRPD) Timespan = 2008–2020 Search language = English	English
WOS	#2	56,988	TOPIC: ("intellectual disability *") OR TOPIC: ("learning disability *") OR TOPIC: ("Intellectual developmental disorder*") OR TOPIC: ("developmental disability *") Timespan = 2008–2020 Search language = English	English
WOS	#3	200	#1 AND #2 Timespan = 2008–2020 Search language = English	English
ProQuest	#1	3787	(Convención OR CDPCD OR CDPD) AND la.Exact("Spanish") Limit to: Peer reviewed, Date: After December 31, 2007	Spanish
ProQuest	#2	404	("discapacidad intelectual" OR "trastorno* del desarrollo" OR "discapacidad* del desarrollo") AND la.Exact("Spanish") Limit to: Peer reviewed, Date: After December 31, 2007	Spanish
ProQuest	#3	52	1 AND 2 Limit to: Peer reviewed, Date: After December 31, 2007	Spanish
Scopus	#1	64	(TITLE-ABS-KEY (convención) OR TITLE-ABS-KEY (cdpd) OR TITLE-ABS-KEY (cdpcd)) AND PUBYEAR > 2007 AND (LIMIT-TO (LANGUAGE, "Spanish"))	Spanish
Scopus	#2	216	(TITLE-ABS-KEY ("discapacidad intelectual") OR TITLE-ABS-KEY ("discapacidad* del desarrollo") OR TITLE-ABS-KEY ("Trastorno* del desarrollo")) AND PUBYEAR > 2007 AND (LIMIT-TO (LANGUAGE, "Spanish"))	Spanish
Scopus	#3	1	1 AND 2	Spanish
N total		253		

2.4. Article Coding and Data Extraction

First, the 65 articles selected for inclusion in this systematic review were grouped into four broad categories: (1) articles that refer to conceptual frameworks (e.g., QOL models) for CRPD monitoring (i.e., they relate to Article 31 "Statistics and data collection" or Article 35 "Reports by States Parties"); (2) articles that propose or use instruments to assess the rights contained in the CRPD (for a specific Article or for several of the Articles from 1 to 50); (3) articles that use or discuss inclusive research (given the solid foundation for ethical, inclusive research with people with disabilities provided for by the CRPD, and particularly the explicit mention in Article 33 "National implementation and monitoring" that "persons with disabilities and their representative organizations must be involved and participate fully in the monitoring process"); and (4) articles that include indicators or personal outcomes associated with one or more of the 26 Articles pertaining to specific rights (i.e., Articles 5 to 30 of the CRPD). Articles assigned to the third category—inclusive research—could simultaneously be classified into one of the other three categories. Categories 1, 2 and 4, on the other hand, were considered mutually exclusive for article coding and categories 1 and 2 were prioritized over category 4. None of the articles could be classified in category 1 and 2 at the same time, but a few could be classified in categories 1 and 4, or categories 2 and 4. In these cases, they were assigned to categories 1 and 2, respectively, but they were also scrutinized in order to identify indicators or personal outcomes.

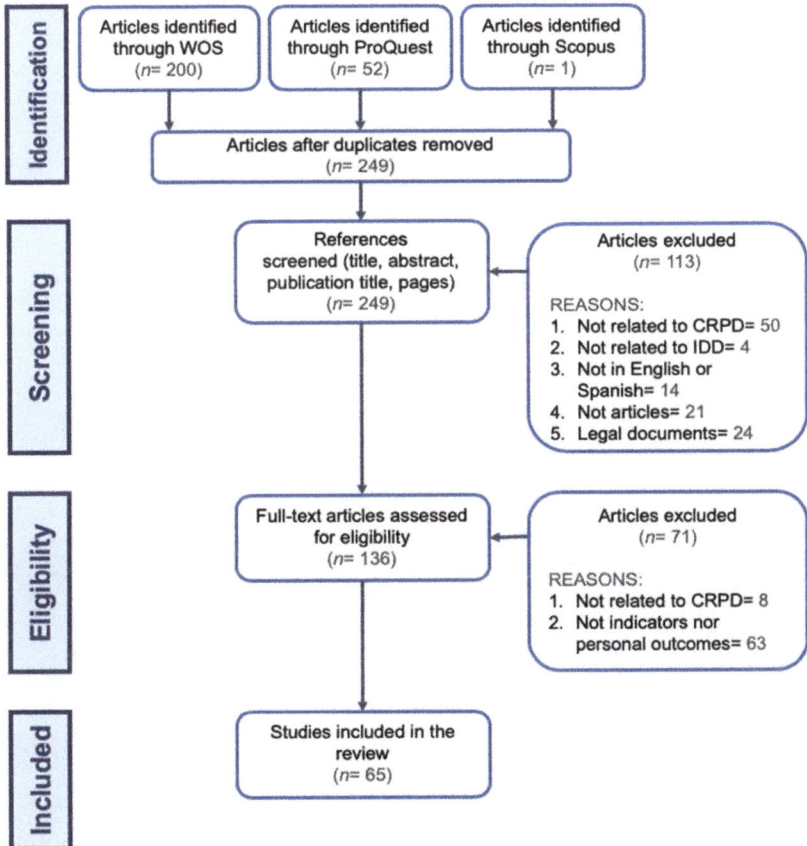

Figure 1. Search and article selection flow diagram.

Secondly, all the articles were coded and subgrouped according to the specific CRPD Article number they referred to. Finally, all articles were classified depending on whether they were: (1) quantitative—descriptive papers; (2) qualitative—descriptive papers; (3) mixed methodology; (4) reviews; (5) position papers; or (6) descriptions or proposals for interventions, programs or practices.

Similar to the process used to test reliability at the article exclusion step, the inter-rater reliability was established for the coding criteria set out above. The first author coded 100% of the articles, and the third author coded 30% ($n = 20$). In the first round, the inter-rater agreement regarding the decision on category (i.e., framework, instrument, specific Article, or inclusive research) was 95% ($n = 1$ disagreement); for the CRPD Article number it was 85% ($n = 3$ partial disagreements; there was total agreement on the main Article being referred to but some disagreement when there were several secondary Articles mentioned); and, finally, for the type of document (i.e., quantitative, qualitative, review, position, intervention), the inter-rater agreement was 85% ($n = 3$ disagreements).

All disagreements were resolved by a discussion among the first four authors and a consensus was reached.

3. Results

A total of 65 articles published between 2008 and 2019 were included in this review. Only four articles were identified for the publication years 2008–2010, with most published after 2017 ($n = 31$; Me = 2016), and the highest publication output recorded in 2019 ($n = 13$). In all, 89.2% of the articles were indexed in WOS, 9.2% in ProQuest, and 1.5% in Scopus. Most of the papers were written in English (86.15%), while only nine were written in Spanish.

These publications involved a total of 348 authors (or 411 including duplicates, where the same author has written more than one paper). With four publications each, the most prolific authors on this subject are J. Fullana, E. García, P. McCallion, M. McCarron, M. Pallisera, and M.A. Verdugo; followed by T. Carney, G. Díaz, L.E. Gómez, M. Redley, N. Salmon, R.L. Schalock, and M. Vila, who have three publications each. The 65 papers were published across a wide variety of journals ($n = 37$), with the largest concentration in the Journal of Policy and Practice in Intellectual Disabilities ($n = 12$), Journal of Intellectual Disability Research ($n = 6$), Journal of Applied Research in Intellectual Disabilities ($n = 4$), British Journal of Learning Disabilities ($n = 4$), Disability and Rehabilitation ($n = 3$), Tizard Learning Disability Review ($n = 3$), International Journal of Law and Psychiatry ($n = 3$), and Disability & Society ($n = 2$). Only one manuscript was published in each the remaining journals.

With regard to the geographical regions covered by the studies, more than half were conducted in Europe (53.8%), and one-quarter each in Oceania (26.2%) and North America (23.1%). There is a lower volume of studies conducted in—or referring to—Asia (10.8%), South America (9.2%), and Africa (6.2%), while only one was carried out in the Middle East (i.e., Israel; 1.5%). Out of a total of 34 countries, the highest number of studies was carried out in Australia ($n = 16$), Spain ($n = 13$), Ireland ($n = 11$), Canada ($n = 8$), England ($n = 6$), and the United States ($n = 6$).

3.1. What is Discussed in the Publications about the CRPD and People with IDD?

The vast majority of the publications ($n = 48$; 73.8%) focused on one or more of the 26 CRPD Articles pertaining to specific rights (i.e., Articles 5 to 30). Only eight papers (12.3%) addressed conceptual frameworks for CRPD monitoring (i.e., they relate to Article 31 "Statistics and data collection" or Article 35 "Reports by States Parties"), and five (7.7%) proposed or applied assessment instruments (for a specific Article or for several of the Articles from 1 to 50). A total of eight (12.3%) used or discussed inclusive research (Article 33).

Most were descriptive studies ($n = 34$)—qualitative (29.2%), quantitative (18.5%), or mixed methodology (4.6%)—and theoretical articles or position papers (27.7%), while 11 were reviews (19.9%), and only four described interventions, programs or practices (6.2%). All referred to people with IDD, although almost one-fifth ($n = 12$; 18.5%) discussed people with disabilities in general, while 6.2% referred specifically to people with Down syndrome ($n = 2$), cerebral palsy ($n = 1$), or neurologic conditions ($n = 1$).

3.2. In the Literature, What Theoretical Frameworks and Assessment Instruments are Proposed to Monitor the Implementation of the CRPD for People with IDD?

Of the eight papers that used or proposed conceptual frameworks to monitor or evaluate the CRPD or its specific Articles, all pointed to the QOL framework and QOL indicators that must be incorporated into comprehensive instruments to assess progress and identify needs and gaps in implementation. The QOL model proposed by Schalock and Verdugo was the most commonly used [1,2,8,9,11]—although the Cummins model [28] is also mentioned—and applications in specific contexts—namely "Educational quality of life" [29]—are also discussed. As shown in Table 3, five of the studies named, applied or proposed specific measurement tools to assess QOL (QOL-Q, Integral Scale, Gencat Scale, Personal Outcomes Scale, Personal Wellbeing Index), self-determination (AIR

Self-Determination Scale), or rights (Rights of Persons with Disabilities ad hoc scale). Only one study used qualitative instruments in the form of focus groups and in-depth interviews [30]. While all of these papers referred to a QOL conceptual framework as a way of evaluating or monitoring the CRPD (Articles 31 and 35), some also focused on other CRPD Articles, the most common being ($n = 2$) Article 7 (children with disabilities), Article 19 (living independently and being included in the community), and Article 24 (education). In the eight studies, the countries where this framework was most used or proposed were Australia, the United States, and Spain.

Table 3. Proposed theoretical frameworks for CRPD monitoring.

Ref	Framework	Proposed/Applied Instruments	Main CRPD Article(s) *	Country
[11]	Quality of life and self-determination	Quality of Life Questionnaire (QOL-Q) AIR Self-Determination Scale Rights of Persons with Disabilities	35	Nepal, Zambia, United States
[28]	Quality of life (satisfaction)	Personal Wellbeing Index - intellectual disability	19, 35	Australia
[29]	Quality of life (educational)	—	7, 24, 35	Australia
[8]	Quality of life	Integral Scale Gencat Scale	6, 12, 19, 23, 24, 29, 35	Spain
[1]	Quality of life	Integral Scale Gencat Scale Personal Outcomes Scale	35	United States, Spain
[2]	Quality of life	—	35	Brazil, Canada, Czech Republic, Germany, Italy, Israel, Portugal, Spain, Taiwan, United States
[9]	Quality of life	—	31, 32	United Kingdom
[30]	Quality of life	Focus groups and interviews	7, 21, 35	Australia

* Main CRPD Article(s) addressed in the publication.

In the five studies that used or proposed specific tools to monitor compliance with the CRPD, a total of five instruments are cited (Table 4). None of them were originally designed with the specific objective of monitoring the CRPD, although the structure of the ITINERIS Scale [31]—while inspired by the Montreal Declaration—was developed by five professionals who independently evaluated the relationship between the items in the scale and the preamble and first 30 Articles of the CRPD. The four other instruments proposed to monitor certain Articles of the CRPD are the rights subscales of QOL scales, comprising the Gencat Scale or the Integral Scale [13]; the National Core Indicators-Adult Consumer Survey (NCI-ACS), aimed at assessing the quality of services [3,32]; and the European Child Environment Questionnaire (ECEQ), which covers physical, social and attitudinal environmental features [33]. The number of items in these five instruments ranges from 8 to 51, and all are designed for adults with ID, save for the ECEQ, which was developed for children with cerebral palsy. In addition, most of the instruments are self-reports administered directly to people with disabilities, while only two are other-reports answered by relatives or professionals. Of the specific CRPD Articles assessed, the range covered by the instruments is limited to the first 30. Articles 21 (freedom of expression and opinion, and access to information) and 22 (respect for privacy) are dealt with in most of the instruments ($n = 4$), followed by ($n = 3$) Articles 3 (general principles), 9 (accessibility), 18 (liberty of movement and nationality), 23 (respect for home and the family), and 27 (work and employment).

Finally, the sociodemographic data gathered in these studies includes the following: (a) personal variables such as gender, age, ethnicity, language, religion, sexual orientation, level of ID, cause of ID, disability onset, civil status, educational level, need of assistive products, mental health diagnosis, problematic behavior, verbal expression, sensory impairment, support needs, residential type, mobility, socioeconomic status, guardianship, advocacy experience; (b) contextual variables such as region, degree of urbanicity, community size, level of involvement and frequency of contact with family or professionals, care and residential setting, type of school setting, employment.

Table 4. Instruments applied or proposed in the studies and their relationship to CRPD Articles and the quality model.

Ref	Instrument(s)	Target Population	Respondents	Construct(s) Assessed	N Items	Related CRPD Article(s)	Region
[33]	European Child Environment Questionnaire (ECEQ)	Children (8–12 years old) with cerebral palsy	Report of others: relatives	Physical environment, Social support, Attitudes	51	9, 18, 21	Europe
[31]	ITINERIS Scale	Adults with ID	Self-report	Rights	30	Preamble 1–30	South America
[32]	National Core Indicators-Adult Consumer Survey (NCI-ACS)	Adults aged 18 or over with IDD	Self-report	Quality of services	35	3, 8, 9, 14, 19, 21, 22, 23, 24, 25, 27, 30	United States
[3]	NCI-ACS				16	3, 8, 14, 21, 22, 23, 27	United States
[13]	Gencat Scale	Adults aged 18 or over with ID	Report of others: professionals	Rights (within the framework of QOL)	10	5, 12, 16, 17, 22, 29	Spain
[13]	Integral Scale (Gómez et al., 2011)		Self-report		8		

It is also important to mention the eight studies that focus on inclusive research, the majority of which were conducted in Ireland (*n* = 5), the others in Spain (*n* = 2) and Australia (*n* = 1). The inclusive research model holds that people with disabilities with relevant experience related to the studied topic should be included in the research, not only as informants but participating and making decisions in all phases. This level of involvement is essential in order to comply with the part of Article 33 where it states that "civil society, in particular persons with disabilities and their representative organizations, shall be involved and participate fully in the monitoring process". Inclusive research incorporates a wide range of research approaches that have traditionally been referred to as "participative", "action", or "emancipatory". Some authors have tried to differentiate between the techniques, arguing that the emancipatory approach is achieved when the initiative and research topic is proposed by people with disabilities, and it is they who control the research, while the participative approach places greater emphasis on the representation of people with disabilities at all stages of the research process [34,35]. The most common ways for people with ID to participate in these studies are by providing their views and opinions through focus groups, structured interviews, and workshops [35–38]; by acting not only as study participants, but also as advisory committee members and co-researchers [39,40], making it essential that they receive research training [41]. The most frequently cited limitations allude to the challenge of remaining inclusive throughout data collection and analysis, together with including people with complex support needs, such as those with profound and multiple disabilities or who use alternative or augmentative communication approaches.

3.3. What Indicators or Personal Outcomes Are Mentioned in the Scientific Literature Discussing the CRPD Articles that Protect Specific Rights for People with IDD?

The indicators and personal outcomes identified in the 48 studies that deal with the specific rights in the CRPD (Arts 5–30) are aligned to the eight QOL domains and presented below.

3.3.1. Personal Development

- Article 24 (education): Nine articles included in this review refer to specific indicators and personal outcomes related to inclusive education [8,42–49] in ordinary settings at all levels of education (preschool, primary, secondary, high school, vocational training, university). The specific indicators mentioned were the right to attend educational establishments near their community; individualized supports within the general education system; assessment of individual support needs in environments that maximize academic and social development; completion of stages and appropriate transitions between them; coordination among the different professionals involved; training about rights; training about sexuality, reproduction and family planning (understanding what sexual relationships are, risks, benefits and alternatives; questions about sexuality can be freely raised and resolved); training and preparation for independent living (in real-life contexts, from compulsory education); vocational guidance; adequate training and qualifications to get a job; individualized educational aids (e.g., teacher's aide, tutors, extended test time, modified course curriculum); appropriate materials; reasonable accommodations; quick access to necessary educational support products (e.g., specialized software, recording or note taking devices, audio/e-book devices); information, care, and guidance services for families (e.g., legislative measures and supports related to the education of their children); participation of the family in the education process; information, care, and guidance services for teachers about disability, supports and special educational needs; attitudes toward the inclusion of family members and teachers; meaningful learning experiences; participation in the activities of the school; the school and its staff enhance the person's self-esteem, satisfaction, autonomy, and self-confidence; friends at school (not only among staff or carers); educational institutions in a holistic perspective of health and care.

3.3.2. Self-Determination

- Article 14 (liberty and security of person): 10 papers [8,38,40,45,48–53] address this Article, specifically freedom of choice (e.g., to choose where and with whom they live, the type of housing, moving house, what to cook, how to spend their free time and with whom); making their own decisions (including decisions about health); personal autonomy (e.g., control of their finances, handling their own money independently, not being overprotected by their family, not being underestimated by their parents or still being perceived as a child); control over life and life events (e.g., social outings, simple events in their daily lives); upbringing experiences focused on developing skills for independence and self-determined behaviors; coping strategies (e.g., impact of health problems on daily life); person-centered approach.
- Article 21 (freedom of expression and opinion, access to information): Seven studies focus on access to—and understanding of—information, as well as opportunities to use information and express their opinion [8,40,48,51,54–56]. From these, the following personal outcomes were extracted: information in accessible formats (e.g., easy-read format); assistive products for communication and cognition (knowledge and awareness; customization); access to the internet, its content and digital services (e.g., adapted applications, internet sites and web browsers; modifying the mouse settings or enlarging the font); technological devices adapted to the person's specific needs (e.g., alternative mice, enlarged keyboards, touch screens, voice synthesis and recognition systems); technical support (e.g., configuring device security, securing the wireless network, installing an antivirus program, setting up the firewall, updating the operating system and software); participation in digital society (educational programs, individualized supports to understand new social interaction rules and conventions); self-advocacy (to have their voice heard, confidence to speak up, defend their health, sexual and emotional options).

3.3.3. Interpersonal Relationships

- Article 23 (respect for home and the family): 10 articles included in the review [8,39,40,49,57–62] refer to the right to have opportunities to meet people, establishing relationships, having friends, meeting the right person, and having a partner relationship (taking risks to be with the person they want, opposing control of the family and restrictive service regulations, receiving support without being treated as children or considered asexual or unable to raise children, choosing their sexual orientation, being listened to about their needs); to marry and found a family (retain their fertility on an equal basis with others, avoiding forced sterilization and covert contraception, making their own reproductive and sexual choices, deciding on the number of children to have); to keep their own children with them (i.e., receiving specific supports for the wellbeing of both children and parents with disabilities, obtaining legal custody of the children in case of divorce, avoiding the separation of children from their parents against their will on the basis of a disability, or denial of their rights as fathers/mothers); to receive sexual information, guidance, and support in caring for their children (e.g., basic care, nutrition, health, education; home-based learning and flexible support services over the long-term that are evidence-based, tailored to individual needs, and built on the strengths of each parent and family; monitoring of new needs); to be able to adopt and foster, and to access assisted reproduction; guidance and training for families and professionals who provide evidence-based methods and non-discriminatory support in sexuality (preventing negative attitudes of professionals and families toward sexuality, such as discouraging marriage and parenting, restricting sexual expression; disapproving relationships, allowing platonic but not intimate relationships); organization policy facilitating sexual experiences and comprehensive sex education programs (not only addressing biological facts but also allowing them to discuss the social and emotional aspects of relationships and sexuality, to learn about abuse and exploitation, to recognize the importance of desire and pleasure).

3.3.4. Social Inclusion

- Article 8 (awareness-raising): Seven articles [8,48,59,63–66] provide indicators and personal outcomes related to advertising campaigns. The specific personal outcomes include giving them visibility; promoting normalization and generating awareness about disabilities; treating their image with respect; sensitizing and ensuring the realization of their rights; promoting equality; improving participation and inclusion; breaking stereotypes. In addition, there was an emphasis on the need for specific awareness campaigns focusing on the reality of women with ID and their capability of parenting (associated with Articles 6 and 23, respectively).
- Article 9 (accessibility): Four studies [46,48,53,67] mention specific elements that could be operationalized with respect to the accessibility of the environment. In particular, they refer to accessibility in health facilities, community centers, educational establishments, and workplaces; accessibility in public infrastructure; accessibility of leisure environments.
- Article 18 (liberty of movement and nationality): Only one article [40] discusses the freedom to use public transport; freedom to move around and have control over their movements; being within walking distance of amenities and shops.
- Article 19 (living independently and being included in the community): 14 papers [8,38–40,42,45,47,49,50,53,63,66,68,69] mention personal outcomes or indicators associated with the right to live independently and be included in the community (i.e., not to be institutionalized in segregated environments, not to be restricted in options for in-home residential and other community support services). To achieve this, the papers highlighted the right to receive the necessary individualized supports (person-centered planning, individualized support to live more independently) for everyday activities to do with autonomy in the home (e.g., getting to appointments, running errands, housework, personal finances, heavy household chores, preparing meals, personal care and medical care); support from professionals (sufficient personal resources) and service providers (to organize preferred housing, help find housemates, forge social connections); in housing, to facilitate flexibility in terms of rules and staff control, freedom to move around and to arrange daily home life, enjoy own space, individualized care, small groups, living with their partner; trust and support from family (role of the family as a source of support and as facilitators of autonomy, opportunities to practice skills, avoiding overprotection); special attention to access supports during and after moving (to organize move, types of support, relationships with supporters, quality of supporters); being within walking distance of amenities and shops; support for older people with disability; control over support arrangements (choose support workers and the kind of support they receive); housing affordability; access to information on independent living experiences.
- Article 20 (personal mobility): Two articles [54,63] include specific aspects related to this right. The indicators and personal outcomes mentioned are a way to be personally mobile (availability of assistive products for mobility; knowledge and awareness about them; customization); and a way to transport across environments (i.e., adapted transport; human support and vehicle available).

- Article 29 (participation in political and public life): Seven studies [8,49,53,66,70–72] consider aspects related to the right of people with ID to vote (e.g., information about the meaning and content of elections and democratic participation; understanding the information from the parties, the electoral procedures, and the voting paper; easy postal votes; accessible local polling stations; using pictures, symbols and logos on the voting paper; courses about voting and elections; easier-to-read election materials; support at polling stations and during the process of voting; treated respectfully by election officials; web accessible guides to voting); to be elected political members; priority on supportive legislation on disability issues in the government and CRPD focus.
- Article 30 (participation in cultural life, recreation, leisure and sport): Measurable indicators and outcomes are found in eight articles [40,47–50,53,66,69]. They refer to being part of society, taking part in all aspects of their community life; having sufficient income to participate in the community; adequate information about community activities for families (e.g., organized social leisure activities); participating in activities with people without ID (e.g., inclusive sports); promotion of active participation and play in their communities; enjoying leisure time (doing a variety of things alone or with others; relaxing and having fun; doing things they enjoy; going to pubs and night life; not being ignored at social events); awareness, positive attitudes and actions of other members of the community.

3.3.5. Rights

- Article 5 (equality and non-discrimination): Five papers [49,50,54,69,73] identify the indicators and personal outcomes of not suffering stigma; not suffering discrimination (e.g., in insurance matters, in access to health care); not experiencing rejection and denial of their individuality, adulthood and capacity.
- Article 6 (women with disabilities): Eight papers refer to the rights of women [8,49,52,58–60,65,74]. Most indicators and personal outcomes were already reflected in other CRPD rights, but there was particular emphasis on the application of these rights—and respect for—women. The most frequently cited aspects in relation to women include prevention and intervention in gender-based violence (knowing their rights, knowing how to deal with acts of aggression perpetrated by men, easy-read guides on gender-based violence, providing information and raising awareness of ID for people working with women who have been victims of gender-based violence, information services and specialist guidance on existing resources and intermediation in the public system, emotional support, legal advice); employment; avoiding overprotection (parents are usually more protective with daughters); taking into account the demands of women with ID; right to participate in decisions about their lives.
- Article 7 (children with disabilities): Six papers focus on the right of children with disabilities to express their views freely on all matters affecting them and to be provided with disability- and age-appropriate assistance to realize that right [8,46,48,67,74,75]. While most of the indicators and personal outcomes matched those already proposed and reflected in other CRPD rights, it was stressed that these must also be fulfilled during childhood and adolescence. Among these are the importance of children participating in civil life and decision-making (including health); the will and preferences of children with disabilities are respected on an equal basis with other children (e.g., children should be asked to express their views and preferences during legal procedures, using all possible ways of communication such as drawing and painting, body language, facial expressions; providing children with accessible information that allows them to express their opinion); promoting inclusion and preventing family vulnerability (e.g., avoiding separation from parents against their will on the basis of a disability and, where this is necessary, providing alternatives within the extended family or in the community in a family environment, child protection services); appropriate transition from child-specific to adult-specific services;

the development of adaptive behavior skills; involving children in advocacy, decision-making or even human rights monitoring.
- Article 10 (right to life): Only two papers give measurable aspects on the right to life [76,77]. Both specifically mention providing supports to make choices about end-of-life: to express their will and preference (using a range of intentional/unintentional and formal/informal behaviors); supporters to listen to the person's expression of preference by acknowledging, interpreting and acting on that preference); intimate or very close relationships between people with ID and their supporters (knowledge of the person's life story; documentation of a person's history and life story through sharing of historical stories, images and video about the person being supported, by those who had known them for a long time, across multiple areas of their life; enjoyment of their company; willingness and ability to see the person "beyond their disability"); person-centered approach (encouraging the use of supports for end-of-life care in home settings, and recognizing variations in what "home" may be like with respect to end-of-life care).
- Article 11 (situations of risk and humanitarian emergencies): States Parties shall take all necessary measures to ensure the protection and safety of persons with disabilities in situations of risk, including situations of armed conflict, humanitarian emergencies and the occurrence of natural disasters. None of the papers included in this review refer to specific indicators or personal outcomes associated with this Article.
- Article 12 (equal recognition before the law): A dozen articles [8,49,71,74–76,78–81] focus on the promotion of supported decision-making strategies. They specifically report on the need to replace guardianship (disapproving of legal incapacity and substituted decision-making) with the supported decision-making model: empower them to exercise their own will and preferences (training about decision-making; providing information about supported decision-making to people with disabilities, their families, and professionals; taking into consideration individual concerns, experiences with legal systems and levels of literacy; identifying communication barriers; implementing measures to enable their voice to be heard); appropriate and ongoing support to exercise decision-making capacity in all areas of their lives (person-centered planning: all forms of support in the exercise of legal capacity must be based on their specific needs, will and preferences, not on what is perceived as being in their objective best interests; support is available at nominal or no cost and lack of financial resources is not a barrier to accessing support in the exercise of legal capacity; safeguards must be established for all processes relating to legal capacity and support in exercising legal capacity); dyad of decision-maker with ID and a decision supporter (legal recognition of the support person(s) formally chosen by the person must be available and accessible, including mechanisms for third parties to verify the identity of a support person and challenge their actions if they believe that the support person is not acting in accordance with the will and preferences of the person concerned; the person has the right to refuse support and terminate or change the support relationship at any time; supporters' respect for rights, values, goals, experiences of individual; having good interpersonal skills and the ability to recognize conflicting interest; responding to the expression of will and preference by acknowledging, interpreting and responding to it; having a close and trusting relationship with the decision-maker or the capacity to build one; using formal decision-making agreements, committing time and providing support for as long as is needed for a decision to be reached; supporting decision makers to take risks, change their minds, make decisions others may not like, and extend their experiences; helping them to access information, discussing available information in understandable ways, and advocating for decisions made to be acted on; showing commitment, familiarity with disability, good communication and advocacy skills, common sense and ethical behavior); the person is encouraged to make their own decision by providing them with a range of options but not imposing choices; the person expresses will and preference, intentionally and unintentionally, using a range of modalities (e.g., behavior, vocalization, vocal pitch, muscle

tone, facial expression, eye movement, self-harm, breath, unintentional physiological functions); the meetings are set up in a comfortable environment with the consent of the person.
- Article 13 (access to justice): Only one paper specifically refers to access to justice (for women with ID who have been victims of gender-based violence) [74]. It points to the need for ways to enable them to successfully engage with the legal system; support from workers and agencies in their interactions with the justice system; supports from police and judicial officers (e.g., adjusting their language, regarding complaints and statements as serious and with the same weight as they would for persons without disabilities, taking time to explain the law and its application, recognizing them as full persons before the law); training police and judicial officers about IDD.
- Article 15 (freedom from torture or cruel, inhuman or degrading treatment or punishment): Only four papers [50,63,73,82] specify indicators or personal outcomes associated with this Article: use of seclusion or solitary confinement (i.e., restrictive interventions, exclusionary practices); restraints (physical, mechanical, chemical); harmful treatments (e.g., inappropriate sedation, forced medication, failure to meet dietary requirements).
- Article 22 (respect for privacy): The four papers [40,49,50,69] that allude to this right identify the following indicators and personal outcomes: respect for privacy by flatmates, parents and caregivers (having their own room and space: private, peace and quiet; privacy of personal and intimate information; privacy related to sexuality).

3.3.6. Emotional Wellbeing

- Article 16 (freedom from exploitation, violence and abuse): 12 articles specify indicators or personal outcomes on this aspect [8,38,40,42,49,57,59,63,65,66,74,82]. Those frequently cited include freedom from concealment, abandonment, abuse or neglect; segregation or exclusion (social and physical isolation); bullying (name calling; cyberbullying) in educational and social settings; experiencing vulnerability and not feeling safe (in relationships, in immediate environment); gender-based violence; sexual abuse (being able to detect abuse), physical violence (violent relationships); economic abuse.
- Article 17 (protecting the integrity of the person): Six papers mention personal outcomes related to indicators of being treated with respect, dignity, and equity [40,47,49,51,52,63]. For professionals, these include providing unconditional support, emotional support, a listening ear, empathy, patience, and trust; and that they know the people with IDD well, understand their perspective, and value and respect them and their family. For the persons with disabilities, these include self-acceptance and self-awareness of disability, not showing low expectations of themselves because of disability; not experiencing exclusionary reactions, such as not being addressed in conversations or being ignored by professionals in different sectors; use of positive behavioral support.

3.3.7. Physical Wellbeing

- Article 25 (health): 10 articles [48,50,51,56,66,67,73,83–85] discuss the right to health, highlighting indicators and personal outcomes associated with good physical health (e.g., healthy weight, absence of weight-related physical problems such as diabetes, gastrointestinal disorders, hypertension); prevention; access to appropriate information on health-related issues; promotion of healthy behaviors in accessible formats; good psychological health (absence of behavioral problems or psychiatric disorders); to have family and disability support worker advocacy (without conflicts of interests between their own needs/vision and those of their son or daughter); early screening and diagnosis (including comorbidities); community programs favoring cognitive, physical, and social development; shared decision-making among health care providers, children and families; supervised, justified and adjusted medication (especially, antipsychotic); rigorous data collection system and epidemiological data on prevalence of IDD and mental illness; existence

- Article 26 (habilitation and rehabilitation): 12 papers [40,48–51,54,66,67,73,83–85] focus on specific elements related to habilitation and rehabilitation, such as accessing quality efficient and specialized physical and mental health care and social care (speech therapists, psychologists, psychiatrists, physiotherapists, dentists, X-ray facilities, primary and tertiary health services); appropriate and affordable early and timely health services, interventions and care; coordination and communication between health, education and social services; health services close to home; appropriate transitions between health services (e.g., from pediatric to adult services); availability, knowledge and use of assistive devices and technologies related to habilitation and rehabilitation; health staff feeling competent to care for patients with IDD (educational curricula for health professionals about disability; availability of specialized training; avoiding misperceptions; well-trained mental health professionals in dual diagnoses); health staff's positive attitudes (looking and directly talking to person with IDD, willing to provide them with care; showing respect); individualized and capability-based services.

3.3.8. Material Wellbeing

- Article 27 (work and employment): Eight papers contain employment-related aspects [39,40,42,46,47,49,59,66]: access to the labor market; having a (local) paid job (not being refused a job, promotion or interview because of disability); safe and suitable employment; satisfaction with the employment and salary (paid on an equal basis to others); adequate provision of accommodation and employment services (e.g., hours, duty, human support); employer and employee attitudes (e.g., aware of work strengths and limitations, not considering the person disadvantaged because of disability; negative attitudes when looking for employment; ongoing disability information and awareness activities for all employees; satisfactory treatment for employees); adequate job information, training and experience (advice on alternative employment; individualized training based on needs, studies, professional experience, interests and availability; skills training to find and keep a job; individual guidance to map out potential professional pathways; assessment and guidance on job options tailored to needs profile; presence of support persons to mediate with the company; tracking recruitment to make adjustments); employment as a way to meet people and friends; work-life balance measures (i.e., childcare while they work).
- Article 28 (adequate standard of living and social protection): 10 studies [8,40,43,47,53,54,59,66,67,69] specify personal outcomes or indicators associated with this Article: financial independence (adequate subsistence base); sufficient financial income to access housing (housing affordability); safe, accessible and suitable housing; aid to cover the additional expenses of supports and specialist care (economic support); having the necessary assistive products for environment and self-care (knowledge and awareness about them; customized); personal assistant when needed; leisure activities in people's home (e.g., listening to the radio, playing instruments, being at home with friends); saving and budgeting (including for holidays); satisfaction with income; assistance with managing money and budgeting; receiving disability benefits (not losing benefits for being employed); easing bureaucracy involved in getting personal assistance and personal budgets; flexibility of support funded; provision of social assistance when needed; existence of personal budgets/personal assistance schemes and awareness of these by people with disability; stability of funding over time; strong supportive legislation.

4. Discussion

This systematic review sought to answer three key questions. The first was to learn about the main themes covered in publications about the CRPD and people with IDD, a broad term that combines the fields of intellectual disability (diagnosis given to individuals who meet the criteria of significant limitations both in intellectual functioning and adaptive behavior as expressed in conceptual, social, and practical skills, and is manifest before age 18) and developmental disabilities (non-categorical label for a chronic disability manifest before age 22 but limited to persons with a specific diagnosis or for those whose disability manifest before age 22 results in substantial functional limitations in three or more major life activity areas and who require long- term services and supports) [86]. The vast majority of the publications focused on one or more of the 26 CRPD Articles pertaining to specific rights (i.e., Articles 5 to 30), while only one-fifth either referred to conceptual frameworks for CRPD monitoring or proposed or applied assessment instruments. While still an emerging approach, inclusive research [34–41], which encourages people with IDD to participate as researchers at all stages of the research process, is increasingly being used or recommended in the scientific literature.

The second research question focused on identifying the conceptual frameworks used to monitor the CRPD or any of its specific Articles. All of the reviewed papers that covered this aspect underscored the relevance of the QOL framework to assess progress and identify needs and gaps in implementation. The most widely used framework was Schalock and Verdugo's eight-domain QOL model (or a variation based on some of its specific domains, such as rights or self-determination). Furthermore, a number of specific assessment instruments developed from this model have been used in studies to explore the implementation of the CRPD (e.g., QOL-Q, Integral Scale, Gencat Scale, Personal Outcomes Scale). Other monitoring instruments used were the Rights of Persons with Disabilities Scale [11], the ITINERIS Scale [31], the National Core Indicators-Adult Consumer Survey (NCI-ACS) [3,32], and the European Child Environment Questionnaire (ECEQ). Although some studies employed qualitative methods (e.g., focus groups), quantitative questionnaires remained the most widely used and recommended approach, particularly in the case of self-report instruments.

The third research question focused on identifying indicators or personal outcome categories. The Article that received the most coverage in the reviewed papers was living independently and being included in the community (Article 19), followed by the right to freedom from exploitation, violence and abuse (Article 16), and habilitation and rehabilitation (Article 26). It is striking, however, that none of the publications referred to specific indicators associated with situations of risk and humanitarian emergencies (Article 11). In light of the global Covid-19 pandemic, this is unlikely to remain the case for much longer, and we would hope that future research will focus on the potential situations of discrimination or particular vulnerability faced by people with IDD in the fight against this pandemic (e.g., if they received appropriate information on how to prevent and treat the infection, if they received the supports they needed during the pandemic, if they were discriminated against by the health services on the grounds of their disability). Similarly, Articles 13 (access to justice) and 18 (liberty of movement and nationality) require further attention. With regard to the latter, it would be important to see studies examining the violation of the rights of people with IDD, where these people are also immigrants in a given country or refugees at a particular border.

The review of the literature and the analysis of the selected studies also revealed some limitations in the conceptual framework used, specifically with regard to the alignment of the CRPD Articles to the QOL domains. In particular, we found that Article 15 (freedom from torture or cruel, inhuman or degrading treatment or punishment), included in the rights domain by Verdugo et al. [1], was closely linked in the literature to the indicators proposed for Article 16 (freedom from exploitation, violence and abuse), assigned to the emotional wellbeing domain. Given this close relationship, and following our review of the scientific literature, we propose that Articles 15 and 16 both be included in the emotional wellbeing domain. In addition, overlaps in the indicators proposed by Lombardi et al. [2] required the removal of some repetitions (e.g., indicators for Article 30 were removed from the interpersonal relationships domain because they had also been included in the social inclusion domain; or the "safe and secure environment" indicators, which in the initial model featured as indicators of Article 14, liberty and security of the person, but also of Article 16, freedom from exploitation, violence and abuse, were finally assigned to the latter). We also reassigned indicators to a different Article where it made more sense, as a result of what we found in our literature review. For example, "dating with persons of choice" was initially included as an indicator of Article 5, equality and non-discrimination, in the rights domain. Since all of the studies included this as an indicator of Article 23, respect for home and the family, in the interpersonal relationships domain, we assigned it accordingly. In this way, as the authors themselves suggested [2], a refinement of their proposal has been made based on an exhaustive review of the literature.

Articles 6 (women with disabilities) and 7 (children with disabilities) deserve particular mention. The literature review revealed that they do not contain additional rights to those already covered in other Articles, but rather they are two cross-cutting Articles that seek to draw attention to these two specific groups in view of their particular vulnerability. Rather than including specific items in any assessment instruments that are developed, we would recommend that this information be collected as sociodemographic variables (i.e., gender, age) in order to verify whether these two conditions can have a significant impact on outcomes.

Finally, this review should be seen as a relevant, critical and necessary step in the development of future instruments to inform people with IDD of their rights, and to inform supporting professionals and family members of these rights, while at the same time to monitor the implementation of the CRPD. This review is just the first step in the process of operationalizing the CRPD through tentative definitions composed of all indicators and outcomes found in the scientific literature. That said, additional steps in each country or culture will be necessary or advisable in order to further refine the pool of indicators and personal outcomes described here, with the aim of achieving a comprehensive list that is relevant to the target group. Such an approach will help enhance the content validity of employing unique indicators to specific Articles and QOL domains. As part of this process, qualitative techniques such as focus groups and consultations with key experts and stakeholders including people with IDD are recommended in order to provide evidences of their quality and validity. Finally, their translation into specific measurable items and testing their psychometric properties will be necessary to determine their validity and utility.

5. Conclusions

The key points that this review highlights are several. First, the relevance of the QOL framework to assess progress and identify needs and gaps in the implementation of the CRPD. Second, the need of specific assessment instruments to explore the implementation of the CRPD. And third, the lack of studies focused on situations of risk and humanitarian emergencies, access to justice, liberty of movement and nationality, women and children with disabilities.

Although it has been more than a decade since the CRPD entered into force in a large number of countries, people with disabilities, especially people with IDD, continue to see their fundamental rights undermined. To fully implement the CRPD, there is an urgent need to operationalize its Articles through the use of a validated conceptual model, such as the QOL model discussed in this article, as a framework to develop and apply reliable and valid instruments that not only allow countries to monitor the fulfillment of the rights set out in the CRPD in the macrosystem, but especially in the microsystem and the mesosystem. It is essential that people with IDD and their support providers (natural and professional) know their rights and that these rights can be evaluated through instruments that demonstrate sufficient levels of validity and reliability. Such a tool would facilitate relating the provision of individualized supports to specific CRPD Articles and implementing evidence-based practices for people with IDD. Such a process would enhance their QOL as full citizens. Based on an analysis of the scientific literature, this study constitutes an essential first step in the operationalization of the CRPD and providing evidence of content validity for the future development of context-focused assessment instruments.

Author Contributions: Conceptualization, L.E.G.; methodology, L.E.G., A.M., M.L.M., and M.Á.A.; writing—original draft preparation, L.E.G.; writing—review and editing, L.E.G., A.M., M.L.M., M.Á.A., M.L., and R.L.S.; funding acquisition and project administration, L.E.G. All authors have read and agreed to the published version of the manuscript.

Funding: This research was funded by the Spanish Ministry of Science, Innovation and Universities, grant number PID2019-105737RB-I00.

Conflicts of Interest: The authors declare no conflict of interest. The funders had no role in the design of the study; in the collection, analyses, or interpretation of data; in the writing of the manuscript, or in the decision to publish the results.

References

1. Verdugo, M.A.; Navas, P.; Gómez, L.E.; Schalock, R.L. The concept of quality of Life and its role in enhancing human rights in the field of intellectual disability. *J. Intellect. Disabil. Res.* **2012**, *56*, 1036–1045. [CrossRef] [PubMed]
2. Lombardi, M.; Vandenbussche, H.; Claes, C.; Schalock, R.L.; De Maeyer, J.; Vandevelde, S. The concept of quality of life as framework for implementing the UNCRPD. *J. Policy Pract. Intellect. Disabil.* **2019**, *16*, 180–190. [CrossRef]
3. Houseworth, J.; Stancliffe, R.J.; Tichá, R. Examining the National Core Indicators' Potential to monitor rights of people with intellectual and developmental disabilities according to the CRPD. *J. Policy Pract. Intellect. Disabil.* **2019**, *16*, 342–351. [CrossRef]
4. United Nations. Convention on the Rights of Persons with Disabilities. Available online: https://www.un.org/development/desa/disabilities/convention-on-the-rights-of-persons-with-disabilities.html (accessed on 31 October 2019).
5. Winzer, M.; Mazurek, K. The convention on the rights of persons with disabilities: Notes on genealogy and prospects. *J. Int. Spec. Needs Ed.* **2014**, *17*, 3–12. [CrossRef]
6. Perlin, M. There must be some way out of here: Why the Convention on the Rights of Persons with Disabilities is potentially the best weapon in the fight against sanism. *Psychiatry Psychol. Law* **2013**, *20*, 462–476. [CrossRef]
7. De Maeyer, J.; Vandenbussche, H.; Claes, C.; Reynaert, D. Human rights, the capability approach and Quality of Life: An integrated paradigm of support in the quest for social justice. *Int. J. Ther. Communities* **2017**, *38*, 1–6. [CrossRef]
8. Navas, P.; Gómez, L.E.; Verdugo, M.A.; Schalock, R.L. Derechos de las personas con discapacidad intelectual: Implicaciones de la Convención de Naciones Unidas [Rights of People with Intellectual Disabilities: Implications of the United Nations Convention]. *Siglo. Cero.* **2012**, *43*, 7–28.
9. Mittler, P. The UN Convention on the rights of persons with disabilities: Implementing a paradigm shift. *J. Policy Pract. Intellect. Disabil.* **2015**, *12*, 79–89. [CrossRef]
10. Shogren, K.A.; Turnbull, H.R. Core concepts of disability policy, the convention on the rights of persons with disabilities, and public policy research with respect to developmental disabilities. *J. Policy Pract. Intellect. Disabil.* **2014**, *11*, 19–26. [CrossRef]
11. Karr, V. A life of quality: Informing the UN convention on the rights of persons with disabilities. *J. Disabil. Policy Stud.* **2011**, *22*, 66–82. [CrossRef]
12. Gómez, L.E.; Verdugo, M.A. Outcomes evaluation. In *Cross-cultural Quality of Life: Enhancing the Lives of Persons with Intellectual Disability*, 2nd ed.; Schalock, R.L., Keith, K.D., Eds.; American Association on Intellectual and Developmental Disabilities: Washington, DC, USA, 2016; pp. 71–80.
13. Gómez, L.E.; Verdugo, M.A.; Arias, B.; Irurtia, M.J. Evaluación de los derechos de las personas con discapacidad intelectual: Estudio preliminar [Assessment of the rights of people with intellectual disabilities: A preliminary study]. *Behav. Psychol.* **2011**, *19*, 207–222.
14. Brown, R.I. Quality of life—Challenges to research, practice and policy. *J. Policy Pract. Intellect. Disabil.* **2017**, *14*, 7–14. [CrossRef]
15. Schalock, R.L.; Gómez, L.E.; Verdugo, M.A.; Claes, C. Evidence and evidence-based practices: Are we there yet? *Intellect. Dev. Disab.* **2017**, *55*, 112–119. [CrossRef] [PubMed]
16. Schalock, R.L.; Verdugo, M.A.; Gómez, L.E. Evidence-based practices in the field of intellectual and developmental disabilities: An international consensus approach. *Eval. Program Plann.* **2011**, *34*, 273–282. [CrossRef]

17. Schalock, R.L.; Verdugo, M.A.; Gómez, L.E. Translating the quality of life concept into practice. In *Handbook of Positive Psychology in Intellectual and Developmental Disabilities: Translating Research into Practice*; Singh, N., Wehmeyer, M.L., Shogren, K., Eds.; Springer: New York, NY, USA, 2017; pp. 115–126.
18. Cummins, R.A. Moving from the quality of life concept to a theory. *J. Intellect. Disabil. Res.* **2005**, *49*, 699–706. [CrossRef]
19. Felce, D.; Perry, J. Quality of life: Its definition and measurement. *Res. Dev. Disabil.* **1995**, *16*, 51–74. [CrossRef]
20. Schalock, R.L.; Verdugo, M.A. *Quality of Life for Human Service Practitioners*; American Association on Mental Retardation: Washington, DC, USA, 2002.
21. Arias, V.B.; Gómez, L.E.; Morán, L.; Alcedo, M.A.; Monsalve, A.; Fontanil, Y. Does quality of life differ for children with autism spectrum disorder and intellectual disability compared to children without autism? *J. Autism. Dev. Disord.* **2018**, *48*, 123–136. [CrossRef]
22. Fernández, M.; Gómez, L.E.; Arias, V.B.; Aguayo, V.; Amor, A.M.; Andelic, N.; Verdugo, M.A. A new scale for measuring quality of life in acquired brain injury. *Qual. Life Res.* **2019**, *28*, 801–814. [CrossRef]
23. Gómez, L.E.; Alcedo, M.A.; Arias, B.; Fontanil, Y.; Arias, V.B.; Monsalve, M.A.; Verdugo, M.A. A new scale for the measurement of quality of life in children with intellectual disability. *Res. Dev. Disabil.* **2016**, *53–54*, 399–410. [CrossRef]
24. Gómez, L.E.; Morán, L.; Alcedo, M.A.; Arias, V.B.; Verdugo, M.A. Addressing quality of life of children with autism spectrum disorder and intellectual disability. *Intellect. Dev. Disab.* **2020**, in press.
25. Gómez, L.E.; Verdugo, M.A.; Rodríguez, M.A.; Morán, L.; Arias, V.B.; Monsalve, A. Adapting a measure of quality of life to children with down syndrome for the development of evidence-based interventions. *Psychosoc. Interv.* **2020**, *29*, 39–48. [CrossRef]
26. Jenaro, C.; Verdugo, M.A.; Caballo, C.; Balboni, G.; Lachapelle, Y.; Otrebski, W.; Schalock, R.L. Cross-cultural study of person-centered quality of life domains and indicators. *J. Intellect. Disabil. Res.* **2005**, *49*, 734–739. [CrossRef] [PubMed]
27. Wang, M.; Schalock, R.L.; Verdugo, M.A.; Jenaro, C. Examining the factor structure and hierarchical nature of the quality of life construct. *AJIDD-AM J. Intellect.* **2010**, *115*, 218–233. [CrossRef] [PubMed]
28. Fisher, K.R.; Lutz, D.; Gadow, F.; Robinson, S.; Gendera, S. A Transformative framework for deinstitutionalisation. *Res. Pract. Intellect. Dev. Disabil.* **2015**, *2*, 60–72. [CrossRef]
29. Faragher, R.; Van Ommen, M. Conceptualising educational quality of life to understand the school experiences of students with intellectual disability. *J. Policy Pract. Intellect. Disabil.* **2017**, *14*, 39–50. [CrossRef]
30. Sheridan, C.; Omalley-Keighran, M.P.; Carroll, C. What are the perspectives of adolescents with Down syndrome about their quality of life? A scoping review. *Br. J. Learn. Disabil.* **2019**, *48*, 98–105. [CrossRef]
31. Aznar, A.; González, D.; Olate, G. The ITINERIS scale on the rights of persons with intellectual disabilities: Development, pilot studies and application at a country level in South America. *J. Intellect. Disabil. Res.* **2012**, *56*, 1046–1057. [CrossRef]
32. Ticha, R.; Qian, X.; Stancliffe, R.J.; Larson, S.A.; Bonardi, A. Alignment between the convention on the rights of persons with disabilities and the national core indicators adult consumer survey. *J. Policy Pract. Intellect. Disabil.* **2018**, *15*, 247–255. [CrossRef]
33. Colver, A.F.; Dickinson, H.O.; Parkinson, K.; Arnaud, C.; Beckung, E.; Fauconnier, J.; Marcelli, M.; McManus, V.; Michelsen, S.I.; Parkes, J.; et al. Access of children with cerebral palsy to the physical, social and attitudinal environment they need: A cross-sectional European study. *Disabil. Rehabil.* **2011**, *33*, 28–35. [CrossRef]
34. Stevenson, M. Flexible and responsive research: Developing rights-based emancipatory disability research methodology in collaboration with young adults with Down syndrome. *Aust. Soc. Work* **2010**, *63*, 35–50. [CrossRef]
35. Fullana, J.; Pallisera, M.; Vilà, M.; Puyalto, C. Discussions, challenges and possibilities of inclusive research. *Empiria* **2016**, *33*, 111–138. [CrossRef]
36. Salmon, N.; Barry, A.; Hutchins, E. Inclusive research: An Irish perspective. *Br. J. Learn. Disabil.* **2018**, *46*, 268–277. [CrossRef]
37. Garcia, E.; O'Brien, P.; Chadwick, D. Involving people with intellectual disabilities within research teams: Lessons learned from an Irish experience. *J. Policy Pract. Intellect. Disabil.* **2014**, *11*, 149–157. [CrossRef]

38. Salmon, N.; Garcia, E.; Donohoe, B.; Murray, L.; Singleton, G.; Barrett, M.; Dillon, M. Our Homes: An inclusive study about what moving house is like for people with intellectual disabilities in Ireland. *Br. J. Learn. Disabil.* **2019**, *47*, 19–28. [CrossRef]
39. Puyalto, C.; Pallisera, M.; Fullana, J.; Diaz, G. Challenges of having a loving partner: The views of adults with intellectual disabilities. *Int. J. Dev. Disabil.* **2019**. [CrossRef]
40. García, E.; O'Brien, P.; McConkey, R.; Wolfe, M.; O'Doherty, S. Identifying the key concerns of Irish persons with intellectual disability. *J. Appl. Res. Intellect.* **2014**, *27*, 564–575. [CrossRef] [PubMed]
41. Salmon, N.; Garcia, E.; Burns, E.Q. Research Active Programme: A pilot inclusive research curriculum in higher education. *Int. J. Res. Method Edu.* **2017**, *40*, 181–200. [CrossRef]
42. Zwicker, J.; Zaresani, A.; Emery, J.C.H. Describing heterogeneity of unmet needs among adults with a developmental disability: An examination of the 2012 Canadian Survey on Disability. *Res. Dev. Disabil.* **2017**, *65*, 1–11. [CrossRef]
43. Echeita, G.; Simon, C.; Verdugo, M.A.; Sandoval, M.; Lopez, M.; Calvo, I.; González-Gil, F. Paradoxes and dilemmas in the inclusive education process in Spain. *Rev. Educ.* **2009**, *349*, 153–178.
44. Judge, S.; Izuzquiza, D. Inclusion in the workforce for students with intellectual disabilities: A case study of a spanish postsecondary education program. *J. Postsecond. Ed. Disabil.* **2015**, *28*, 121–127.
45. Symeonidou, S. Rights of people with intellectual disability in cyprus: Policies and practices related to greater social and educational inclusion. *J. Policy Pract. Intellect. Disabil.* **2015**, *12*, 120–131. [CrossRef]
46. Figueroa, M.; Vázquez, G.; Castro, G.J. Theoretical and practical contributions, aimed at the social and labor insertion of children, adolescents and young people with disabilities from Milagro State University (UNEMI). *Dilem. Contemp. Ed. Polít. Valor* **2018**. Available online: https://search.proquest.com/openview/80b299a4f3ca522bd4aaa2c2784b6c02/1?pq-origsite=gscholar&cbl=4400984 (accessed on 15 July 2020).
47. Pallisera, M.; Fullana, J.; Puyalto, C.; Vila, M.; Valls, M.J.; Diaz, G.; Castro, M. Retos para la vida independiente de las personas con discapacidad intelectual. Un estudio basado en sus opiniones, las de sus familias y las de los profesionales [Challenges for independent living of people with intellectual disabilities. A study based on their opinions, opinions of their families and professionals]. *Rev. Esp. Discap.* **2018**, *6*, 7–29. [CrossRef]
48. Shikako-Thomas, K.; Shevell, M. Promoting the human rights of children with neurologic conditions. *Semin. Pediatr. Neurol.* **2018**, *27*, 53–61. [CrossRef]
49. Steinert, C.; Steinert, T.; Flammer, E.; Jaeger, S. Impact of the UN convention on the rights of persons with disabilities (UN-CRPD) on mental health care research-a systematic review. *BMC Psychiatry* **2016**, *16*, 166. [CrossRef]
50. O'Donovan, M.A.; Mannan, H.; McVeigh, J.; Mc Carron, M.; McCallion, P.; Byrne, E. Core human rights concepts in Irish health and housing policy documents: In search of equity for people with ID. *J. Policy Pract. Intellect. Disabil.* **2018**, *15*, 307–313. [CrossRef]
51. Brolan, C.E.; Boyle, F.M.; Dean, J.H.; Taylor, M.; Ware, R.S.; Lennox, N.G. Health advocacy: A vital step in attaining human rights for adults with intellectual disability. *J. Intellect. Disabil. Res.* **2012**, *56*, 1087–1097. [CrossRef]
52. Strnadova, I.; Evans, D. Older women with intellectual disabilities: Overcoming barriers to autonomy. *J. Policy Pract. Intellect. Disabil.* **2015**, *12*, 12–19. [CrossRef]
53. Siska, J.; Beadle-Brown, J.; Kanova, S.; Sumnikova, P. Social inclusion through community living: Current situation, advances and gaps in policy, practice and research. *Soc. Incl.* **2018**, *6*, 94–109. [CrossRef]
54. Boot, F.H.; MacLachlan, M.; Dinsmore, J. Are there differences in factors influencing access and continues use of assistive products for people with intellectual disabilities living in group homes? *Disabil. Rehabil. Assist. Technol.* **2019**, *15*, 173–182. [CrossRef]
55. Lussier-Desrochers, D.; Normand, C.L.; Romero, A.; Lachapelle, Y.; Godin-Tremblay, V.; Dupont, M.E.; Roux, J.; Pepin-Beauchesne, L.; Bilodeau, P. Bridging the digital divide for people with intellectual disability. *Cyberpsychol: J. Psychosoc. Res. Cyberspace* **2017**, *11*, 1. [CrossRef]
56. Feldman, M.A.; Owen, F.; Andrews, A.; Hamelin, J.; Barber, R.; Griffiths, D. Health self-advocacy training for persons with intellectual disabilities. *J. Intellect. Disabil. Res.* **2012**, *56*, 1110–1121. [CrossRef] [PubMed]
57. Polanco, M.; Martín, J.L. Conocimientos, actitudes y prácticas de familias de adolescentes con discapacidad cognitiva en sexualidad y afectividad [Knowledge, attitudes and practices of families of teenagers with cognitive disabilities in sexuality and affectivity]. *Diversitas* **2017**, *13*, 187–199. [CrossRef]

58. Kong, C. Constructing female sexual and reproductive agency in mental capacity law. *Int. J. Law Psychiatry* **2019**, *66*, 101488. [CrossRef] [PubMed]
59. Villaró, G.; Galindo, L. Intellectual disability and gender violence: Comprehensive intervention program. *Acción Psicol.* **2012**, *9*, 101–114.
60. Azzopardi-Lane, C. Intimate relationships and persons with learning disability. *Tizard Learn. Disabil. Rev.* **2017**, *22*, 24–27. [CrossRef]
61. McConnell, D. Parents labelled with intellectual disability: Position of the IASSID SIRG on parents and parenting with intellectual disabilities. *J. Appl. Res. Intellect.* **2008**, *21*, 296–307. [CrossRef]
62. Kelly, G.; Crowley, H.; Hamilton, C. Rights, sexuality and relationships in Ireland: 'It'd be nice to be kind of trusted'. *Br. J. Learn. Disabil.* **2009**, *37*, 308–315. [CrossRef]
63. Chan, J. Challenges to realizing the Convention on the Rights of Persons with Disabilities (CRPD) in Australia for people with intellectual disability and behaviours of concern. *Psychiatry Psychol. Law* **2016**, *23*, 207–214. [CrossRef]
64. Del Castillo, S.; Martín, R. Comunicación inclusiva: Una experiencia en creación de campañas sobre discapacidad intelectual [Inclusive Communication: An Experience in Creation of Campaigns on Intellectual Disability]. *Area. Abierta.* **2012**, *31*, 1–18.
65. Fraser, V.; Llewellyn, G. Good, Bad or absent: Discourses of parents with disabilities in Australian news media. *J. Appl. Res. Intellect.* **2015**, *28*, 319–324. [CrossRef]
66. McKenzie, J.; McConkey, R.; Adnams, C. Residential facilities for adults with intellectual disability in a developing country: A case study from South Africa. *J. Intellect. Dev. Dis.* **2014**, *39*, 45–54. [CrossRef]
67. Conceição, D.B.; Vázquez, V.; Costa da Cunha, C.; López, O. Accesibilidad en salud: Revisión sobre niños y niñas con discapacidad en Brasil-Perú-Colombia. *Rev. Lat. Cienc. Soc. Niñez* **2019**, *17*, 1–20. [CrossRef]
68. Fullana, J.; Pallisera, M.; Vila, M.; Valls, M.J.; Diaz-Garolera, G. Intellectual disability and independent living: Professionals' views via a Delphi study. *J. Intellect. Disabil.* **2019**. [CrossRef] [PubMed]
69. Fisher, K.R.; Purcal, C.; Jones, A.; Lutz, D.; Robinson, S.; Kayess, R. What place is there for shared housing with individualized disability support? *Disabil. Rehabil.* **2019**. [CrossRef]
70. James, E.; Harvey, M.; Hatton, C. Participation of adults with learning disabilities in the 2015 UK General Election. *Tizard Learn. Disabil. Rev.* **2018**, *23*, 65–71. [CrossRef]
71. Redley, M.; Maina, E.; Keeling, A.; Pattni, P. The voting rights of adults with intellectual disabilities: Reflections on the arguments, and situation in Kenya and England and Wales. *J. Intellect. Disabil. Res.* **2012**, *56*, 1026–1035. [CrossRef]
72. Van Hees, S.G.M.; Boeije, H.R.; de Putter, I. Voting barriers and solutions: The experiences of people with disabilities during the Dutch national election in 2017. *Disabil. Soc.* **2019**, *34*, 819–836. [CrossRef]
73. Brehmer-Rinderer, B.; Zigrovic, L.; Naue, U.; Weber, G. Promoting health of persons with intellectual disabilities using the UN Convention on the Rights of Persons with Disabilities: Early implementation assessment in Spain and Hungary. *J. Policy Pract. Intellect. Disabil.* **2013**, *10*, 25–36. [CrossRef]
74. Douglas, H.; Harpur, P. Intellectual disabilities, domestic violence and legal engagement. *Disabil. Soc.* **2016**, *31*, 305–321. [CrossRef]
75. Gabor, P. Children with learning disabilities and their participation in judicial procedures-what can disability advocacy offer? *Tizard Learn. Disabil. Rev.* **2017**, *22*, 10–15. [CrossRef]
76. Watson, J.; Wilson, E.; Hagiliassis, N. Supporting end of life decision making: Case studies of relational closeness in supported decision making for people with severe or profound intellectual disability. *J. Appl. Res. Intellect.* **2017**, *30*, 1022–1034. [CrossRef] [PubMed]
77. Watchman, K.; Janicki, M.P.; Asante, C.; Berankova, A.; Bishop, K.; Cadovius, N.; Cooper, S.A.; Coppus, T.; Crowe, J.; Dodd, K.; et al. The intersection of intellectual disability and dementia: Report of The International Summit on Intellectual Disability and Dementia. *Gerontol.* **2019**, *53*, 411–419. [CrossRef] [PubMed]
78. Bigby, C.; Douglas, J.; Carney, T.; Then, S.N.; Wiesel, I.; Smith, E. Delivering decision making support to people with cognitive disability-What has been learned from pilot programs in Australia from 2010 to 2015. *Aus. J. Soc. Issues* **2017**, *52*, 222–240. [CrossRef]
79. Werner, S.; Chabany, R. Guardianship law versus supported decision-making policies: Perceptions of persons with intellectual or psychiatric disabilities and parents. *Am. J. Orthopsychiatr.* **2016**, *86*, 486–499. [CrossRef] [PubMed]

80. Devi, N.; Prodinger, B.; Pennycott, A.; Sooben, R.; Bickenbach, J. Investigating supported decision-making for persons with mild to moderate intellectual disability using institutional ethnography. *J. Policy Pract. Intellect. Disabil.* **2019**, *17*, 143–156. [CrossRef]
81. Davidson, G.; Kelly, B.; Macdonald, G.; Rizzo, M.; Lombard, L.; Abogunrin, O.; Clift-Matthews, V.; Martin, A. Supported decision making: A review of the international literature. *Int. J. Law Psychiatry* **2015**, *38*, 61–67. [CrossRef]
82. McSherry, B. Regulating seclusion and restraint in health care settings: The promise of the Convention on the Rights of Persons with Disabilities. *Int. J. Law Psychiatry* **2017**, *53*, 39–44. [CrossRef]
83. Ramsay, H.; Mulryan, N.; McCallion, P.; McCarron, M. Geographical Barriers to Mental Health Service Care Among Individuals with an Intellectual Disability in the Republic of Ireland. *J. Policy Pract. Intellect. Disabil.* **2016**, *13*, 261–268. [CrossRef]
84. Werner, S.; Levav, I.; Stawski, M.; Polakiewicz, Y. Israeli Psychiatrists Report on Their Ability to Care for Individuals with Intellectual Disability and Psychiatric Disorders. *Isr. J. Psychiatry Relat. Sci.* **2013**, *50*, 202–209.
85. Evans, E.; Howlett, S.; Kremser, T.; Simpson, J.; Kayess, R.; Trollor, J. Service development for intellectual disability mental health: A human rights approach. *J. Intellect. Disabil. Res.* **2012**, *56*, 1098–1109. [CrossRef]
86. Schalock, R.L.; Luckasson, R.; Tassé, M.J. The contemporary view of intellectual and developmental disabilities: Implications for psychologists. *Psicothema* **2019**, *31*, 223–228. [CrossRef] [PubMed]

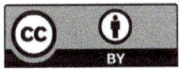

© 2020 by the authors. Licensee MDPI, Basel, Switzerland. This article is an open access article distributed under the terms and conditions of the Creative Commons Attribution (CC BY) license (http://creativecommons.org/licenses/by/4.0/).

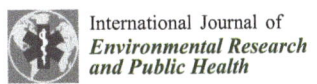

Perspective

The Importance of Self-Determination to the Quality of Life of People with Intellectual Disability: A Perspective

Michael L. Wehmeyer

Department of Special Education, School of Education and Human Sciences, Joseph R. Pearson Hall, University of Kansas, 1122 W. Campus Road, Room 521, Lawrence, KS 66045-3101, USA; wehmeyer@ku.edu; Tel.: +1-785-864-0723

Received: 20 August 2020; Accepted: 27 September 2020; Published: 29 September 2020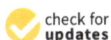

Abstract: There is both an intuitive and theoretical link between self-determination and quality of life for people with intellectual and developmental disabilities. Theoretically, definitions of self-determination have framed the construct with regard to its contribution to a person's overall quality of life, while theoretical frameworks of quality of life have included self-determination among the core dimensions contributing to enhanced quality of life. These theoretical linkages have been supported by research on the quality of life and self-determination of people with intellectual and developmental disabilities and the relationships between these constructs. This article provides an overview of theoretical frameworks of self-determination, their relationship with theoretical frameworks of quality of life, and research pertaining to these constructs with people with intellectual and developmental disabilities. It is concluded that self-determination and quality of life are important constructs in designing supports that enable people with intellectual and developmental disabilities and that an important means to enhance the quality of life of people with intellectual and developmental disabilities is to promote and enable people to be self-determined.

Keywords: self-determination; quality of life; intellectual disability; causal agency; volitional action; agentic action; action-control beliefs; choice

1. Introduction

There has been building, over the past four decades, a movement toward the application of strengths-based approaches to supporting people with intellectual and developmental disabilities [1]. It can be argued that the earliest contributions to this movement came with the application of the quality of life construct to the field [2]. The quality-of-life construct has evolved from one that was tied only to subjective perceptions of people to one in which the field "had ... embraced the QOL concept as a sensitizing notion and an overarching principle for service delivery" [3] (p. 3). Schalock and Keith defined quality of life as "a multidimensional phenomenon composed of core domains influenced by personal characteristics and environmental factors" [3] (p. 11). The quality-of-life conceptual model that has driven the application of this construct as an overarching principle for service delivery, as forwarded by Schalock and Keith, consists of eight domains, or core dimensions, namely personal development, self-determination, interpersonal relations, social inclusion, rights, emotional well-being, physical well-being, and material well-being [3,4].

However, another construct that has been instrumental in the shift from a deficits approach to intellectual and developmental disabilities to a strengths-based approach is the self-determination construct [5,6]. In fact, the first mention of the importance of self-determination to the lives of people with intellectual and developmental disabilities occurred in a 1972 chapter by Swedish philosopher Bengt Nirje, who argued for the right of people with intellectual disability to live 'normalized' lives and experience self-determination [7]. It was another 20 years, however, before a focus on self-determination and people with intellectual and developmental disabilities returned [5], and that focus emerged along with the recognition of the importance of the quality-of-life construct as an overarching principle for services and supports [6]. Too often over the years, however, the contribution of self-determination to quality of life has been taken as a given. The purpose of this Perspective is to provide a theoretical basis for understanding self-determination that has utility for, in turn, understanding it as a core dimension of quality of life and, further, in understanding the importance of self-determination as contributing to quality of life of people with intellectual disability in public health and human rights domains. The article begins with a brief introduction to the quality of life framework, followed by an overview of self-determination as it has been conceptualized within the field of intellectual disability. That, in turn, is followed by consideration of the research that has examined relationships between self-determination and quality of life. Finally, suggestions for future research are discussed.

2. Quality of Life

There is no intent to provide a comprehensive overview of quality of life in this article, in part because that will be evident to readers of this topical issue from other articles and because there is insufficient space to do this justice. In our work, we have adopted the quality-of-life framework forwarded by Robert Schalock [1]. Schalock and Verdugo [8] identified five overarching ways in which a focus on quality of life in the field of intellectual disability has, in fact, benefitted people with intellectual and developmental disabilities, and several of these speak to the ongoing importance of quality of life in moving toward strengths-based approaches to intellectual disability. Quality of life, argued Schalock and Verdugo, has provided a framework for a service delivery system that is "based on the values of dignity, equality, empowerment, self-determination, non-discrimination, and inclusion" [8] (p. 46). Quality of life is not a "thing" that people have; it is a multidimensional construct that provides a means to design and evaluate supports for people in service systems [9]. Research using this framework has identified eight core quality-of-life dimensions: emotional well-being, interpersonal relationships, material well-being, personal development, physical well-being, self-determination, social inclusion, and rights [10]. However, it is also worth noting that, in addition to being a core dimension of quality of life, self-determination with Schalock's framework is also a value upon which services are based and, presumably, an outcome of such services and supports.

3. Self-Determination

The self-determination construct was first applied to the intellectual disability context in the early 1990s [11]. Through the 20th century, the construct had been applied within personality and motivational psychology and in the field of social work and welfare. The common themes in how the construct has been used across these disparate fields was that self-determination fundamentally refers to people acting as causal agents; that is, as acting volitionally to make or cause things to happen in one's life [12]. Within the field of intellectual disability, Wehmeyer defined self-determination as "acting as the primary causal agent in one's life and making choices and decisions regarding one's quality of life free from undue external influence or interference [13] (p. 30). It is important to note that, even at the earliest stage of the application of the self-determination construct to the field of intellectual disability, it was, by definition, linked to quality of life.

The most recent iteration of the theoretical framework introduced by Wehmeyer is Causal Agency Theory [14]. Briefly, Causal Agency Theory was proposed to explain how people become self-determined and to explicate the development of self-determination [15]. Causal Agency Theory defined self-determination as follows:

> ... a dispositional characteristic manifested as acting as the causal agent in one's life. Self-determined people (i.e., causal agents) act in service to freely chosen goals. Self-determined actions function to enable a person to be the causal agent in his or her life. [14] (p. 258)

Acting as a causal agent implies that a person makes or causes things to happen in their life. Self-determined people act to accomplish specific ends or to cause or create change in their lives. Acting in a self-determined manner implies that people make or causes things to happen in their own lives, rather than someone or something else making them act in other ways. Self-determined action is goal-oriented, driven by preferences and interests, and ultimately serves to enable people to enhance the quality of their lives [16].

Causal Agency Theory is grounded in human agentic theories that assume that action is self-caused and that people want to be the origin of their own behavior [17]. Self-determined action refers to the degree to which action is volitional and agentic, driven by beliefs about the relationships between actions (or means) and ends. Causal Action Theory posits three essential characteristics of self-determined action—volitional action, agentic action, and action-control beliefs—that contribute to causal agency and the development of self-determination. These essential characteristics refer not to specific actions performed or the beliefs that drive action, but to the function the action serves for the person; that is, whether the action enabled the person to act as a causal agent and enhances the development of self-determination [18].

Volitional action is based on conscious choices that reflect one's preference. That is, volitional actions are self-initiated and function to enable a person to act autonomously and to engage in self-governed action. Volitional actions involve the initiation and activation of causal capabilities—the capacity to cause something to happen—in one's life. Agentic actions refer to the means by which something is done or achieved; they are self-directed and goal-focused. When acting agentically, self-determined people identify pathways that lead to a specific end or cause or create change. The identification of pathways, or pathways thinking, is a proactive, purposive process. Agentic action is self-regulated, self-directed, and enables progress toward freely chosen goals. Volitional actions involve the initiation and activation of agentic capabilities—the capacity to sustain action toward a goal [18].

Finally, in acting volitionally and agentically, self-determined people develop a sense of personal empowerment and a belief that they have what it takes to achieve their freely chosen goals. They perceive linkages between their actions and the outcomes they want to experience; they develop adaptive action-control beliefs. To account for these beliefs and actions, Causal Agency Theory incorporates basic tenets of Action-Control Theory [19], which posits three types of action-control beliefs: beliefs about the link between the self and the goal (control expectancy beliefs; "When I want to do ____, I can"); beliefs about the link between the self and the means for achieving the goal (capacity beliefs; "I have the capabilities to do ____"); and beliefs about the utility or usefulness of a given means for attaining a goal (causality beliefs; "I believe my effort will lead to goal achievement" vs. "I believe other factors—luck, access to teachers, or social capital—will lead to goal achievement"). As adaptive action-control beliefs emerge, people are better able to act with self-awareness and self-knowledge in a goal-directed manner [19].

Through each iteration of this theoretical work and research in self-determination, the relationship between self-determination and quality of life has remained a critical feature. Self-determination, in Causal Agency Theory, is seen as contributing to one's overall quality of life. In the following section, the role of self-determination within theories of quality of life is discussed, followed be a look at the research pertaining to quality of life and self-determination in the disability context.

4. Quality of Life and Self-Determination

Schalock and Verdugo [20] pointed out that the quality-of-life concept has provided an outcomes-based evaluation framework associated with specific domains (including self-determination) that enable both the consideration of personally valued life outcomes and the design of large systems of supports. However, we do not have to take the relationship between quality of life and self-determination as a theoretical supposition only. There has been some research examining the relationship among these two constructs or as part of the examination of relative contributions of all the core dimensions of quality of life. Schalock and colleagues [20] conducted a study examining the core dimensions of quality of life across five geographical groups (Spain, Central/South America, Canada, Mainland China, and the United States). The purpose of the study was to identify properties of these core dimensions across geographically and culturally diverse populations. More than 750 respondents completed a survey that asked questions about relative importance of each of eight core dimension (including self-determination) and 24 indicators of those dimensions, and the degree to which each indicator was available to the person/supported by the system. Respondents indicated importance and availability on a four-point scale, with 1 indicating not important or never and 4 indicating very important or always. Participants included people with intellectual and developmental disabilities, professionals in the field, and families of people with intellectual and developmental disabilities. Across type of respondents and geographical regions, all dimensions scored high (around 3 out of 4 up to 3.5 out of 4) on ratings of the importance of each of these. Interestingly, when reporting on the importance of the core dimension of self-determination, people with disabilities themselves rated it higher than did either professionals or family members. Based upon analyses of variance by group (person with disability, professional, parent) and geographic region (Spain, Central/South America, Canada, Mainland China, and the United States), there were significant differences in reports of importance of self-determination as a function of group (with, as previously noted, people with disability reporting the highest importance and professionals reporting the lowest) as well as geographic regions (with importance of self-determination generally lower (though still at or around 3 out of 4) in China and highest in Spain and North America.

Two studies have directly measured quality of life and self-determination to examine relationships among people with intellectual and developmental disabilities. Wehmeyer and Schwartz [21] measured the self-determination and quality of 50 adults with an intellectual disability. Quality of life was measured by using the Quality of Life Questionnaire [22], and self-determination status was measured by The Arc's Self-Determination Scale [23]. The number of choices available to each participant was measured by using the Life Choices Survey [24]. These researchers hypothesized that individual self-determination status and choice opportunity would predict high- or low-quality-of-life group membership. Based on a discriminant function analysis, it was determined that self-determination scores predicted membership in the high-quality-of-life group, and that such scores correlated significantly with choice opportunities. Lachapelle and colleagues [25] replicated this study, though measuring only self-determination and quality of life, with a sample of people with intellectual and developmental disabilities in four countries: Canada, the United States, Belgium, and France. Those findings mirrored those of Wehmeyer and Schwartz, indicating that overall self-determination as well as subdomains of self-determined behavior (including autonomous functioning) predicted membership in the higher quality of life group.

Choice and choice opportunity have been linked with self-determination and quality of life. Research has established that the environments in which many people with an intellectual disability live or work—and particularly congregate settings—restrict opportunities for choice-making and the expression of preferences [26]. Wehmeyer and Metzler [27] conducted a secondary analysis of data from a nationwide US survey of more than 4500 people with intellectual disability, finding that participants had limited choice opportunities across virtually every aspect of their lives, from whom they lived with to where they ate or worked. Stancliffe and Wehmeyer [28] used the Life Choices Survey [24] with nearly 400 people with an intellectual disability, and they found that living arrangement impacted choice opportunity with more inclusive living arrangements supporting enhanced choice opportunities, but, that, in general, beyond mundane day-to-day tasks, people with intellectual disability were provided very few opportunities to make choices, particularly when it came to more meaningful choices such as where to work. Two studies examining the relationship between choice opportunity, self-determination, and living/working arrangements directly confirmed the link between choice and self-determination, as well as to lifestyle satisfaction. Wehmeyer and Bolding [29] conducted a matched-samples study of adults with intellectual disability who were matched by age and intelligence level but varied as to whether they lived or worked in a large congregate, community-based congregate, or community-based setting. Level of self-determination, choice opportunity, and lifestyle satisfaction varied by living or working setting, with people living or working in more typical community-based settings higher in all those areas. In a subsequent study, these researchers [30] measured the self-determination and choice opportunities of people with intellectual disability who were moving from a more restrictive (congregate) work or living situation to an integrated, community-based work or living situation. There were significant positive changes in self-determination and choice opportunity as a function of moving from the more restrictive to the community-based setting. Finally, there are several studies of people with intellectual and developmental disabilities who have moved from institutions into the community that document the connection between choice opportunity and quality of life. Kozma and colleagues [31] summarized this literature, finding that people who moved to the community had, among other factors, increased opportunities for choice and experienced better quality of life and life satisfaction.

5. Discussion

There is both an intuitive and theoretical link between self-determination and quality of life for people with intellectual and developmental disabilities. Intuitively, it makes sense that greater autonomy and volitional action would enhance one's quality of life. Theoretically, definitions of self-determination have framed the construct with regard to its contribution to a person's overall quality of life, while theoretical frameworks of quality of life have included self-determination as among the core dimensions contributing to enhanced quality of life. These theoretical linkages have been supported by research, discussed previously, on the quality of life and self-determination of people with intellectual and developmental disabilities and the relationship between those constructs. There are several implications from this knowledge base that warrant consideration. First, most of this research has been survey research or quasi-experimental, and there is a need for more rigorous examinations of the two constructs. Both constructs can only be measured by using self-report assessments, and thus such research is labor-intensive. Nevertheless, it would be important to have larger-scale studies that employ randomized trial designs to establish these relationships. Second, the field of positive psychology has expanded research in areas pertaining to well-being, happiness, optimism, and life satisfaction, all of which pertain to quality of life and with which self-determination interacts to improve life outcomes for people. For example, Shogren and colleagues [32] conducted a structural equation modeling analysis of the relationships among the psychological constructs of hope, optimism, locus of control, and self-determination in predicting life satisfaction of adolescents with and without cognitive disabilities. Hope and optimism predicted life satisfaction directly, but those effects were mediated (positively) by self-determination and locus of control. Thus, there is a need to examine the interrelatedness among and between self-determination, quality of life, and other closely associated constructs. Third, we know very little about the quality of life and self-determination of people with intellectual and developmental disabilities who cannot reliably complete self-report measures. There are some larger-scale, statewide surveys, such as the National Core Indicators project in the United States (https://www.nationalcoreindicators.org/), that use proxy reporting to provide indicators of quality of life, but there is a need for validated measures of self-determination and quality of life that do not rely on self-report. Finally, most of this research has been in the domains of education, independent living, or employment. There is a need to examine issues of self-determination and quality of life of people with an intellectual disability in the public-health domain. Issues of autonomy and volition are critically important in the public-health domain, and, obviously, greater opportunity to act as a causal agent in one's health-related life should contribute to improved quality of life. However, that research has yet to be conducted and is needed.

6. Conclusions

It goes without saying that, individually, self-determination and quality of life are important constructs, particularly in designing supports that enable people with intellectual and developmental disabilities to live, learn, work, and play in their communities. Being self-determined—that is, acting volitionally and making things to happen in one's life—has been linked to multiple positive outcomes, including, importantly, enhanced quality of life and life satisfaction. Therefore, one means to enhance the quality of life of people with intellectual and developmental disabilities is to promote and enable people to be self-determined.

Author Contributions: Conceptualization, writing, and editing by M.L.W. The author has read and agreed to the published version of the manuscript.

Funding: This research received no external funding.

Conflicts of Interest: The author declares no conflict of interest.

References

1. Wehmeyer, M.L. *The Oxford Handbook on Positive Psychology and Disability*; Oxford University Press: Oxford, UK, 2013.
2. Schalock, R.L. *Quality of Life: Perspectives and Issues*; American Association on Mental Retardation: Washington, DC, USA, 1990.
3. Schalock, R.L.; Keith, K.D. The evolution of the quality-of-life concept. In *Cross-cultural Quality of Life: Enhancing the Lives of People with Intellectual Disability*, 2nd ed.; Schalock, R.L., Keith, K.D., Eds.; American Association on Intellectual and Developmental Disabilities: Washington, DC, USA, 2016; pp. 3–12.
4. Schalock, R.L. *Quality of Life: Vol. 1. Conceptualization and Measurement*; American Association on Mental Retardation: Washington, DC, USA, 1996.
5. Wehmeyer, M.L.; Schalock, R.L. Self-determination and quality of life: Implications for special education services and supports. *Focus Except. Child.* **2001**, *33*, 1–16.
6. Wehmeyer, M.L. Self-determination and the education of students with mental retardation. *Educ. Train. Ment. Retard.* **1992**, *27*, 302–314.
7. Nirje, B. The right to self-determination. In *The Principle of Normalization in Human Services*; Wolfensberger, W., Ed.; Canadian National Institute on Mental Retardation: Toronto, CA, Canada, 1972; pp. 176–193.
8. Schalock, R.L.; Verdugo, M.A. The impact of the quality of life concept on the field of intellectual disability. In *The Oxford Handbook of Positive Psychology and Disability*; Wehmeyer, M., Ed.; Oxford University Press: Oxford, UK, 2013; pp. 37–47.
9. Schalock, R.L. Quality of life, quality enhancement, and quality assurance: Implications for program planning and evaluation in the field of mental retardation and developmental disabilities. *Eval. Program Plan.* **1994**, *17*, 121–131. [CrossRef]
10. Schalock, R.L. Reconsidering the conceptualization and measurement of quality of life. In *Quality of Life: Vol. I: Conceptualization and Measurement*; Schalock, R.L., Ed.; American Association on Mental Retardation: Washington, DC, USA, 1996; pp. 3–21.
11. Wehmeyer, M.L.; Kelchner, K.; Richards, S. Essential characteristics of self-determined behavior of individuals with mental retardation. *Am. J. Ment. Retard.* **1996**, *100*, 632–642. [PubMed]
12. Wehmeyer, M.L.; Mithaug, D. Self-determination, causal agency, and mental retardation. In *International Review of Research in Mental Retardation: Vol. 31 Current Perspectives on Individual Differences in Personality and Motivation in Persons with Mental Retardation and Other Developmental Disabilities*; Glidden, L.M., Switzky, H., Eds.; Academic Press: San Diego, CA, USA, 2006; pp. 31–71.
13. Wehmeyer, M.L. Self-determination and mental retardation. In *International Review of Research in Mental Retardation*; Glidden, L., Ed.; Academic Press: San Diego, CA, USA, 2001; pp. 1–48.
14. Shogren, K.A.; Wehmeyer, M.L.; Palmer, S.B.; Forber-Pratt, A.; Little, T.; Lopez, S. Causal Agency Theory: Reconceptualizing a functional model of self-determination. *Educ. Train. Ment. Retard.* **2015**, *50*, 251–263.
15. Wehmeyer, M.L.; Shogren, K.A.; Little, T.D.; Lopez, S.J. *Development of Self-determination Through the Life-course*; Springer: New York, NY, USA, 2017.
16. Wehmeyer, M.L.; Shogren, K.A. Goal setting and attainment and self-regulation. In *Handbook of Positive Psychology in Intellectual and Developmental Disabilities: Translating Research into Practice*; Shogren, K.A., Wehmeyer, M.L., Singh, N.N., Eds.; Springer: New York, NY, USA, 2017; pp. 231–245.

17. Wehmeyer, M.L.; Little, T.; Sergeant, J. Self-Determination. In *Handbook of Positive Psychology*, 2nd ed.; Lopez, S., Snyder, R., Eds.; Oxford University Press: Oxford, UK, 2009; pp. 357–366.
18. Shogren, K.A.; Wehmeyer, M.L.; Palmer, S.B. Causal Agency Theory. In *Development of Self-Determination through the Life-Course*; Wehmeyer, M.L., Shogren, K.A., Little, T.D., Lopez, S., Eds.; Springer: New York, NY, USA, 2017; pp. 55–67.
19. Little, T.D.; Hawley, P.H.; Henrich, C.C.; Marsland, K. Three views of the agentic self: A developmental synthesis. In *Handbook of Self-Determination Research*; Deci, E.L., Ryan, R.M., Eds.; University of Rochester Press: Rochester, NY, USA, 2002; pp. 389–404.
20. Schalock, R.L.; Verdugo, M.A.; Jenaro, C.; Wang, M.; Wehmeyer, M.; Jiancheng, X.; Lachapelle, Y. Cross-cultural study of quality of life indicators. *Am. J. Ment. Retard.* **2005**, *110*, 298–311. [CrossRef]
21. Wehmeyer, M.L.; Schwartz, M. The relationship between self-determination, quality of life, and life satisfaction for adults with mental retardation. *Educ. Train. Ment. Retard.* **1998**, *33*, 3–12.
22. Schalock, R.; Keith, K.D. *Quality of Life Questionnaire*; IDS Publishers: Worthington, OH, USA, 1993.
23. Wehmeyer, M.L.; Kelchner, K.A. *The Arc's Self-Determination Scale*; The Arc of the United States: Arlington, TX, USA, 1996.
24. Kishi, G.; Teelucksingh, B.; Zollers, N.; Park-Lee, S.; Meyer, L. Daily decision-making in community residences: A social comparison of adults with and without mental retardation. *Am. J. Ment. Retard.* **1988**, *92*, 430–435. [PubMed]
25. Lachapelle, Y.; Wehmeyer, M.L.; Haelewyck, M.-C.; Courbois, Y.; Keith, K.D.; Schalock, R.; Verdugo, M.A.; Walsh, P.N. The relationship between quality of life and self-determination: An international study. *J. Intellect. Disabil. Res.* **2005**, *49*, 740–744. [CrossRef] [PubMed]
26. Stancliffe, R. Living with supports in the community: Predictors of choice and self-determination. *Ment. Retard. Dev. Disabil. Res. Rev.* **2001**, *7*, 91–98. [CrossRef] [PubMed]
27. Wehmeyer, M.L.; Stancliffe, R. How self-determined are people with mental retardation? The National Consumer Survey. *Ment. Retard.* **1995**, *33*, 111–119. [PubMed]
28. Stancliffe, R.; Wehmeyer, M.L. Variability in the availability of choice to adults with mental retardation. *J. Vocat. Rehabil.* **1995**, *5*, 319–328. [CrossRef]
29. Wehmeyer, M.L.; Bolding, N. Self-determination across living and working environments: A matched samples study of adults with mental retardation. *Ment. Retard.* **1999**, *37*, 353–363. [CrossRef]
30. Wehmeyer, M.L.; Bolding, N. Enhanced self-determination of adults with mental retardation as an outcome of moving to community-based work or living environments. *J. Intellect. Disabil. Res.* **2001**, *45*, 1–13. [CrossRef] [PubMed]
31. Kozma, A.; Mansell, J.; Beadle-Brown, J. Outcomes in different residential settings for people with intellectual disability: A systemic review. *Am. J. Intellect. Dev. Disabil.* **2009**, *114*, 193–222. [CrossRef] [PubMed]
32. Shogren, K.A.; Lopez, S.J.; Wehmeyer, M.L.; Little, T.D.; Pressgrove, C.L. The role of positive psychology constructs in predicting life satisfaction in adolescents with and without cognitive disabilities: An exploratory study. *J. Posit. Psychol.* **2006**, *1*, 37–52. [CrossRef]

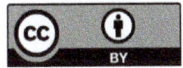

© 2020 by the author. Licensee MDPI, Basel, Switzerland. This article is an open access article distributed under the terms and conditions of the Creative Commons Attribution (CC BY) license (http://creativecommons.org/licenses/by/4.0/).

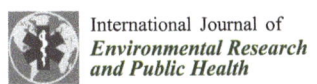

Article

Self-Determination in People with Intellectual Disability: The Mediating Role of Opportunities

Eva Vicente [1,*], Cristina Mumbardó-Adam [2], Verónica M. Guillén [3], Teresa Coma-Roselló [4], María-Ángeles Bravo-Álvarez [1] and Sergio Sánchez [5]

[1] Department of Psychology and Sociology, University of Zaragoza, C./Pedro Cerbuna, 12, 50009 Zaragoza, Spain; marian@unizar.es
[2] Psychology and Educational Sciences Studies, Open University of Catalonia, Rambla del Poblenou, 156, 08018 Barcelona, Spain; cmumbardoa@uoc.edu
[3] Department of Education, University of Cantabria, Av./de los Castros, 52, 39005 Santander, Spain; guillenvm@unican.es
[4] Department of Education, University of Zaragoza, C./Pedro Cerbuna, 12, 50009 Zaragoza, Spain; tcoma@unizar.es
[5] Department of Developmental and Educational Psychology, Autonomous University of Madrid, C./Francisco Tomas y Valiente, 3, 28049 Madrid, Spain; sergio.sanchezfuentes@uam.es
* Correspondence: evavs@unizar.es; Tel.: +34-878554816

Received: 30 July 2020; Accepted: 23 August 2020; Published: 26 August 2020

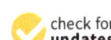

Abstract: The Convention on the Rights of Persons with Disabilities have proclaimed the basic right of people to make one's own choices, have an effective participation and inclusion. Research in the field of disability have stressed self-determination as a key construct because of its impact on their quality of life and the achievement of desired educational and adulthood related outcomes. Self-determination development must be promoted through specific strategies and especially, by providing tailored opportunities to practice those skills. Providing these opportunities across environments could be especially relevant as a facilitator of self-determination development. This manuscript aims to ascertain if opportunities at home and in the community to engage in self-determined actions are mediating the relationship between people intellectual disability level and their self-determination. Results have confirmed direct effects of intellectual disability level on self-determination scores. Indirect effects also predicted self-determination and almost all its related components (self-initiation, self-direction, self-regulation, self-realization, and empowerment) through opportunities in the community and at home. Autonomy was predicted by the intellectual disability level through an indirect effect of opportunities at home, but not in the community. These results highlight the need for further research to better operationalize and promote contextually rooted opportunities for people with intellectual disability to become more self-determined.

Keywords: intellectual disability; self-determination; opportunities; mediation analysis

1. Introduction

Current trends in self-determination research and promotion highlight it as a key construct in the lives of people with intellectual disability (ID). For both adolescents and adults, self-determination related skills are determinant to face curricular, transition to adulthood, and also job-related challenges and situations [1], but also to stand for their right to live a life of quality and to reach personal goals. In fact, that self-determination related skills, such as choice-making, problem solving or goal-setting and goal-attainment skills are useful abilities that serve multiple goals and have a positive impact in people with disabilities life has largely been proved [2]. These abilities are not only useful to navigate daily life situations and challenges, but perhaps more importantly, are necessary to fight for one's rights such as living independently, being included and fully participate in one's community or having access to information so as to take well-informed decisions, as described in the Convention on the Rights of Persons with Disabilities [3]. For this main reason and given the importance and scope of self-determination related components in the lives of people with disabilities, self-determination research has constantly endeavored to better understand its development so as to build responsive contexts for people to engage in self-determined actions.

Research under the Causal Agency Theory has propelled a deeper understanding of self-determination development by reconceptualizing it according to the newest knowledge stemming from positive psychology frameworks and from the strengths-based approach through which disability is currently understood [4]. Under this framework, self-determined action is embodied and operationalized by three essential characteristics: volitional action, agentic action, and action-control beliefs [5]. Volitional action refers to the extent to which a person makes intentional, conscious choices based on individual preferences and interests. Agentic action involves self-directing and managing actions in service of a freely chosen goal and implies identifying different ways to solve a problem, engaging in self-directed action, and managing, self-regulating and evaluating the actions taken. In being engaged in volitional and agentic actions, people develop adjusted action-control beliefs about their own performance and abilities [6]. Action-control beliefs include control-expectancy, that is believing one's skills and resources will enable goal attainment, psychological empowerment, and self-knowledge of strengths and weakness to reach goals. When people act in a self-determined manner engaging in volitional and agentic actions mediated by action-control beliefs, they respond to environmental challenges (opportunities or threats); thus, propelling self-determination to develop [6]. Causal Agency Theory defines self-determination "as a dispositional characteristic manifested as acting as the causal agent in one's life" [5] (p. 257). In this sense, self-determination must be understood as a tendency to act in a certain way, which is a frame of reference through which a person evaluates a situation and acts accordingly. Importantly though, this personal tendency might not be wrongly assimilated to a static trait, but it is contrarily shaped by contextual variables both across and within individuals, as this disposition interacts with situational characteristics of contexts that can either propel or thwart self-determined actions [6].

For this main reason, self-determination must not be understood in isolation of the context where self-determined actions occur, but must instead be comprehended across contexts that can have an impact, influence and be part of self-determination development. The opportunities provided in those contexts may act as catalyzers or barriers of self-determined actions [7]. As facilitating elements, opportunities provide context embedded situations to put into practice self-determination related skills, which implies evaluating and gauging the appropriateness of engaging in self-determined actions and acting in a self-determined way by navigating challenges as they occur. For instance, in educational contexts, it has been proved that, besides teaching self-determination related skills, instruments as the Self-Determined Model of Instruction [8] may guide the provision of opportunities to practice these skills along the school day and in a wide array of learning situations, maximizing thus self-determination related learning [9]. Too often though, people with disabilities are barely provided with enough opportunities in the community [10], at home or at school [11]. Professionals working with adolescents, but also with adults with intellectual disability, claim for further opportunities for them to engage in self-determined actions at a microsystem level, but perhaps more importantly, at a macrosystem level as well, to maximize its effect in learning to act in a self-determined manner [7]. In fact, teaching people self-determination related skills and providing them with opportunities to act in this way in the contexts where they live or develop (e.g., home, school job places, and community) are undoubtedly helpful strategies but still not enough sustainable ones. To this aim, social environments need to warrant mechanisms for people with intellectual disability to act as causal agents in their communities as well.

Given the importance of self-determination and its promotion, it is important to explore the impact of both personal characteristics and contextual variables on people self-determination. These personal and contextual variables are likely to serve as predicting, moderating, and mediating variables influencing the effect of self-determination and, as such, must be considered in the design and implementation of specific interventions. Several studies have identified personal characteristics that are associated with self-determination. Research has shown that students with ID are less self-determined than their peers without disabilities [12], or with learning and other disabilities [13], and that there is a positive correlation between intellectual functioning, as measured by IQ tests or other estimations, and self-determination [14–16]. However, research has also shown that other factors, particularly environmental and contextual factors, are stronger predictors of self-determination status than intellectual level [15,17,18], suggesting that all individuals can enhance self-determination when appropriate supports [19] and opportunities to engage in self-determined actions are provided. Wehmeyer and Bolding [20,21] demonstrated that the placement where a person with ID disability lived or worked (i.e., restrictive or inclusive setting) strongly predicted higher or lower self-determination. The provision of opportunities to engage in self-determined actions might though be influenced by contextual variables. For instance, in congregate or restrictive settings, opportunities to choose and act as the causal agent in one's life are likely to be restricted [16]. These findings clearly underline that while intellectual functioning may be related with the level of support a person will need to become fully self-determined, the degree to which this person will finally engage in self-determined actions basically depends on the opportunities provided in his or her environment and the supports available to succeed in this environment [22].

There is a clear need to investigate the specific role of opportunities in these contexts where people live or develop as catalyzers of self-determination, given the different roles and influences that these opportunities might have on self-determination development. For instance, opportunities at home may have a strong impact in adolescents with intellectual disability volitional actions, whereas opportunities at school influenced action control beliefs [23]. Moreover, the impact of contextual opportunities on self-determination dimensions differed according to the presence of disability. Higher support needs, and specifically the intellectual disability level, has traditionally been associated with self-determination, with lower levels of self-determination being reported for people with severe and profound intellectual disability [24]. Seeing people as more or less capable of acting in a self-determined manner can clearly determine the frequency and quality of opportunities given in their contexts; thus, aligning with an understanding of the context as interactive amongst multilevel (involving micro, meso, and macro level) and multifactor variables such as culture or family embedded conceptions and dynamics [25]. Setting the environment for the person with intellectual disability to act in a self-determined manner might not be enough if the levels and factors influencing opportunities are not identified and manipulated to enhance self-determination. Following Schalock, Luckasson, and Shogren [25], in order to identify and create appropriate opportunities, several models such as quality of life, human rights, human functioning and multidimensional context model should be combined together. However, to the best of our knowledge, there is still scarce research on this topic, and given its complexity, an in-depth approach of the role of environmental opportunities in self-determination development urges. In line with recent studies that have recognized the relevance of testing moderator and/or mediator variables that may be influencing people with disabilities quality of life [26], the aim of this study is to ascertain if opportunities to engage in self-determined actions are mediating the relationship between the person ID level and their level of other-reported self-determination, that is, if opportunities to act in a self-determined manner actually explain the relationship amongst intellectual disability and self-determination levels. Our results will have thus the potential to better inform the design and implementation of interventions to promote self-determination [22].

2. Materials and Methods

2.1. Participants

As self-determination of people with intellectual disability was not reported by themselves but by professionals working with them, throughout this section we will refer to the former as participants and to the latter as informants. The recruitment criteria were (1) people with intellectual disability; and (2) being aged between 11 and 40 years. No exclusion criteria were established. The final sample of participants included 541 evaluated participants with intellectual disability, the majority being men ($n = 334$; 61.7%), and with an average age of 26.28 years (SD = 8.28). The distribution according to gender and age was non-homogeneous ($\chi^2_{(30)} = 47.23$, $p < 0.05$). Information about age, gender, and the level of intellectual disability is provided in Table 1. Furthermore, informants were required to provide associated conditions and possible specific etiologies. Behavioral problems were reported in 25.9% ($n = 140$) and communication problems in 18.1% ($n = 98$); motor disability 16.3% ($n = 88$); epilepsy 14% ($n = 76$); autism spectrum disorder up to 8.7% ($n = 47$); cerebral palsy 6.9% ($n = 32$); visual impairment 3.7% ($n = 20$); and hearing impairment 2.4% ($n = 13$). It should also be noted that in 12.2% of the sample ($n = 66$), intellectual disability was associated with Down syndrome. Participants information was gathered through an initial questionnaire (see below).

Table 1. Characteristics of participants (% (N)).

Variable		Participants ($n = 541$)			Total
Age Range		11–21 Years % (N)	22–30 Years % (N)	31–40 Years % (N)	
Gender	Male	66.7 (116)	57.8 (104)	61.3 (114)	61.7 (334)
	Female	33.3 (58)	42.2 (76)	38.7 (72)	38.1 (206)
	Missing Data	-	-	-	0.2 (1)
ID level	Mild ID	31.6 (51)	51.1 (92)	36.0 (67)	38.8 (210)
	Moderate ID	46.0 (75)	32.8 (59)	43.5 (81)	39.7 (215)
	Severe ID	17.2 (28)	12.2 (22)	14.0 (26)	14.1 (76)
	Profound ID	5.5 (9)	3.9 (7)	6.5 (12)	5.2 (28)
	Missing Data	-	-	-	2.2 (12)

The sample recruitment was incidental, with the voluntary participation of multiple organizations. Professionals of these institutions and organizations collected the data, only when potential participants (or their legal representatives) provided informed consent to participate.

The assessment was carried out by 181 informants from 33 Spanish agencies that provide support to people with intellectual and developmental disabilities. In this case, the number of women (75.1%) was higher in comparison to the number of male informants (24.9%). All were professionals, with diverse profiles, including teachers (21%), professional caregivers (20.4%), psychologists (9.9%), occupational therapists (3.9%), directors of centers or services (2.8%), speech therapists (2.8%), social workers (2.8%), and educators (2.8%). Informants had known participants for at least four months (with a mean of five years and four months). Almost all of them (74.8%) had daily contact with the participant or at least several times per week.

2.2. Measures

2.2.1. Sociodemographic Data

An initial questionnaire was used to collect sociodemographic data from both respondents and participants, including variables such as gender and age. Informants also had to classify the appropriate participants severity level of ID giving an estimate of their intellectual functioning (i.e., mild, moderate, severe, and profound) based on the current International Statistical Classification of Diseases [27] at the moment when the study was held. Informants were asked to use available reports in their organizations with information about Intellectual Quotient (IQ) or other clinical judgments to classify participants.

2.2.2. Self-Determination Opportunities

For the purpose of this study, a brief scale was elaborated to measure opportunities for self-determination, with 12 items divided into two subscales that measure their opportunities at (1) home (six items) and (2) in the community (six items) to perform self-determined actions. These subscales gathered data on the other-reported opportunities to engage in self-determined actions. Scores are rated on a Likert scale from 1 (Never) to 4 (Always). Items details and psychometric properties of the instruments are in the first results part.

2.2.3. Personal Self-Determination

The AUTODDIS Scale is addressed to assess self-determination of adolescents and adults from 11 to 40 years old with ID. The scale is composed of six subscales, which can be assembled into three domains of self-determination according to the most recent theoretical model [5]. The first domain, volitional characteristics (autonomous and volitional actions), is made up of two subscales: autonomy (7 items) and self-initiation (6 items). The second domain, agentic characteristics (self-managed actions), includes the subscales of self-direction (12 items) and self-regulation (3 items). Finally, the action-control beliefs domain is structured around two subscales: self-realization (6 items), and empowerment (12 items). All items must be answered in a four-point Likert scale based on level of agreement (i.e., strongly disagree, disagree, agree, and strongly agree) by an external respondent who knows the person with ID well (for at least 4 months).

This scale has been developed following a solid elaboration process based on (1) a Delphi method [28]; (2) a pilot study [29]; and (3) a rigorous analysis of the reliability and validity evidences [30,31]. The final version of the scale shows Cronbach's alpha values close to or greater than 0.95 as well as evidences of concurrent validity [31]. Results also confirmed the internal structure of this instrument and its equivalence and measurement invariance in adolescents and adults [30].

2.3. Procedures

The collection of information has been carried out with the collaboration of 33 organizations working with people with intellectual disabilities spread over 11 of the 17 autonomous communities in Spain. Since the objective was for the largest number of organizations to participate, in addition to sending an email invitation directly, the study was disseminated on the website of the Institute for Community Integration (INICO) of the University of Salamanca. Subsequently, the research team contacted the reference person at each participant organization and continued support was established for the research process.

The Ethics Committee of the Community of Aragon (CEICA) approved this study, indicating that it complied with the principles for research development set out in the Declaration of Helsinki. The research team kept all the informed consents that were collected through participating organizations. Identification codes were used, replacing the name and surname, to guarantee confidentiality and anonymity.

It is important to highlight the organizations valued contribution to the process, as their knowledge of participants eligibility to take part of the study was crucial to identify potential participants. Given that it is a third-party evaluation, organizations had also a relevant role in assigning a professional to act as informant. This informant had to know the person well (for at least 4 months with frequent contact) and be familiar with the self-determination construct.

Data collection consisted of three blocks: firstly sociodemographic data was collected; then informants should provide information about opportunities at home and in the community of the participants to engage in self-determined actions, and; finally they had to complete the AUTODDIS Scale. Participants' organizations could decide upon online or paper format data collection. Most of them were conducted online (88%) and only 12% on paper.

2.4. Data Processing and Analyses

Previous to main analysis, psychometric properties of the Self-Determination Opportunities instrument were reported. Then, in a first stage, descriptive statistics, internal consistency scores and correlations among study variables were examined. Correlations were determined to be weak (r < 0.30), moderate (r = 0.30–0.60), or strong (r > 0.60) based on established criteria [32]. In the second stage, preliminary associations between sociodemographic variables (i.e., gender and age range) and opportunities and level of self-determination were explored to identify confounding variables for statistical control before the main analyses. Mann–Whitney U and Kruskal–Wallis H tests (nonparametric tests for continuous variables) were carried out at this stage to examine differences in study variables by gender and age range. For the main analyses, several simple mediation models (model 4) of the PROCESS Macro version 3.3 by Andrew F. Hayes for SPSS [33] were performed to examine the direct relationship between ID level and self-determination and their components (measured with AUTODDIS Scale), as well as the indirect effect of opportunities at home and community on these relationships. These models reflect a causal sequence in which X_1 affects Y_n indirectly through mediator variables M_n (see in Figure 1). The data analytic strategy utilized [34,35] allows for estimation and significance testing of the total indirect (mediation) effects through bootstrapping. Bootstrapping generates an empirical representation of the sampling distribution of the indirect effect from which a confidence interval can be generated [34]. Conservative confidence intervals (99%) were specified to adjust for Type I error rate inflation [36]; the confidence intervals (CIs) for the indirect effects were estimated with bootstrapped analyses (10,000 resamples) as recommended [34,35]. In other words, this conditional process analysis (CPA) produces CIs, based on bootstrapped sampling distribution, and it can be assumed that the indirect effects are significant, and that mediation occurs if zero falls outside the 99% confidence interval [37].

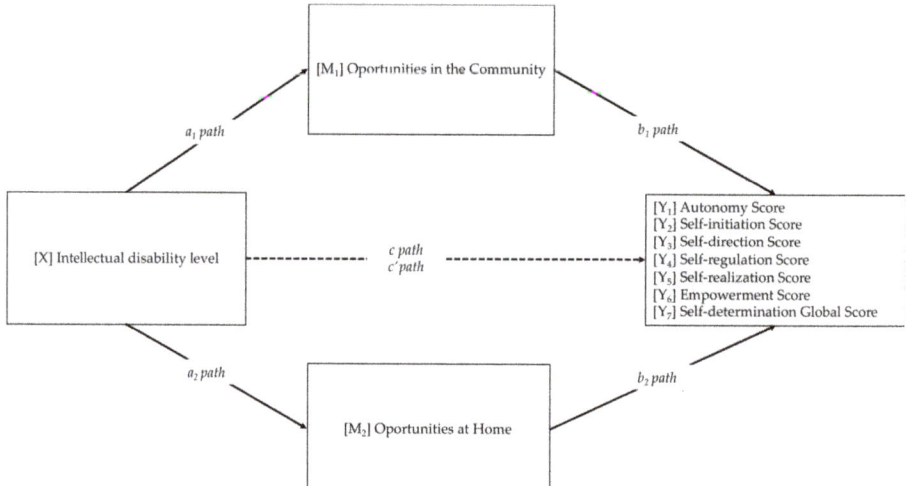

Figure 1. Conceptual diagram of the mediation analysis. Note: a_1 path = effect of X on M_1; b_1 paths = effect of M_1 on Y_i; a_2 path = effect of X on M_2; b_2 paths = effect of M_2 on Y_i; c paths = total effect of X on Y_i; and c′ paths = direct effect of X on Y_i controlling for M. Seven separate paths were conducted (Y_{1-4}) with the predictor (X).

3. Results

3.1. Psychometric Properties of Self-Determination Opportunities Instrument

To guarantee the reliability of the Self-Determination Opportunities instrument, internal consistency was assessed by calculating Cronbach's alpha and item-subscale correlation matrix was performed to identify low-discrimination items. The scale showed strong internal consistency (Cronbach's alpha = 0.955). In turn, data yielded good values for Opportunities in the Community (0.958) and at Home (0.933) subscales. All items showed significant item-subscale correlations higher than 0.60 (ranging from 0.677 to 0.841).

In terms of validity, an exploratory factor analysis based on covariances matrix was conducted, using the principal axis factoring as a retention factor criteria and oblique rotation (oblimin). The aim was to check the dimensionality of the scale and the items factor loading, considering the following criteria: (a) explained variance based on eigenvalues; and (b) the rule 0.40, 0.30, and 0.20 [38]. Results supported a two-factor structure explaining 81.32% of the instrument variance, and all items following the rule 0.40, 0.30, and 0.20 and loaded in the proposed factor (Table 2).

Table 2. Exploratory factor analysis.

	Exploratory Factor Analysis Results Item by Item	Factor 1	Factor 2
	Eigenvalue	7.255	1.316
	% of Variance	67.64	12.27
	Cumulative % of Variance	67.064	79.92
	ROTATED LOADING MATRIX	Factor 1	Factor 2
Item 1	He/She has opportunities in the community to express his/her own interests and wishes.	-	0.621
Item 2	He/She has opportunities in the community to set his/her own goals.	-	0.573
Item 3	He/She has opportunities in the community to learn about making plans to achieve his/her own goals.	-	0.748
Item 4	People in the community encourage him/her to carry out own plans.	-	0.884
Item 5	People in the community tell him/her if he/she is achieving own goals.	-	0.883
Item 6	People in the community give advice and encourage him/her to change plans if they are not working.	-	0.818
Item 7	He/She has opportunities at home to express his/her own interests and wishes.	0.762	-
Item 8	He/She has opportunities at home to set his/her own goals.	0.787	-
item 9	He/She has opportunities at home to learn about making plans to achieve his/her own goals.	0.897	-
Item 10	People at home encourage him/her to carry out own plans.	0.882	-
Item 11	People at home tell him/her if he/she is achieving own goals.	0.894	-
Item 12	People at home give advice and encourage him/her to change plans if they are not working.	0.943	-

3.2. Descriptive Statistics, Internal Consistency and Correlations

Descriptive statistics, correlations, and internal reliability scores are presented in Table 3. Internal reliability scores among study variables were deemed excellent (range = 0.842–0.982). Pearson and Spearman correlation analyses revealed moderate and strong associations (all significant, $p < 0.01$) among all variables. As expected, ID level was negatively correlated with all variables, showing a moderate inverse relation with the opportunities at home and community; and strong inverse associations with self-determination subscales and scale.

3.3. Preliminary Analysis

In terms of contrast statistics, nonparametric tests (i.e., Mann–Whitney U and Kruskal–Wallis H tests) were used to identify confounding variables for statistical control before conducting the main analyses (Table 4). These analyses revealed self-determination subscales and opportunities scores were not associated with gender, except for the autonomy score. Males and females showed similar levels of self-initiation ($p = 0.817$), self-direction ($p = 0.562$), self-regulation ($p = 0.456$), self-realization ($p = 0.440$) and empowerment ($p = 0.900$). However, females showed more autonomy than males ($p = 0.005$). Regarding self-determination opportunities, no significant differences were found by gender (at home, $p = 0.359$; and in the community, $p = 0.524$).

Secondly, the analyses revealed that opportunities at home and community, as well as the scores in two of the self-determination subscales (i.e., self-regulation and self-realization) were not associated with age ranges. In contrast, participants between 22 and 30 years old reported more autonomy ($p = 0.009$) and self-direction ($p = 0.014$) levels than the other two age ranges; and more self-initiation ($p = 0.006$) and empowerment ($p = 0.042$) than younger ones.

Therefore, to control for any possible effects, age range and gender were entered as covariates in the subsequent mediation (Table 4).

Table 3. Descriptive statistics, internal reliability and Pearson and Spearman's correlations.

Variables		AUT	SIN	SDI	SRE	REA	EMP	SDGS	OH	OC	ID
SIN	P	0.812	-	-	-	-	-	-	-	-	-
	S	0.764	-	-	-	-	-	-	-	-	-
SDI	P	0.767	0.792	-	-	-	-	-	-	-	-
	S	0.726	0.745	-	-	-	-	-	-	-	-
SRE	P	0.653	0.643	0.770	-	-	-	-	-	-	-
	S	0.618	0.590	0.725	-	-	-	-	-	-	-
REA	P	0.721	0.757	0.785	0.681	-	-	-	-	-	-
	S	0.639	0.672	0.741	0.628	-	-	-	-	-	-
EMP	P	0.757	0.808	0.862	0.728	0.799	-	-	-	-	-
	S	0.694	0.740	0.824	0.685	0.748	-	-	-	-	-
SDGS	P	0.877	0.895	0.943	0.800	0.871	0.944	-	-	-	-
	S	0.845	0.850	0.926	0.768	0.814	0.924	-	-	-	-
OH	P	0.475	0.588	0.488	0.400	0.444	0.488	0.545	-	-	-
	S	0.428	0.530	0.457	0.369	0.373	0.432	0.497	-	-	-
OC	P	0.424	0.535	0.544	0.463	0.454	0.532	0.562	0.692	-	-
	S	0.408	0.519	0.537	0.453	0.436	0.535	0.565	0.700	-	-
ID	P	−0.595	−0.580	−0.597	−0.485	−0.544	−0.660	−0.656	−0.314	−0.390	-
	S	−0.527	−0.503	−0.544	−0.424	−0.413	−0.556	−0.566	−0.269	−0.353	-
i		7	6	12	3	6	12	46	6	6	1
n		541	541	541	541	541	540	540	494	449	530
Missing		0	0	0	0	0	1	1	47	92	11
M		18.34	16.40	25.86	6.74	15.81	29.77	113.00	18.79	15.66	1.85
Median		19	17	26	7	16	31	117	20	16	2
SD		5.56	4.29	8.34	2.06	3.69	8.45	29.37	4.70	5.31	0.86
Min		7	6	12	3	6	12	46	6	6	1
Max		28	24	48	12	24	48	184	24	24	4
Sk		−0.458	−0.488	−0.054	−0.118	−0.622	−0.540	−0.500	−0.742	−0.006	0.791
Ku		−0.460	0.045	−0.432	−0.417	0.747	−0.168	−0.029	−0.342	−0.979	−0.037
α		0.916	0.903	0.961	0.841	0.909	0.949	0.982	0.933	0.958	-

Note: AUT = autonomy score; SIN = self-initiation score; SDI = self-direction score; SRE = self-regulation score; REA = self-realization score; EMP = empowerment score; SDGS = Self-determination AUTODDIS Global Score; HO = Opportunities at home Score; CO = Opportunities in the community Score; ID = Intellectual Disability Level; P = Pearson correlations; S = Spearman Correlation; i = number of items; n = sample; M = mean; SD; Standard Deviation; Min = minimum; Max = maximum; sk = symmetry; ku = kurtosis; α = Cronbach alpha.

Table 4. Contrast statistics.

	Age Ranges					Gender			
Variables	11–21 M(SD)	22–30 M(SD)	31–40 M(SD)	H	p	Female M(SD)	Male M(SD)	U	p
AUT	18.03(0.44)	19.59(0.43)	18.73(0.43)	9.416	0.009	18.92(0.28)	18.24(0.54)	29622.5	0.005
SIN	15.88(0.34)	17.31(0.33)	17.17(0.30)	10.321	0.006	16.86(0.21)	16.52(0.45)	34161	0.817
SDI	25.91(0.67)	27.79(0.66)	26.57(0.64)	8.519	0.014	26.79(0.42)	26.69(0.87)	33546	0.562
SRE	7.07(0.18)	6.97(0.16)	6.73(0.15)	2.099	0.350	6.90(0.10)	7.02(0.22)	33267.5	0.456
REA	15.88(0.32)	16.17(0.26)	16.27(0.26)	0.837	0.658	16.11(0.18)	16.09(0.38)	33215	0.440
EMP	29.53(0.68)	31.53(0.64)	31.14(0.58)	6.336	0.042	30.72(0.41)	30.86(0.85)	34180	0.900
OH	18.43(0.40)	19.01(0.40)	18.65(0.37)	1.595	0.450	18.82(0.24)	18.18(0.57)	27416.	0.359
OC	15.56(0.44)	16.01(0.45)	15.42(0.42)	0.777	0.670	15.68(0.27)	15.62(0.62)	22869.5	0.524

Note: AUT = autonomy score; SIN = self-initiation score; SDI = self-direction score; SRE = self-regulation score; REA = self-realization score; EMP = empowerment score; SDGS = Self-determination AUTODDIS Global Score; OH = Opportunities at home Score; OC = Opportunities in the community Score; M = mean; SD; Standard Deviation; H = Kruskal–Wallis H; U = Mann–Whitney U.

3.4. Mediation Analysis

As depicted in Figure 1, seven multiple mediation analyses were conducted with the ID level as a dependent variable (X) and opportunities at home (M_1) and in the community (M_2) as mediators. The independent variables were the six subscales of the AUTODDIS Scale (autonomy, self-initiation, self-direction, self-regulation, self-realization, and empowerment) and the global self-determination score (Y_1–Y_7). Indirect effects results are presented in Table 5.

In terms of the autonomy score, the results of this first mediation analysis showed that the full model with opportunities at home and community was significant ($R^2 = 0.396$, $F(4, 443) = 56.95$, $p < 0.001$). The standardized parameter estimates of this model included a statistically significant direct effect of ID level on the autonomy score (i.e., $c_1 = -2.631$, $SE = 0.276$, $CI\ (-3.467, -1.917)$). Testing indirect effect, results indicated that ID level was associated with the autonomy score, which indirectly occurred through the effect of the opportunities at home (i.e., $a_2 * b_2 = -0.657$, $SE = 0.157$; $CI\ (-1.102, -0.308)$), but no through the effect of the opportunities in the community (i.e., $a_1 * b_1 = -0.190$, $SE = 0.144$; $CI\ (-0.575, 0.191)$).

For the rest of the subscales scores, the full models with opportunities at home and in the community were significant (R^2 ranged from 0.318 to 0.512, all $p < 0.001$). The standardized parameter estimates included a statistically significant direct effects of ID level on the self-initiation score (i.e., $c_2 = -1.571$, $SE = 0.192$, $CI\ (-2.067, -1.076)$); self-direction score (i.e., $c_3 = -3.696$, $SE = 0.394$, $CI\ (-4.715, -2.678)$); self-regulation score (i.e., $c_4 = -0.725$, $SE = 0.111$, $CI\ (-1.015, -0.440)$); self-realization score (i.e., $c_5 = -1.310$, $SE = 0.187$, $CI\ (-1.793, -0.827)$); and empowerment score (i.e., $c_6 = -4.084$, $SE = 0.360$, $CI\ (-5.015, -3.154)$). The test of the indirect effect indicated that ID level were associated with these self-determination subscales, which indirectly through the effect of both opportunities at home and in the community (Table 5).

Finally, with regards to Self-determination Global Score, the full model with opportunities at home and in the community as mediators accounted for significant variance ($R^2 = 0.541$, $F(5, 434) = 102.39$, $p < 0.001$). Although direct effects of ID level on the self-determination score was also significant (i.e., $c_7 = -13.022$, $SE = 1.239$, $CI\ (-17.228, -10.916)$), and, in terms of indirect effects, ID level predicted self-determination indirectly through opportunities at the community (i.e., $a_2 * b_2 = -3.368$, $SE = 0.701$, $CI\ (-5.237, -1.685)$) and home (i.e., $a_1 * b_1 = -2.977$, $SE = 0.713$, $CI\ (-4.978, -1.347)$).

Table 5. Indirect effects.

M	Y	Mediators	Path	b	SE	LLCI	ULCI
M1	Y_1	OC—Opportunities in the Community	($a_1 * b_1$) ID-OC-AUT	*-0.190*	*0.144*	*-0.575*	*0.191*
		OH—Opportunities at Home	($a_2 * b_2$) ID-OH-AUT	-0.657	0.157	-1.110	-0.308
M2	Y_2	OC—Opportunities in the Community	($a_1 * b_1$) ID-OC-SIN	-0.336	0.097	-0.593	-0.087
		OH—Opportunities at Home	($a_2 * b_2$) ID-OH-SIN	-0.628	0.128	-0.972	-0.327
M3	Y_3	OC—Opportunities in the Community	($a_1 * b_1$) ID-OC-SDI	-1.224	0.249	-1.914	-0.617
		OH—Opportunities at Home	($a_2 * b_2$) ID-OH-SDI	-0.606	0.185	-1.157	-0.189
M4	Y_4	OC—Opportunities in the Community	($a_1 * b_1$) ID-OC-SRE	-0.223	0.066	-0.429	-0.087
		OH—Opportunities at Home	($a_2 * b_2$) ID-OH-SRE	-0.131	0.050	-0.280	-0.017
M5	Y_5	OC—Opportunities in the Community	($a_1 * b_1$) ID-OC-REA	-0.363	0.092	-0.613	-0.125
		OH—Opportunities at Home	($a_2 * b_2$) ID-OH-REA	-0.293	0.097	-0.573	-0.076
M6	Y_6	OC—Opportunities in the Community	($a_1 * b_1$) ID-OC-EMP	-1.002	0.199	-1.563	-0.533
		OH—Opportunities at Home	($a_2 * b_2$) ID-OH-EMP	-0.663	0.191	-1.201	-0.238
M7	Y_7	OC—Opportunities in the Community	($a_1 * b_1$) ID-OC-SD	-3.368	0.701	-5.237	-1.685
		OH—Opportunities at Home	($a_2 * b_2$) ID-OH-SD	-2.977	0.713	-4.978	-1.347

Note 1: N for analyses is 541 cases. The standard error and 99% CI for the indirect effects (a * b) are obtained through bootstrapping with 10,000 re-samples. Note 2: b = Standardized Coefficients; SE = Standard Error; LLCI = lower 99% level confidence interval; ULCL = upper 99% level confidence interval; M_i = Mediation Models; ($a_i * b_i$) = indirect effect; Y_1 = AUT = autonomy score; Y_2 = SIN = self-initiation score; Y_3 = SDI = self-direction score; Y_4 = SRE = self-regulation score; Y_5 = REA = self-realization score; Y_6 = EMP = empowerment score; Y_7 = SD = Self-determination AUTODDIS Global Score; ID = Intellectual Disability Level. Note 3: Values in italics correspond to non-significant results

4. Discussion

The current study contributed to the literature by examining whether the role of opportunities at home and in the community explained, in part, the relationship between ID and self-determination level and its components in people with ID. Consistent with the theorical framework, the results of the present study showed that when professionals' reports were used, opportunities at home and in the community mediated the association between intellectual functioning and self-determination level, as well as between intellectual functioning and five self-determination components (i.e., self-initiation; self-direction; self-regulation; self-realization, and empowerment). In contrast, opportunities at home, but not in the community, mediated the association between ID level and autonomy. A higher level of ID was associated with lower opportunities at home (the a_n path), which in turn was associated with lower level of autonomy, self-initiation, self-direction, self-regulation, self-realization, empowerment, and the global self-determination score (the b_n path). Notably, the observed indirect effects (the $a_n * b_n$ path) were evident for all criterion variables, after adjusting for the influence of covariates (such as, age and gender). The same results have been found with opportunities in the community, except for autonomy subdomain.

These findings align with other studies that found a positive correlation between intellectual functioning and self-determination, but also affirmed that this relationship might be influenced and explained by other variables [14,16]. Research has shown that other factors, particularly contextual variables (i.e., instructional factors, support needs, or choice opportunities) act as stronger predictors of self-determination than the intellectual level. [15–18] made a discriminant function analysis of predictors of self-determination scores, showing that only perception of choice opportunity (from among four variables, including IQ) predicted membership in the group of participants with high self-determination scores. Likewise, previous studies [39–43] have also described opportunities for self-determination as significant predictors of self-determined actions. Interestingly, the autonomy domain has been shown to be influenced by opportunities at home but not in other environments, in line with recent studies where data was collected directly amongst participants with ID [23]; thus, stressing this shared perspective. Engaging in volitional actions, that is initiating autonomous actions (with the required supports), is the necessary first step for then regulating and directing agentic actions by navigating challenges and problems as they occur, while nurturing a personal sense of empowerment and self-knowledge about one's skills and resources to attain goals (action-control beliefs). It makes then sense that closer environments of the person, such as home, might be promoting autonomous actions in first place, though further research is required to design opportunities, in the community, to act in an autonomous way as well. All in all, these considerations must be understood with caution and without assimilating the provision of opportunities to leaving the person at his or her expense, but rather to providing tailored supports for the person to act autonomously and in an agentic manner, watching over his or her safety.

Consistently with the aim of this study, the analysis of self-determination of people with ID and related personal and environmental variables should be considered from a more sophisticated perspective, rather than simply focusing on relationships. No previous studies have considered incorporating these factors into a mediational analysis. Identifying mediator variables allow for a more in-depth understanding of the process by which two variables are related [26], and thus guide the decision making processes towards interventions and programs improvement, but also to evaluate the process of change achieved through an intervention, among others [44,45]. That opportunities to engage in self-determined actions both at home and in the community stand as key components in self-determination promotion seems undeniable, in the light of the presented results. Further, more sustainable and tailored opportunities to act in a self-determined manner not only at a microsystem level, but also in the community is exactly what professionals working both with adolescents but also with adults with ID in Spain are claiming for [23]. In other words, self-determination promotion should start by enhancing opportunities (mediating variables) so as to cause changes in the expected outcome, which is in the level of self-determination. However, further work is needed to operationalize how these contextual opportunities have to be built, considering the interaction between the different levels and factors [25] in order to propel self-determination development.

Further, and perhaps more importantly, more severe levels of ID were associated with less opportunities both at home and in the community to act in a self-determined manner which, in turn, ended in lower levels of global self-determination and self-determination components. As previously stated, people with more limitations in intellectual functioning (and other competences such as adaptive behavior), and commonly with higher support needs, tend to be offered with less opportunities to make their choices and act in a self-determined manner [24]. However, conversely, people with higher support needs will probably need additional opportunities to practice self-determined related abilities in a wide array of environments to reach higher self-determination levels. People with higher support needs have the right to be provided with as much opportunities as needed to develop self-determination and its related components, and the environments where they live and develop embody the best scenarios for contextual opportunities onset. Further efforts must be then devoted to providing support to services providers, stakeholders, professionals and families for them to create contextualized and relevant opportunities for people with ID at home and in the community.

Despite its contribution to the existing body of knowledge and its implications on self-determination promotion, the present study is not exempt from some limitations. First, the study design was cross-sectional and correlational, and causality therefore cannot be discerned from the data. More randomized controlled trials are needed to test opportunities efficacy in improving self-determination of people with ID. In addition, longitudinal studies are required to determine the underpinnings of this relationship and its directionality and strength (i.e., ID level, opportunities and self-determination). Second, the present study measured ID level as an estimation reported by professionals, and although this represents a common practice in our context where ID assessments might not be homogeneously reported, results have to be interpreted taking it into account. We were not able to collect data on students' levels of intelligence (IQ). Likewise, opportunities at home and community were measured as specific variables, using no standardized questionnaires. Although, data indicates that it possesses adequate reliability and validity; the understanding of contextual opportunities as the interaction amongst multiple levels and factors might require other measurement alternatives. The operationalization and evaluation of opportunities to engage in self-determined actions stand as a necessary line of future research in the field, as undoubtedly, these opportunities will need to vary and be tailored to the person developmental stage (early adolescence, transition to adulthood period, etc.). Third, a narrow set of variables were incorporated for analysis in terms of their influence on self-determination. We focused only on ID level and opportunities at home and in the community but, other personal and contextual variables may also play a mediational role on the development and expression of self-determination. More complex models should be tested to clarify how multiple factors may influence people with ID to become self-determined. Finally, the convenience sample was recruited from organizations that agreed to participate in this project, so the results might be interpreted within the context where the sample was drawn and taking into account it is not necessarily representative of the population of people with ID in Spain.

5. Conclusions

The mediating role of contextual opportunities (at home and in the community) was observed in the relationship between ID level and self-determination as well as most of their specific domains (i.e., self-initiation; self-direction; self-regulation; self-realization, and empowerment). Interestingly, the autonomy domain has been shown to be influenced by opportunities at home but not in the community. This study contributes to increase the understanding of self-determination of people with ID and related personal and environmental variables from a more sophisticated perspective, rather than simply focusing on relationships. Hopefully, these findings will have implications in fostering the incorporation of contextual opportunities into self-determination promotion and intervention programs.

Author Contributions: Conceptualization, E.V. and C.M.-A.; methodology, E.V., V.M.G., T.C.-R., M.-Á.B.-Á., and S.S.; software, E.V.; formal analysis, E.V., C.M.-A., and V.M.G.; investigation, E.V., C.M.-A., V.M.G., T.C.-R., M.-Á.B.-Á., and S.S.; resources, T.C.-R., M.-Á.B.-Á., and S.S.; data curation, E.V., C.M.-A., and V.M.G.; writing—original draft preparation, T.C.-R., M.-Á.B.-Á., and S.S.; writing—review and editing, E.V. and C.M.-A.; visualization and supervision, E.V. and V.M.G.; project administration, E.V., C.M.-A., V.M.G., T.C.-R., M.-Á.B.-Á., and S.S.; and funding acquisition, E.V., C.M.-A., V.M.G., T.C.-R., M.-Á.B.-Á., and S.S. All authors have read and agreed to the published version of the manuscript.

Funding: This research was funded by the Spanish Ministry of Economy and Competitiveness, grant number PSI2016-75826-P. AEI/FEDER, UE.

Acknowledgments: We gratefully acknowledge the support of the organizations, professionals, people with intellectual disability, and families on this study.

Conflicts of Interest: The authors declare no conflict of interest. The funders had no role in the design of the study; in the collection, analyses, or interpretation of data; in the writing of the manuscript, or in the decision to publish the results.

References

1. Lee, S.H.; Wehmeyer, M.L.; Soukup, J.H.; Palmer, S.B. Impact of curriculum modifications on access to the general education curriculum for students with disabilities. *Except. Child.* **2010**, *76*, 213–233. [CrossRef]
2. Burke, K.M.; Raley, S.K.; Shogren, K.A.; Hagiwara, M.; Mumbardó-Adam, C.; Uyanik, H.; Behrens, S. A meta-analysis of interventions to promote self-determination for students with disabilities. *Remedial Spec. Educ.* **2020**, *41*, 176–188. [CrossRef]
3. United Nations. Convention on the Rights of Persons with Disabilities. 2006. Available online: https://www.un:disabilities/documents/convention/convoptprot-s.pdf (accessed on 10 July 2020).
4. Shogren, K.A.; Wehmeyer, M.L.; Buchanan, C.L.; Lopez, S.J. The application of positive psychology and self-determination to research in intellectual disability: A content analysis of 30 years of literature. *Res. Pract. Pers. Sev. Disabil.* **2006**, *31*, 338–345. [CrossRef]
5. Shogren, K.A.; Wehmeyer, M.L.; Palmer, S.B.; Forber-Pratt, A.J.; Little, T.J.; Lopez, S. Causal agency theory: Reconceptualizing a functional model of self-determination. *Educ. Train. Autism Dev. Disabil.* **2015**, *50*, 251–263.
6. Shogren, K.A.; Wehmeyer, M.L.; Palmer, S.B. Causal agency theory. In *Development of Self-Determination through the Life-Course*; Wehmeyer, M.L., Shogren, K.L., Little, T.D., Lopez, S.J., Eds.; Springer: Dordrecht, The Netherlands, 2017; pp. 55–67.
7. Mumbardó-Adam, C.; Vicente, E.; Simon, D.; Coma, T. Understanding practitioners' needs in supporting self-determination in people with intellectual disability. *Prof. Psychol. Res. Pract.* **2020**, *51*, 341. [CrossRef]
8. Wehmeyer, M.L.; Palmer, S.B.; Agran, M.; Mithaug, D.E.; Martin, J.E. Promoting causal agency: The self-determined learning model of instruction. *Except. Child.* **2000**, *66*, 439–453. [CrossRef]
9. Raley, S.K.; Shogren, K.A.; Mumbardó-Adam, C.; Simó-Pinatella, D.; Gine, C. Curricula to teach skills associated with self-determination: A review of existing research. *Educ. Train. Autism Dev. Disabil.* **2018**, *53*, 353–362. [CrossRef]
10. Robertson, J.; Emerson, E.; Hatton, C.; Gregory, N.; Kessissoglou, S.; Hallam, A.; Walsh, P.N. Environmental opportunities and supports for exercising self-determination in community-based residential settings. *Res. Dev. Disabil.* **2001**, *22*, 487–502. [CrossRef]
11. Carter, E.W.; Lane, K.L.; Pierson, M.R.; Glaeser, B. Self-determination skills and opportunities of transition-age youth with emotional disturbance and learning disabilities. *Except. Child.* **2006**, *72*, 333–346. [CrossRef]
12. Mumbardó-Adam, C.; Guàrdia-Olmos, J.; Giné Giné, C.; Shogren, K.; Vicente, E. Psychometric properties of the Spanish version of the Self-Determination Inventory Student Self-Report: A structural equation modeling approach. *Am. J. Intellect. Dev. Disabil.* **2018**, *123*, 545–557. [CrossRef]
13. Wehmeyer, M.L.; Schwartz, M. The relationship between self-determination and quality of life for adults with mental retardation. *Educ. Train. Ment. Retard. Dev. Disabil.* **1998**, *33*, 3–12.
14. Nota, L.; Ferrari, L.; Soresi, S.; Wehmeyer, M.L. Self-determination, social abilities, and the quality of life of people with intellectual disabilities. *J. Intellect. Disabil. Res.* **2007**, *51*, 850–865. [CrossRef] [PubMed]

15. Vicente, E.; Verdugo, M.A.; Gómez-Vela, M.; Fernández-Pulido, R.; Wehmeyer, M.L.; Guillén, V.M. Personal characteristics and school contextual variables associated with student self-determination in Spanish context. *J. Intellect. Dev. Disabil.* **2019**, *44*, 23–34. [CrossRef]
16. Wehmeyer, M.L.; Garner, N.W. The impact of personal characteristics of people with intellectual and developmental disability on self-determination and autonomous functioning. *J. Appl. Res. Intellect. Disabil.* **2003**, *16*, 255–265. [CrossRef]
17. Lee, Y.; Wehmeyer, M.L.; Palmer, S.B.; Williams-Diehm, K.; Davies, D.K.; Stock, S.E. Examining individual and instruction-related predictors of the self-determination of students with disabilities: Multiple regression analyses. *Remedial Spec. Educ.* **2012**, *33*, 150–161. [CrossRef] [PubMed]
18. Stancliffe, R.J.; Abery, B.H.; Smith, J. Personal control and the ecology of community living settings: Beyond living-unit size and type. *Am. J. Ment. Retard.* **2000**, *105*, 431–454. [CrossRef]
19. Shogren, K.A.; Wehmeyer, M.L.; Palmer, S.B.; Paek, Y. Exploring personal and school environment characteristics that predict self-determination. *Exceptionality* **2013**, *21*, 147–157. [CrossRef]
20. Wehmeyer, M.L.; Bolding, N. Self-determination across living and working environments: A matched samples study of adults with mental retardation. *Ment. Retard.* **1999**, *37*, 353–363. [CrossRef]
21. Wehmeyer, M.L.; Bolding, N. Enhanced self-determination of adults with intellectual disability as an outcome of moving to community-based work or living environments. *J. Intellect. Disabil. Res.* **2001**, *45*, 371–383. [CrossRef]
22. Wehmeyer, M.L.; Abery, B.H.; Zhang, D.; Ward, K.; Willis, D.; Hossain, W.A.; Heller, T. Personal Self-Determination and Moderating Variables that Impact Efforts to Promote Self-Determination. *Exceptionality* **2011**, *19*, 19–30. [CrossRef]
23. Mumbardó-Adam, C.; Guàrdia-Olmos, J.; Giné Giné, C. An integrative model of self-determination and related contextual variables in adolescents with and without disabilities. *J. Appl. Res. Intellect. Disabil.* **2020**, *33*, 856–864. [CrossRef]
24. Simões, C.; Santos, S.; Biscaia, R.; Thompson, J.R. Understanding the relationship between quality of life, adaptive behavior and support needs. *J. Dev. Phys. Disabil.* **2016**, *28*, 849–870. [CrossRef]
25. Schalock, R.L.; Luckasson, R.; Shogren, K.A. Going beyond environment to context: Leveraging the power of context to produce change. *Int. J. Environ. Res. Public Health* **2020**, *17*, 1885. [CrossRef]
26. Gómez, L.E.; Schalock, R.L.; Verdugo, M.A. The role of moderators and mediators in implementing and evaluating intellectual and developmental disabilities-related policies and practices. *J. Dev. Phys. Disabil.* **2020**, *32*, 375–393. [CrossRef]
27. WHO. ICD-10 Version: 2016. Available online: https://icd.who.int/browse10/2016/en#/F70-F79 (accessed on 21 August 2020).
28. Vicente, E.; Guillén, V.M.; Gómez, L.E.; Ibáñez, A.; Sánchez, S. What do stakeholders understand by self-determination? Consensus for its evaluation. *J. Appl. Res. Intellect. Disabil.* **2019**, *32*, 206–218. [CrossRef] [PubMed]
29. Vicente, E.; Guillén, V.M.; Fernández-Pulido, R.; Bravo, M.Á.; Vived, E. Avanzando en la evaluación de la Autodeterminación: Diseño de la Escala AUTODDIS. *Aula Abierta* **2019**, *48*, 301–310. [CrossRef]
30. Vicente, E.; Verdugo, M.A.; Guillén, V.M.; Martinez, A.; Gómez, L.E.; Ibáñez, A. Advances in the assessment of self-determination: Internal structure of a scale for people with intellectual disabilities aged 11 to 40. *J. Intellect. Disabil. Res.* **2020**, *64*, 700–712. [CrossRef] [PubMed]
31. Verdugo, M.A.; Vicente, E.; Guillén, V.M.; Sánchez, S.; Ibáñez, A.; Gómez, L.E. A measurement of self-determination for people with intellectual disability: Description of the AUTODDIS Scale and evidences of reliability and external validity. *Behav. Psychol.* **2020**. manuscript submitted for publication.
32. Pagano, M.; Gauvreau, K. *Principles of Biostatistics*, 2nd ed.; Brooks/Cole, Cengage Learning: Belmont, CA, USA, 2000.
33. Hayes, A.F. *An Introduction to Mediation, Moderation, and Conditional Process Analysis: A Regression-Based Approach*; Guilford Press: New York, NY, USA, 2013.
34. Hayes, A.F. Beyond Baron and Kenny: Statistical mediation analysis in the new millennium. *Commun. Monogr.* **2009**, *76*, 408–420. [CrossRef]
35. Preacher, K.J.; Hayes, A.F. SPSS and SAS procedures for estimating indirect effects in simple mediation models. *Behav. Res. Methods Instrum. Comput.* **2004**, *36*, 717–731. [CrossRef]

36. Hayes, A.F.; Preacher, K.J. Statistical mediation analysis with a multicategorical independent variable. *Br. J. Math. Stat. Psychol.* **2014**, *67*, 451–470. [CrossRef] [PubMed]
37. Preacher, K.J.; Hayes, A.F. Asymptotic and resampling strategies for assessing and comparing indirect effects in multiple mediator models. *Behav. Res. Methods* **2008**, *40*, 879–891. [CrossRef] [PubMed]
38. Howard, M.C. A review of exploratory factor analysis decisions and overview of current practices: What we are doing and how can we improve? *Int. J. Hum.-Comput. Interact.* **2016**, *32*, 51–62. [CrossRef]
39. Carter, E.W.; Owens, L.; Trainor, A.A.; Sun, Y.; Swedeen, B. Self-determination skills and opportunities of adolescents with severe intellectual and developmental disabilities. *Am. J. Intellect. Dev. Disabil.* **2009**, *114*, 179–192. [CrossRef]
40. Cavendish, W. The Role of Gender, Race/Ethnicity, and Disability Status on the Relationship between Student Perceptions of School and Family Support and Self-determination. *Career Dev. Transit. Except. Individ.* **2017**, *40*, 113–122. [CrossRef]
41. Mason, C.; Field, S.; Sawilowsky, S. Implementation of self-determination activities and student participation in IEPs. *Except. Child.* **2004**, *70*, 441–451. [CrossRef]
42. Mumbardó-Adam, C.; Shogren, K.A.; Guàrdia-Olmos, J.; Giné, C. Contextual predictors of self-determined actions in students with and without intellectual disability. *Psychol. Sch.* **2017**, *54*, 183–195. [CrossRef]
43. Pierson, M.R.; Carter, E.W.; Lane, K.L.; Glaeser, B.C. Factors influencing the self-determination of transition-age youth with high-incidence disabilities. *Career Dev. Except. Individ.* **2008**, *31*, 115–125. [CrossRef]
44. MacKinnon, D.P. *Introduction to Statistical Mediation Analysis*; Erlbaum: New York, NY, USA, 2008.
45. MacKinnon, D.P. Integrating mediators and moderators in research design. *Res. Soc. Work Pract.* **2011**, *21*, 675–681. [CrossRef]

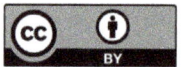

© 2020 by the authors. Licensee MDPI, Basel, Switzerland. This article is an open access article distributed under the terms and conditions of the Creative Commons Attribution (CC BY) license (http://creativecommons.org/licenses/by/4.0/).

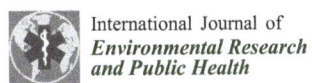

Article

Chronic Health Conditions in Aging Individuals with Intellectual Disabilities

Laura García-Domínguez, Patricia Navas *, Miguel Ángel Verdugo and Víctor B. Arias

Institute for Community Inclusion, University of Salamanca, 37005 Salamanca, Spain; lauragarciad@usal.es (L.G.-D.); verdugo@usal.es (M.Á.V.); vbarias@usal.es (V.B.A.)
* Correspondence: patricianavas@usal.es

Received: 3 April 2020; Accepted: 27 April 2020; Published: 30 April 2020

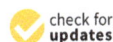

Abstract: Life expectancy of people with intellectual disability (ID) has increased in recent decades. However, there is little evidence of whether these extra years of life are spent in good health. The aim of this study, conducted in Spain, is to obtain information about the prevalence of chronic health conditions in people with ID over the age of 44 and compare it with that of their peers without disability. Twenty health conditions were analyzed in 1040 people with ID and 12,172 people without ID through a study of their prevalence. The findings show that chronic constipation, urinary incontinence, thyroid disorders and obesity are the most prevalent chronic diseases among individuals with ID. In addition, this population group suffers these health conditions more frequently than older adults without ID. Detection and early intervention in these health conditions will improve adequate access to social health services and subsequent treatment of aging adults with ID.

Keywords: chronic health conditions; health; intellectual disability; aging

1. Introduction

The significant increase in life expectancy is one of the major achievements of our society during the past century. By 2050, one in six people will be over the age of 65 [1] due to a number of factors that are contributing to a decrease in mortality and birth rates [2]. In developed countries, life expectancy increases by at least two years per decade [3], and the World Health Organization [4] estimates that the average number of years that a person who reaches the age of 60 is expected to live will be of around 20 years more. Life expectancy in Spain, the country where this study is carried out, is 83.19 years [5].

The reality of a greater longevity also translates to individuals with intellectual disability (ID). In the late 1970s and early 1980s [6–8], the scientific literature started to report an unprecedented growth in the life expectancy of individuals with ID as a result of different factors such as improvements in care provision. At the present time, the number of adults with intellectual and developmental disabilities over the age of 60 is expected to grow from around 641,860 in 2000 to 1.2 million in 2030 [9]. Moreover, people over the age of 65 in Europe already account for 45% of people with disabilities [10]. Regarding the current situation in Spain, more than 60% of the people with ID will be older than 45 in half a decade's time [11].

In summary, people with ID can currently expect to live almost as long as their peers without disability [12–15], although the scientific literature points out certain differences in the aging process between the two groups.

Thus, people with ID (considering the broad variability within this group) can experience aging-related health conditions earlier than the general population [16–19]. In this regard, it has been pointed out that the beginning of the aging period in this population group could start at the age of 45 [20]. This premature aging can have a negative impact on their quality of life [21], and also increases their mortality rate [13,22].

Apart from experiencing premature aging, individuals with ID are more frequently affected throughout their life by certain chronic health conditions than their peers without disability, which could affect their quality of life as they age. These conditions include cardiovascular diseases [23,24], obesity [25,26], diabetes [27,28], epilepsy [29–31], gastrointestinal tract anomalies such as constipation [32], kidney disease [33], osteoarticular disorders [16,34], and thyroid disorders [32,35].

Although the concept of health is broad and difficult to be captured by one single measure, the presence of chronic health conditions can precipitate early health decline in aging people with ID and greater levels of frailty [36]. However, adequate prevention and identification is complex in individuals with ID due to several factors. Some of them are related to the disability itself, like the existence of communication difficulties that complicate the diagnosis [37], but there are also contextual factors that could contribute to a higher prevalence of chronic health conditions within this group. Outstanding among the latter are difficulties to access healthcare services [38], high poverty rates [39] that are related to poorer nutrition [40], residential care settings where physical inactivity might prevail [41], high rates of polypharmacy [42], or a lack of healthcare standards for people with ID in general, and for those who are aging in particular [43]. Such factors, among others, can have a negative impact not only on the incidence of health-related problems, but also on their progression and severity through the last stage of people with ID's lifespan.

Despite the aforementioned situation, research literature comparing the prevalence of chronic health conditions among aging individuals with and without ID is scarce. Prominent in this regard are the publications from The Irish Longitudinal Study on Ageing (TILDA) and its Disability Supplement (IDS)-TILDA, a high-impact longitudinal study carried out in Ireland [44]. Most of the scientific literature, however, has focused on describing the health status of adults with ID [28,45] or comparing the health of young adults with ID with that of their peers without disability [24,29,46]. In Spain, we have data from the POMONA-Spain study [32] on the health of people with ID over the age of 18, but does not pay specific attention to the elderly population.

Thus, the present study is carried out considering the demographic changes that are taking place in our country, as well as the paucity of literature regarding the prevalence of chronic health conditions among older adults with ID. A deeper understanding of the prevalence rates of health related problems can lead to their early prevention and detection through improvements in healthcare practices and access to health care [17]. It could also have a positive impact on the functioning and wellbeing of people with ID who are aging.

In the light of the above, the purpose of this study is to analyze the presence of chronic health conditions in elderly population with ID. The data obtained will also be compared to national-level data from adults without disabilities reported by the Spanish National Health Survey [47]. This comparison furthers our understanding of the health risks and associated chronic health problems of older individuals with ID.

2. Method

2.1. Participants

A survey aimed at gathering information on the health status of people with ID over the age of 44 was designed. These data encompass the first sample of this study, which consists of 1040 people with ID (Table 1). Men and women are equally represented in the ID population, ranging in age from 44 to 88 years old (M = 55.29; SD = 7.34). The diagnosis of the individuals assessed was intellectual disability of unknown etiology in 64.9% of the cases, 25.5% of the sample having mild ID, 42.4% moderate ID, and 32.1% severe/profound ID. Almost half (45.8%) of the sample required extensive and generalized support.

Data on the non-ID population (Table 1) were taken from the Spanish National Health Survey 2011/12 [47]. This large-scale survey is carried out in Spain around every five years with the purpose of gathering information on citizens' health at the national and regional level, and to plan and assess healthcare procedures. It provides information on 21,007 adults, among whom 12,172 are individuals without disability over the age of 44.

Table 1. Sociodemographic information of the participants in the study.

Sociodemographic Data	ID (n = 1040) % (n)	Non-ID (n = 12,172) % (n)
Age		
44–64	87.2 (907)	54.8 (6669)
65 and over	12.8 (133)	45.2 (5503)
Gender		
Male	49.5 (515)	43.3 (5265)
Female	50.5 (525)	56.7 (6907)
Place of residence		
Residential settings	53.5 (554)	-
Family home	37.7 (15)	100 (12,172)
Supported living	8.2 (85)	-
Other places of residence	0.6 (6)	-

Data corresponding to the ID population were obtained from assessments carried out by 362 informants. They were mostly reference professionals for people with ID and/or their relatives, belonging to 83 disability support organizations in 34 of the 50 Spanish provinces. Their main characteristics are detailed in Table 2.

Table 2. Sociodemographic data of informants.

Sociodemographic Data	% (n)
Gender	
Male	24.3 (88)
Female	75.7 (274)
Relationship with the person evaluated	
Professionals	58.3 (211)
Mean age	40.7
Professional position	
Management or technical positions	35.9
Caregivers	21.4
Psychologists	19.4
Educators	13.1
Social workers	6.8
Occupational therapists	1.9
Doctors	1.5
Relatives	40.0 (145)
Mean age	64.7
Family relationship	
Siblings	48.3
Parents	41.4
Other relatives	10.3
Other relationships	1.7 (6)
Frequency of contact with the person evaluated	
Daily	74.3
Weekly	22.0
Several times per month	3.7

2.2. Instrument

Data on the health of people with ID over the age of 44 were collected by means of a survey that was designed using information extracted from three types of document: (1) scientific literature in the area of ID, health and aging published between 2000 and 2016, which was accessed through specialized databases such as PsycINFO and PubMed; (2) already existing assessment tools on health in the general and in the ID population, such as the National Core Indicators Survey [48], the SF-36 Health Survey [49], the HoNOS scales [50] and the scale used by the research team of the Carlos III Health Institute within the framework of the POMONA-Spain project [51]; and (3) the National Health Survey of the National Statistics Institute 2011/2012 [47].

These three sources were used as a basis to draft a first version of the survey consisting of a total of 55 questions. The survey was then sent to 13 experts in the area of intellectual and developmental disabilities so that they could submit their observations and comments on the questions included. After this first round, a further 20 items that were considered relevant by the experts were added, covering aspects related to mental health and difficulties in accessing healthcare services. In a second round, the survey, consisting now of 75 items, was again assessed by the team of experts. Three questions related to women's health during pregnancy that were regarded as too specific were removed, and the items were grouped according to the structure of the National Health Survey: (a) sociodemographic data; (b) health status of the person with ID over the age of 44 (i.e., questions related to chronic diseases, mental health and behavioral problems); (c) number of accidents; (d) health-related quality of life as measured by the EuroQol five-dimensional, EQ- [52]; (e) participation restrictions; (f) limitations in daily life activities; (g) hearing and sight characteristics; (h) use of healthcare services; (i) hospitalizations, use of emergency services and healthcare insurance; (j) medication intake; (k) preventive practices; and (l) other determinants of health (e.g., tobacco and alcohol use).

The final instrument was composed of 72 questions. Examples of items within each section are presented in Table 3.

This study was focused on the analysis of chronic health conditions diagnosed by a healthcare professional that could affect people with ID during their aging process.

Table 3. Examples of questions included in the survey.

Survey Section	Examples of Questions
Health status of the person with ID over the age of 44	Does the individual present any of the following chronic health diseases as diagnosed by a healthcare professional? Hypertension Myocardial infarction Other heart diseases Osteoarticular diseases Chronic back pain Allergy Asthma Lung diseases Diabetes Stomach ulcer Urinary incontinence Hypercholesterolemia Cataract Chronic constipation Cerebrovascular accidents or CVAs Migraines Malignant tumors Osteoporosis Thyroid disorders Obesity
Number of accidents	During the last twelve months, has the person with intellectual disability suffered an accident of any kind, including poisoning or burns?

Table 3. Cont.

Survey Section	Examples of Questions
Participation restrictions	During the past two weeks, has the person had to reduce or limit his or her usual activities because of any pain or symptoms?
Limitations in daily life activities	Thinking about the last six months, to what extent has the person been limited in carrying out the activities that people usually do because of a healthcare problem?
Hearing and sight characteristics	Does he or she need glasses or contact lenses? Does he or she need a hearing aid?
Use of healthcare services	How long has it been since the person have his or her last health check?
Hospitalizations, use of emergency services and healthcare insurance	In the last twelve months, has the person used an emergency service for any problem or illness? In the last twelve months, have the person not received medical assistance the he or she needed?
Medication intake	Please list all medications the person is taking, indicating which one has been prescribed by a physician
Preventive practices	Has the person ever visited a gynecologist or urologist?
Other determinants of health	Does the person smoke?

2.3. Procedure

Initially, all the organizations (N = 1068) that are part of the four main service providers for people with ID in Spain were approached. A total of 227 (21%) showed an interest in participating in the study. Finally, 83 organizations that provide support for aging people with ID in 34 different Spanish provinces took part in the study. The survey described in the previous section was sent to the organizations either via regular post or via email, along with two other documents: an informed consent form to be returned by the professionals or relatives before their participation in the study, and an information letter stating the research objectives, method, funding sources and other relevant information concerning the study, as well as contact information where requests for further information should be sent.

This study was approved by the Bioethics Committee of the University of Salamanca, and all procedures performed in this research were in accordance with the 1964 Helsinki Declaration and its later amendments or comparable ethical standards.

Data on the non-ID population were extracted from the website of the Ministry of Health, Social Services and Equality of Spain, which gathers the microdata and syntax of the National Health Survey of the National Statistics Institute 2011/2012 [47]. The cases of people under the age of 45 were excluded.

2.4. Data Analysis

First, data regarding the prevalence of chronic health conditions diagnosed by a healthcare professional were obtained (Table 3).

Chi-square tests were used to estimate the statistical significance of the relationship between the likelihood of developing a chronic disease and the presence of ID, alongside Cramer's V to measure effect size: V > 0.25 being very strong effect, V > 0.15 strong effect, V > 0.10 moderate effect, V > 0.05 weak effect, and V < 0.05 no effect [53].

Due to the difference in size between the ID sample (N = 1040) and the non-ID sample (N = 12,172), the latter was divided into 10 random subsamples so that the sample size of both groups would be similar when making comparisons, and to ensure the replicability and power of the analysis conducted. Since the contrasts performed for the 10 subsamples yielded similar results, this study only reports those of the analysis based on the total data. Finally, the analysis was again carried out between the two subsamples matched on age and sex.

Data were analyzed using IBM SPSS Statistics version 25. The significance level set by the researchers to conduct the statistical analyses was $\alpha = 0.05$.

3. Results

Table 4 gathers the frequency of occurrence of the health conditions analyzed in people with and without ID over the age of 44. The results of the analysis on the matching samples are shown in parentheses. The most frequent chronic diseases among the aging population with ID were obesity (25.3%; $n = 263$), urinary incontinence (18.7%; $n = 192$), osteoarticular problems (16.9%; $n = 168$), hypercholesterolemia (16.6%; $n = 166$), hypertension (16.6%; $n = 166$), chronic constipation (16.2%; $n = 165$) and thyroid disorders (12.4%; $n = 122$).

When comparing the prevalence of chronic health conditions between groups, we observe that the ID population was more likely to experience urinary incontinence (18.7% vs. 6.4%; $\chi^2 = 205.81$; $p < 0.001$; OR = 3.34) and chronic constipation (16.2% vs. 6.5%; $\chi^2 = 128.69$; $p < 0.001$; OR = 2.77), the strength of the association between the study variables being moderate in both cases.

Although individuals with ID experienced a higher prevalence than the general population of thyroid disorders ($\chi^2 = 25.84$; $p < 0.001$; OR = 1.69) and obesity ($\chi^2 = 17.32$; $p < 0.001$; OR = 1.37), the effect size of the association was weak in both cases (V = 0.05 y V = 0.04).

As for the remaining health conditions, there was a higher prevalence among the general population, which was especially significant and reported moderate effect sizes in the case of osteoarticular disorders (16.9% vs. 36.9%; $\chi^2 = 161.47$; $p < 001$; V = 0.11); hypertension (16.6% vs. 38.4%; $\chi^2 = 185.2$; $p < 0.001$; V = 0.12) and chronic back pain (10.4% vs. 35.3%; $\chi^2 = 258.20$; $p < 001$; V = 0.14).

When carrying out the analysis with the matching samples, different results were found for some chronic health conditions. Small differences observed in the beginning, suggesting a higher prevalence among individuals without ID, were no longer significant. This was the case for cataracts (9.9% vs. 9%; $\chi^2 = 0.09$; $p = 0.342$; V = 0), diabetes (8.9% vs. 10.4%; $\chi^2 = 2.15$; $p = 0.142$; V = 0.01), and other heart diseases (7.2% vs. 7.1%; $\chi^2 = 0.03$; $p = 0.84$; V = 0). In urinary incontinence, the initially moderate difference between groups became stronger (18.7% vs. 3.8%; $\chi^2 = 396$; $p < 0.001$; V = 0.20; OR = 5.77), indicating a higher prevalence within the ID group.

In the remaining conditions, no substantial changes were observed, although differences tended to be slightly less pronounced.

Table 4. Prevalence of chronic health conditions in people over 44 years with intellectual disability (ID) and without ID.

Chronic Health Condition	Power (1-β)	Intellectual Disability (%)	General Population (%)	x^2	p-Value	V Cramer	Odds Ratio (ID/No ID)
Allergy	1.00	5.7	11.3 (11.7)	29.6 (33.1)	<0.001 (<0.001)	0.05 (0.05)	0.47 (0.45)
Asthma	1.00	1.9	4.9 (4.5)	17.6 (14.8)	<0.001 (<0.001)	0.04 (0.04)	0.38 (0.42)
Cataract	1.00	9.9	17.3 (9)	36.34 (0.09)	<0.001 (**0.342**)	0.05 (0)	0.52 (1.1)
Chronic back pain	0.94	10.4	35.3 (33.4)	258.2 (223)	<0.001 (<0.001)	0.14 (0.15)	0.21 (0.23)
Chronic constipation	0.97	16.2	6.5 (5)	128.69 (196)	<0.001 (<0.001)	0.1 (0.14)	2.77 (3.67)
CVAs	1.00	1.6	1.9 (1.3)	0.2 (0.5)	**0.655 (0.483)**	0.01 (0)	0.86 (1.21)
Diabetes	1.00	8.9	13.4 (10.4)	17.2 (2.15)	<0.001 (**0.142**)	0.04 (0.01)	0.62 (0.85)
Hypercholesterolemia	1.00	16.6	31.2 (29.1)	94.2 (70.5)	<0.001 (<0.001)	0.09 (0.08)	0.43 (0.48)
Hypertension	1.00	16.6	38.4 (31.7)	185.2 (95.6)	<0.001 (<0.001)	0.12 (0.10)	0.32 (0.42)
Lung disease	1.00	3.9	7.2 (5.8)	15.44 (6.4)	<0.001 (0.011)	0.04 (0.02)	0.52 (0.65)
Malignant tumors	0.98	2.4	5.2 (4.3)	14.4 (8.1)	<0.001 (0.004)	0.03 (0.02)	0.45 (0.54)
Myocardial infarction	1.00	0.6	3.4 (2.4)	22.81 (13.4)	<0.001 (<0.001)	0.04 (0.03)	0.38 (0.25)
Migraines	0.90	5.3	11 (11.1)	31.09 (31.5)	<0.001 (<0.001)	0.05 (0.05)	0.45 (0.44)
Obesity	1.00	25.3	19.8 (20.3)	17.3 (13.8)	<0.001 (<0.001)	0.04 (0.037)	1.37 (1.33)
Osteoarticular disorders	0.86	16.9	36.9 (28.7)	161.47 (63.3)	<0.001 (<0.001)	0.11 (0.08)	0.34 (0.50)
Osteoporosis	1.00	6.8	8.6 (6.5)	3.44 (0.08)	**0.064 (0.76)**	0.02 (0)	0.77 (1.00)
Other heart diseases	0.57	7.2	10.7 (7.1)	11.78 (0.03)	<0.001 (**0.84**)	0.03 (0)	0.65 (1.03)
Stomach ulcer	1.00	2.3	6.9 (6.5)	32.2 (28.2)	<0.001 (<0.001)	0.05 (0.05)	0.31 (0.33)
Thyroid disorders	0.77	12.4	7.7 (7.7)	25.84 (26)	<0.001 (<0.001)	0.05 (0.05)	1.69 (1.70)
Urinary incontinence	1.00	18.7	6.4 (3.8)	205.81 (396)	<0.001 (<0.001)	0.13 (0.20)	3.34 (5.77)

Note: The results of the analysis on the matching samples are shown in parentheses. Non-significant relationships are highlighted in bold.

4. Discussion

The first goal of this study was to analyze the prevalence of chronic health conditions in people with ID over the age of 44. According to the results, the most prevalent diseases among the ID population are obesity, urinary incontinence, osteoarticular disorders, hypercholesterolemia, hypertension, chronic constipation and thyroid disorders. The remaining chronic health conditions studied yielded prevalence results below 10%.

The second part of the study compared the health of older adults with ID with that of their peers without disability. The scientific literature includes several references to the higher prevalence of obesity in the adult population with ID as compared to the general population [25,28,31,32,54,55]. These data seem to be replicated in elderly individuals with ID, with their probability of presenting obesity being 1.33 times higher than in the general population (25.3% vs. 20.3%). Other chronic conditions that are mentioned in the literature as being more frequent in people with ID than in those without ID are chronic constipation [32,55,56] and urinary incontinence [32]. The data of this study reflect that the probability of suffering from chronic constipation and urinary incontinence is also higher in aging individuals with ID, with the odds being 3.67 and 5.77 times greater, respectively. Other conditions, such as thyroid disorders, also occur more often in individuals with ID who are aging (12.4% vs. 7.7%), which is consistent with the findings of other studies [24,29,32,33,46].

Other diseases (e.g., allergy, asthma, chronic back pain, diabetes, hypercholesterolemia, hypertension, lung diseases, malignant tumors, migraines, myocardial infarction, osteoarticular disorders, and stomach ulcer) report lower rates of prevalence in older adults with ID. This result is also observed in other studies that analyze the risks for hypercholesterolemia [32,45,57], lung diseases [29,35,58,59] or malignant tumors [33,45,59] in this population group.

Our data, unlike those reported by other studies [24,28,31,44,60–64], suggest that older adults with ID are at a lower risk of suffering from diabetes or hypercholesterolemia than the general population. After controlling for age and sex, differences between the ID and non-ID population regarding diabetes disappear. Nevertheless, further research into variables that might mediate in the development of other conditions such as hypercholesterolemia is required, since other studies support the idea that the prevalence rate is similar in both population groups [28,29,31,44,57,65].

This work is the first study conducted in Spain where the health of older adults with and without ID is compared. The higher prevalence of certain chronic health conditions among older adults with ID could contribute to explaining the increased morbidity and early mortality reported within this group [13]. These health conditions may be potentially preventable with quality medical care [33]. However, research has indicated that individuals with ID are three times more likely than the general population to die from causes that could have been easily avoided [66]. Furthermore, the scientific literature has reported that older adults with ID encounter different barriers that hinder access to appropriate medical care, among which the absence of healthcare protocols focused on their aging process stands out [38,67,68]. There is therefore an urgent need to develop preventive healthcare plans to improve the health-related quality of life of older persons with ID. These healthcare plans should be accompanied by a better understanding of the patterns of medical care use and non-use among people with and without ID [47] so possible difficulties using healthcare services can be foreseen and prevented.

This study has certain limitations that should be considered. One of them is related to the contrast statistic used, chi-square, a comparison index that is sensitive to sample size, in the same way as statistical power.

A further limitation concerns the differences observed between the two sample groups. All the individuals that made up the sample without ID lived in their own home, while a large part of the ID sample lived in residential facilities. As is stated by different authors, living in residential settings may have a strong impact on people with ID's health [69] and quality of life [70]. Also, and given the difficulties associated with self-report for people with intellectual disability [71], the survey was completed by professionals or family members who had known the person with intellectual disability for at least 12 months. This could be a limitation to the study as the knowledge of each group on the health status of the person with ID they are evaluating may differ. Furthermore, individuals without

ID completed the National Health Survey by themselves, so possible bias related to different sources of information should be also taken into account.

5. Conclusions

This study has assessed the health status of 1040 aging individuals with ID and has compared it with that of 12,172 older adults without ID living in Spain. This pioneering study in our country suggests that the main health problems of people with ID are chronic constipation, obesity, thyroid disorders, and urinary incontinence. These conditions are more frequently observed in this population group than in older adults without disabilities. Early detection and intervention in the case of these health conditions should be a priority for public health organizations and administrations, ensuring that elderly people with ID have adequate access to appropriate healthcare services and subsequent treatment.

This research seeks to generate scientific knowledge that can help healthcare professionals to approach the services they provide for this population group more efficiently. The ultimate goal is to succeed in ensuring that the increased life expectancy of people with ID may be accompanied by the best state of health possible and that they can therefore spend their last years with better quality of life.

Author Contributions: Conceptualization, P.N.; Methodology, L.G.-D., P.N. and V.B.A.; Writing—original draft, L.G.-D., P.N., M.Á.V. and V.B.A.; Writing—review & editing, L.G.-D., P.N., M.Á.V. and V.B.A. All authors have read and agreed to the published version of the manuscript.

Funding: Spanish Ministry of Economy and Competitiveness, Grant/Award Number: PSI2015-64157-R and the University of Salamanca and Banco Santander 463A.B.01, 2016.

Acknowledgments: The authors would like to thank professionals and family members who participated in the study.

Conflicts of Interest: The authors declare no conflict of interest.

References

1. United Nations. *World Population Prospects 2019, Highlights*; United Nations Department for Economic and Social Affairs: New York, NY, USA, 2019.
2. Yasobant, S. Comprehensive public health action for our aging world: The quintessence of public health policy. *J. Int. Med. Res.* **2018**, *46*, 555–556. [CrossRef] [PubMed]
3. Mathers, C.D.; Stevens, G.A.; Boerma, T.; White, R.A.; Tobias, M.I. Causes of international increases in older age life expectancy. *Lancet* **2015**, *385*, 540–548. [CrossRef]
4. World Health Organization. *World Report on Ageing and Health*. Available online: https://www.who.int/ageing/publications/world-report-2015/en/ (accessed on 12 January 2016).
5. Instituto Nacional de Estadística. *Indicadores de Mortalidad Resultados Nacionales*. Available online: https://www.ine.es/jaxiT3/Datos.htm?t=1414#!tabs-tabla (accessed on 13 June 2018).
6. Balakrishnan, T.R.; Wolf, L.C. Life expectancy of mentally retarded persons in Canadian institutions. *Am. J. Ment. Defic.* **1976**, *80*, 650–662. [PubMed]
7. Carter, G.; Jancar, J. Mortality in the mentally handicapped: A 50 year survey at the Stoke Park group of hospitals (1930–1980). *J. Ment. Defic. Res.* **1983**, *27*, 143–156. [PubMed]
8. Fryers, T. Current Topic Survival in Down's Syndrome. *J. Intellect. Disabil. Res.* **1986**, *30*, 101–110. [CrossRef]
9. Heller, T. People with Intellectual and Developmental Disabilities Growing Old: An Overview. *Impact Feature Issue Aging People Intellect. Dev. Disabil.* **2010**, *23*, 2–3.
10. Grammenos, S. European Comparative Data on Europe 2020 & People with Disabilities. Available online: https://digitalcommons.ilr.cornell.edu/cgi/viewcontent.cgi?article=1569&context=gladnetcollect (accessed on 9 October 2019).
11. Baroja, H. *Envejecimiento y Discapacidad Intelectual*; FEVAS: Bilbao, Spain, 2014; p. 24.
12. Bowers, B.; Webber, R.; Bigby, C. Health issues of older people with intellectual disability in group homes. *J. Intellect. Dev. Disabil.* **2014**, *39*, 261–269. [CrossRef]
13. Hahn, J.E.; Fox, S.; Janicki, M.P. Aging among Older Adults with Intellectual and Developmental Disabilities: Setting National Goals to Address Transitions in Health, Retirement, and Late-Life. *Inclusion* **2015**, *3*, 250–259.

14. Lin, J.-D.; Lin, L.-P.; Hsu, S.-W. Aging People with Intellectual Disabilities: Current Challenges and Effective Interventions. *Rev. J. Autism Dev. Disord.* **2016**, *3*, 266–272. [CrossRef]
15. Dolan, E.; Lane, J.; Hillis, G.; Delanty, N. Changing Trends in Life Expectancy in Intellectual Disability over Time. *Ir. Med. J.* **2019**, *112*, P1006.
16. Haveman, M.; Heller, T.; Lee, L.; Maaskant, M.; Shooshtari, S.; Strydom, A. Major health risks in aging persons with intellectual disabilities: An overview of recent studies. *J. Policy Pract. Intellect. Disabil.* **2010**, *7*, 59–69. [CrossRef]
17. Heller, T.; Sorensen, A. Promoting healthy aging in adults with developmental disabilities. *Dev. Disabil. Res. Rev.* **2013**, *18*, 22–30. [CrossRef]
18. Sandberg, M.; Ahlstrom, G.; Axmon, A.; Kristensson, J. Somatic healthcare utilisation patterns among older people with intellectual disability: An 11-year register study. *BMC Health Serv. Res.* **2016**, *16*, 642. [CrossRef] [PubMed]
19. Wark, S.; Hussain, R.; Edwards, H. The main signs of ageing in people with intellectual disability. *Aust. J. Rural Health* **2016**, *24*, 357–362. [CrossRef] [PubMed]
20. Barrio del Campo, J.A.; Árias, M.; Ruiz Fernández, M.I.; Vicente Castro, F. Envejecimiento y Discapacidad Intelectual; La nueva etapa. *Int. J. Dev. Educ. Psychol.* **2007**, *1*, 43–56.
21. Reppermund, S.; Trollor, J.N. Successful ageing for people with an intellectual disability. *Curr. Opin. Psychiatry* **2016**, *29*, 149–154. [CrossRef]
22. Hosking, F.J.; Carey, I.M.; Shah, S.M.; Harris, T.; DeWilde, S.; Beighton, C.; Cook, D.G. Mortality Among Adults With Intellectual Disability in England: Comparisons With the General Population. *Am. J. Public Health* **2016**, *106*, 1483–1490. [CrossRef]
23. Erickson, S.R.; Spoutz, P.; Dorsch, M.; Bleske, B. Cardiovascular risk and treatment for adults with intellectual or developmental disabilities. *Int. J. Cardiol.* **2016**, *221*, 371–375. [CrossRef]
24. Morin, D.; Mérineau-Côté, J.; Ouellette-Kuntz, H.; Tassé, M.J.; Kerr, M. A comparison of the prevalence of chronic disease among people with and without intellectual disability. *Am. J. Intellect. Dev. Disabil.* **2012**, *117*, 455–463. [CrossRef]
25. Hsieh, K.; Rimmer, J.H.; Heller, T. Obesity and associated factors in adults with intellectual disability. *J. Intellect. Disabil. Res.* **2014**, *58*, 851–863. [CrossRef]
26. Salehi, S.; Nassadj, G.; Shakhi, K.; Hossein, M.; Javadipour, S. The prevalence of overweight and obesity among adults with Intellectual and developmental disabilities in Ahvaz, Iran. *Biosci. Biotechnol. Res. Commun.* **2017**, *10*, 1–6.
27. Axmon, A.; Ahlström, G.; Höglund, P. Prevalence and treatment of diabetes mellitus and hypertension among older adults with intellectual disability in comparison with the general population. *BMC Geriatr.* **2017**, *17*, 272. [CrossRef] [PubMed]
28. Emerson, E.; Hatton, C.; Baines, S.; Robertson, J. The physical health of British adults with intellectual disability: Cross sectional study. *Int. J. Equity Health* **2016**, *15*, 11. [CrossRef] [PubMed]
29. Cooper, S.-A.; Hughes-McCormack, L.; Greenlaw, N.; McConnachie, A.; Allan, L.; Baltzer, M.; McArthur, L.; Henderson, A.; Melville, C.; McSkimming, P.; et al. Management and prevalence of long-term conditions in primary health care for adults with intellectual disabilities compared with the general population: A population-based cohort study. *J. Appl. Res. Intellect. Disabil.* **2018**, *31*, 68–81. [CrossRef] [PubMed]
30. Robertson, J.; Hatton, C.; Emerson, E.; Baines, S. Prevalence of epilepsy among people with intellectual disabilities: A systematic review. *Seizure* **2015**, *29*, 46–62. [CrossRef]
31. Wong, C.W. Adults with Intellectual Disabilities Living in Hong Kong's Residential Care Facilities: A Descriptive Analysis of Health and Disease Patterns by Sex, Age, and Presence of Down Syndrome. *J. Policy Pract. Intellect. Disabil.* **2011**, *8*, 231–238. [CrossRef]
32. Folch, A.; Salvador-Carulla, L.; Vicens, P.; Cortés, M.J.; Irazábal, M.; Muñoz, S.; Rovira, L.; Orejuela, C.; González, J.A.; Martínez-Leal, R. Health indicators in intellectual developmental disorders: The key findings of the POMONA-ESP project. *J. Appl. Res. Intellect. Disabil.* **2019**, *32*, 23–34. [CrossRef]
33. Carey, I.M.; Shah, S.M.; Hosking, F.J.; DeWilde, S.; Harris, T.; Beighton, C.; Cook, D.G. Health characteristics and consultation patterns of people with intellectual disability: A cross-sectional database study in English general practice. *Br. J. Gen. Pract.* **2016**, *66*, E264–E270. [CrossRef]
34. Sinai, A.; Bohnen, I.; Strydom, A. Older adults with intellectual disability. *Curr. Opin. Psychiatry* **2012**, *25*, 359–364. [CrossRef]

35. Cooper, S.-A.; McLean, G.; Guthrie, B.; McConnachie, A.; Mercer, S.; Sullivan, F.; Morrison, J. Multiple physical and mental health comorbidity in adults with intellectual disabilities: Population-based cross-sectional analysis. *BMC Fam. Pract.* **2015**, *16*, 110. [CrossRef]
36. Evenhuis, H.; Schoufour, J.; Echteld, M. Frailty and intellectual disability: A different operationalization? *Dev. Disabil. Res. Rev.* **2013**, *18*, 17–21. [CrossRef]
37. Domínguez, J.; Navas, P. Deterioro cognitivo y trastorno neurodegenerativo en personas con discapacidad intelectual. *Siglo Cero* **2018**, *49*, 53–67. [CrossRef]
38. Navas, P.; Llorente, S.; García, L.; Tassé, M.J.; Havercamp, S.M. Improving healthcare access for older adults with intellectual disability: What are the needs? *J. Appl. Res. Intellect. Disabil.* **2019**, *32*, 1453–1464. [CrossRef] [PubMed]
39. Emerson, E.; Hatton, C. *Health Inequalities and People with Intellectual Disabilities*; University Press: Cambridge, UK, 2014.
40. Robertson, J.; Emerson, E.; Baines, S.; Hatton, C. Obesity and health behaviours of British adults with self-reported intellectual impairments: Cross sectional survey. *BMC Public Health* **2014**, *14*, 219. [CrossRef] [PubMed]
41. Schepens Niemiec, S.L.; Blanchard, J.; Vigen, C.L.P.; Martínez, J.; Guzmán, L.; Concha, A.; Fluke, M.; Carlson, M. Evaluation of ¡*Vivir Mi Vida!* to improve health and wellness of rural-dwelling, late middle-aged Latino adults: Results of a feasibility and pilot study of a lifestyle intervention. *Prim. Health Care Res. Dev.* **2018**, *19*, 448–463. [CrossRef]
42. Robertson, J.; Emerson, E.; Gregory, N.; Hatton, C.; Kessissoglou, S.; Hallam, A. Receipt of psychotropic medication by people with intellectual disability in residential settings. *J. Intellect. Disabil. Res.* **2000**, *44*, 666–676. [CrossRef]
43. Bigby, C. *Ageing with a Lifelong Disability: A Guide to Practice, Program, and Policy Issues for Human Services Professionals*; Jessica Kingsley Publishers: London, UK, 2004.
44. McCarron, M.; Cleary, E.; McCallion, P. Health and Health-Care Utilization of the Older Population of Ireland: Comparing the Intellectual Disability Population and the General Population. *Res. Aging* **2017**, *39*, 693–718. [CrossRef]
45. Cocks, E.; Thomson, A.; Thoresen, S.; Parsons, R.; Rosenwax, L. Health status and use of medications by adults with intellectual disability in Western Australia. *J. Intellect. Dev. Disabil.* **2016**, *41*, 87–96. [CrossRef]
46. Hughes-McCormack, L.A.; Rydzewska, E.; Henderson, A.; MacIntyre, C.; Rintoul, J.; Cooper, S.-A. Prevalence and general health status of people with intellectual disabilities in Scotland: A total population study. *J. Epidemiol. Community Health* **2018**, *72*, 78–85. [CrossRef]
47. Instituto Nacional de Estadística. *Encuesta Nacional de Salud 2011–2012*. Available online: https://www.mscbs.gob.es/estadEstudios/estadisticas/encuestaNacional/encuesta2011.htm (accessed on 23 March 2018).
48. Human Services Research Institute (HSRI); The National Association of State Directors of Developmental Disabilities Services (NASDDDS). *National Core Indicators Survey*. Available online: https://www.nationalcoreindicators.org/resources/ (accessed on 28 April 2016).
49. López-García, E.; Banegas, J.R.; Pérez-Regadera, A.G.; Gutiérrez-Fisac, J.L.; Alonso, J.; Rodríguez-Artalejo, F. Valores de referencia de la versión española del Cuestionario de Salud SF-36 en población adulta de más de 60 años. *Med. Clín.* **2003**, *120*, 568–573. [CrossRef]
50. Ausín Benito, B.; Muñoz López, M.; Quiroga Estévez, M.A. Adaptación española de las escalas de resultados para personas mayores HoNOS65+ (Health of the Nation Outcome Scales for Older Adults). *Rev. Esp. Geriatr. Gerontol.* **2007**, *42*, 88–95. [CrossRef]
51. Perry, J.; Allen, D.G.; Pimm, C.; Meek, A.; Lowe, K.; Groves, S.; Cohen, D.; Felce, D. Adults with intellectual disabilities and challenging behaviour: The costs and outcomes of in- and out-of-area placements. *J. Intellect. Disabil. Res.* **2013**, *57*, 139–152. [CrossRef] [PubMed]
52. Herdman, M.; Gudex, C.; Lloyd, A.; Janssen, M.F.; Kind, P.; Parkin, D.; Bonsel, G.; Badia, X. Development and preliminary testing of the new five-level version of EQ-5D (EQ-5D-5L). *Qual. Life Res.* **2011**, *20*, 1727–1736. [CrossRef] [PubMed]
53. Akoglu, H. User's guide to correlation coefficients. *Turk. J. Emerg. Med.* **2018**, *18*, 91–93. [CrossRef] [PubMed]
54. Havercamp, S.M.; Scott, H.M. National health surveillance of adults with disabilities, adults with intellectual and developmental disabilities, and adults with no disabilities. *Disabil. Health J.* **2015**, *8*, 165–172. [CrossRef]

55. Martinez-Leal, R.; Salvador-Carulla, L.; Ruiz, M.; Nadal, M.; Novell-Alsina, R.; Martorell, A.; Gonzalez-Gordon, R.G.; Reyes, M.; Angel, S.; Milagrosa-Tejonero, L.; et al. Health among persons with intellectual disability in Spain: The European POMONA-II study. *Rev. Neurol.* **2011**, *53*, 406–414. [PubMed]
56. Hermans, H.; Evenhuis, H.M. Multimorbidity in older adults with intellectual disabilities. *Res. Dev. Disabil.* **2014**, *35*, 776–783. [CrossRef]
57. de Winter, C.F.; Bastiaanse, L.P.; Hilgenkamp, T.I.M.; Evenhuis, H.M.; Echteld, M.A. Cardiovascular risk factors (diabetes, hypertension, hypercholesterolemia and metabolic syndrome) in older people with intellectual disability: Results of the HA-ID study. *Res. Dev. Disabil.* **2012**, *33*, 1722–1731. [CrossRef]
58. Axmon, A.; Sandberg, M.; Ahlström, G. Gender differences in psychiatric diagnoses in older people with intellectual disability: A register study. *BMC Psychiatry* **2017**, *17*, 192. [CrossRef]
59. Janicki, M.P.; Davidson, P.W.; Henderson, C.M.; McCallion, P.; Taets, J.D.; Force, L.T.; Sulkes, S.B.; Frangenberg, E.; Ladrigan, P.M. Health characteristics and health services utilization in older adults with intellectual disability living in community residences. *J. Intellect. Disabil. Res.* **2002**, *46*, 287–298. [CrossRef]
60. de Winter, C.F.; Magilsen, K.W.; van Alfen, J.C.; Penning, C.; Evenhuis, H.M. Prevalence of cardiovascular risk factors in older people with intellectual disability. *Am. J. Intellect. Dev. Disabil.* **2009**, *114*, 427–436. [CrossRef] [PubMed]
61. Lin, J.-D.; Lin, L.-P.; Lee, J.-T.; Liou, S.-W.; Chen, Y.-J.; Hsu, S.-W.; Liu, C.-T.; Leu, Y.-R.; Wu, C.-L. Prevalence and risk factors associated with fasting blood glucose levels in adults aged 30 years and older with disabilities: The results from an annual health check-up. *Int. J. Dev. Disabil.* **2014**, *60*, 57–64. [CrossRef]
62. MacRae, S.; Brown, M.; Karatzias, T.; Taggart, L.; Truesdale-Kennedy, M.; Walley, R.; Sierka, A.; Northway, R.; Carey, M.; Davies, M. Diabetes in people with intellectual disabilities: A systematic review of the literature. *Res. Dev. Disabil.* **2015**, *47*, 352–374. [CrossRef] [PubMed]
63. McVilly, K.; McGillivray, J.; Curtis, A.; Lehmann, J.; Morrish, L.; Speight, J. Diabetes in people with an intellectual disability: A systematic review of prevalence, incidence and impact. *Diabet. Med.* **2014**, *31*, 897–904. [CrossRef] [PubMed]
64. Wee, L.E.; Koh, G.C.; Auyong, L.S.; Cheong, A.; Myo, T.T.; Lin, J.; Lim, E.; Tan, S.; Sundaramurthy, S.; Koh, C.W.; et al. Screening for cardiovascular disease risk factors at baseline and post intervention among adults with intellectual disabilities in an urbanised Asian society. *J. Intellect. Disabil. Res.* **2014**, *58*, 255–268. [CrossRef] [PubMed]
65. van de Louw, J.; Vorstenbosch, R.; Vinck, L.; Penning, C.; Evenhuis, H. Prevalence of hypertension in adults with intellectual disability in the Netherlands. *J. Intellect. Disabil. Res.* **2009**, *53*, 78–84. [CrossRef]
66. Jaques, H. Premature death in people with learning disabilities. *Nurs. Times* **2014**, *110*, 19.
67. Ali, A.; Scior, K.; Ratti, V.; Strydom, A.; King, M.; Hassiotis, A. Discrimination and Other Barriers to Accessing Health Care: Perspectives of Patients with Mild and Moderate Intellectual Disability and Their Carers. *PLoS ONE* **2013**, *8*, e70855. [CrossRef]
68. Schepens, H.R.M.M.; Van Puyenbroeck, J.; Maes, B. How to improve the quality of life of elderly people with intellectual disability: A systematic literature review of support strategies. *J. Appl. Res. Intellect. Disabil.* **2019**, *32*, 483–521. [CrossRef]
69. Martínez-Leal, R.; Salvador-Carulla, L.; Linehan, C.; Walsh, P.; Weber, G.; Van Hove, G.; Määttä, T.; Azema, B.; Haveman, M.; Buono, S.; et al. The impact of living arrangements and deinstitutionalisation in the health status of persons with intellectual disability in Europe: A study using a health survey in 14 EC countries. *J. Intellect. Disabil. Res.* **2011**, *55*, 858–872. [CrossRef]
70. Sáenz, I. Influencia del tipo de vivienda en la calidad de vida de las personas mayores con discapacidad intelectual o del desarrollo. *Siglo Cero* **2018**, *49*, 89–106.
71. Lunsky, Y.; Emery, C.F.; Benson, B.A. Staff and self-reports of health behaviours, somatic complaints, and medications among adults with mild intellectual disability. *J. Intellect. Dev. Disabil.* **2002**, *27*, 125–135. [CrossRef]

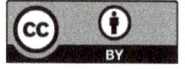

© 2020 by the authors. Licensee MDPI, Basel, Switzerland. This article is an open access article distributed under the terms and conditions of the Creative Commons Attribution (CC BY) license (http://creativecommons.org/licenses/by/4.0/).

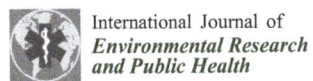

Article

Improving Environmental Capacities for Health Promotion in Support Settings for People with Intellectual Disabilities: Inclusive Design of the DIHASID Tool

Kristel Vlot-van Anrooij [1,*], Thessa I.M. Hilgenkamp [2,3], Geraline L. Leusink [1], Anneke van der Cruijsen [1], Henk Jansen [1], Jenneken Naaldenberg [1] and Koos van der Velden [4]

[1] Department of Primary and Community Care, Intellectual Disabilities and Health, Radboud Institute for Health Sciences, Radboud University Medical Center, P.O box 9101, 6500 HB Nijmegen, The Netherlands; geraline.leusink@radboudumc.nl (G.L.L.); anneke.vandercruijsen@radboudumc.nl (A.v.d.C.); Henk.jansen@radboudumc.nl (H.J.); Jenneken.Naaldenberg@radboudumc.nl (J.N.)

[2] Department of Physical Therapy, University of Nevada, Las Vegas, NV 89154-3029, USA; thessa.hilgenkamp@unlv.edu

[3] Department of General Practice, Intellectual Disability Medicine, Erasmus University Medical Center, Rotterdam, P.O box 2040, 3000 CA Rotterdam, The Netherlands

[4] Department of Primary and Community Care, Radboud Institute for Health Sciences, Radboud University Medical Center, P.O box 9101, 6500 HB Nijmegen, The Netherlands; koos.vandervelden@radboudumc.nl

* Correspondence: kristel.vananrooij@radboudumc.nl; Tel.: +31-24-361-8181

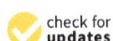

Received: 20 December 2019; Accepted: 24 January 2020; Published: 28 January 2020

Abstract: People with intellectual disabilities (ID) have unhealthier lifestyles than the general population. To sustainably improve their lifestyle and health status, a whole-system approach to creating healthy environments is crucial. To gain insight into how support for physical activity and healthy nutrition can be embedded in a setting, asset mapping can be helpful. Asset mapping involves creating a bottom–up overview of promoting and protective factors for health. However, there is no asset mapping tool available for ID support settings. This study aims to develop an asset mapping tool in collaboration with people with ID to gain insight into assets for healthy nutrition and physical activity in such settings. The tool is based on previous research and development continued in an iterative and inclusive process in order to create a clear, comprehensive, and usable tool. Expert interviews ($n = 7$), interviews with end-users ($n = 7$), and pilot testing ($n = 16$) were conducted to refine the tool. Pilot participants perceived the tool as helpful in pinpointing perceived assets and in prompting ideas on how to create inclusive environments with support for physical activity and healthy nutrition. This overview of assets can be helpful for mobilizing assets and building the health-promoting capacities of ID support settings.

Keywords: health promotion; lifestyle; settings approach; health assets; intellectual disability; community participation; inclusive research; context-based interventions; empowerment; inclusion

1. Introduction

People with intellectual disabilities (ID) have unhealthier lifestyles than people without disabilities, with more physical inactivity and unhealthy dietary habits [1–4], and their lifestyles contribute to many of their health problems [1,5]. The promotion of physical activity and healthy nutrition may help to decrease the health inequities faced by people with ID. However, people with ID are more dependent on their environment to live healthily. In a previous study on health promotion, people with ID expressed the need for a supportive social and physical environment to be able to live healthily [6]. This is supported by the growing evidence of environmental factors associated with lifestyle, such as the association between the presence of convenience stores and fast-food restaurants and nutrition intake, and the association between the accessibility of facilities, street safety, aesthetic attributes, and physical activity [7–10]. ID support settings are specialized in providing long-term residential, community living arrangements, and day activities for people with ID, who face limitations in intellectual functioning and adaptive behavior [11]. In the Netherlands, about 68,000 people live in facilities from ID support settings, ranging from clustered group homes to small-group living in apartments or single-family homes in neighborhoods [12,13]. People with ID spend a lot of time in these settings where they receive support with personal, daily, social, and home health tasks, mainly provided by daily care professionals trained in behavior aspects and/or assisted nursing [14]. So, environmental support for health promotion could contribute to sustainable improvement in the health status of people with ID and achieve more equality for this population in which ID support settings can play a crucial role.

Despite the efforts of ID support organizations to improve the lifestyle of people with ID, the sustainable embedment of health promotion in daily support faces challenges [6,15,16]. On the one hand, many interventions developed by researchers in program settings are challenged by difficulties in implementing them in practice [15]. On the other hand, many of the interventions developed in practice focus mostly on the individual, consist of stand-alone activities, and lack embedment in policy [17,18]. Moreover, they lack sustainability as they are not embedded in the daily support system of ID support organizations [17,18]. To sustainably improve the lifestyles of people with ID in settings where they engage, a whole-system approach has been identified as a way forward [19].

Taking a whole-system approach is complex, as it requires health promotion to be embedded in the day-to-day practices of ID care organizations. This whole-system approach has been successfully implemented using the healthy settings approach [20,21]. This healthy settings approach is a whole-system approach where stakeholders are given the capacity to address behavioral and environmental factors and embed health within the routines and the culture of a setting [20,21]. It has been successfully implemented in hospitals and schools as healthy school and healthy hospital projects. These have resulted in transformed policies, organizational structures, and community action to facilitate healthy living [22,23]. Due to these successes in other settings, this approach might also be beneficial for health promotion in ID support settings.

Co-creating healthy settings is key, as the people who actually use a setting know best which of the existing resources can be useful and how health promotion can be made part of the whole-system in a certain setting [24]. Asset mapping is a bottom–up process for creating an overview of those resources (promoting and protective factors) that maintain and sustain health and well-being in a defined setting. In this approach, people who use the setting are actively involved, as they have essential knowledge and experiences about living in a place and the resources available. Therefore, asset mapping can be used to provide input for the whole-system approach. In general, there is a lack of asset mapping techniques [25]. Although existing tools can help assess resources for health promotion in the environment [26–36], these tools fit poorly with an assets mapping approach due to the lack of a whole-system focus, the lack of a positive approach, or a scope that is too narrow. Furthermore, making a tool that can be used by people with ID themselves requires a clear structure and language with instructions to create meaningful engagement by people with ID.

This study aimed to develop a comprehensive, clear, and usable inclusive tool for environmental asset mapping for ID support settings that can also be used by people with ID themselves. The tool, developed in Dutch, provides insight into perceived environmental assets and points for improvements regarding support for healthy nutrition and physical activity for people with moderate to profound ID in settings where they engage. These insights can be used to create inclusive and health-promoting environments. This article describes the iterative and inclusive development process of creating the tool using expert interviews, cognitive interviews, and pilot testing. The inclusive research team used this input to create a functional tool that can be used by people with ID and care professionals.

2. Materials and Methods

2.1. Development Phases

This study used an iterative process in which end-users were involved to develop the asset mapping tool named DIscovering Health-promoting Assets in Settings for people with Intellectual Disabilities (DIHASID). End-users include people who engage in a living or day-activity location, e.g., people with mild to moderate ID, proxy respondents for people with severe/profound ID, and care professionals. The three development steps are visualized in Table 1 and described below.

Table 1. Development of the DIHASID tool: phases, action, results, and participants. ID: intellectual disabilities.

Phase	Action	Result	Participants
Make the DIHASID tool comprehensive	Check the extent to which the DIHASID tool represents all facets of a given construct	Based on expert feedback, the DIHASID tool is adjusted to make it comprehensive	Experts on physical activity, nutrition, and health promotion for people with ID ($n = 7$)
Make the DIHASID tool clear	Check the readability, clarity of language, and consistency of style of the questions and format of the DIHASID tool	Points of attention deduced in the cognitive interviews are used to improve the clarity of the DIHASID tool	End-users: people with mild/moderate ID, proxy respondents for people with severe/profound ID, and care professionals ($n = 7$)
Make the DIHASID tool usable	Pilot test the DIHASID tool to test the usability of the scan in settings where people with ID live, work, and engage	Pilot testing improves the tool's usability, and the final DIHASID tool is developed	End-users from three pilot locations ($n = 16$)

The DIHASID tool is underpinned by an ecological model and the theory of salutogenesis. This implicates a focus on multiple environmental levels and on protective or promotive factors rather than on barriers and needs, and a focus on assets [37,38].

The research team developed a draft asset mapping tool based on the Healthy Settings for People with Intellectual Disabilities (HeSPID) framework. This framework was built on two studies in which academics, people with ID, and proxies for people with ID developed a framework of themes and assets relevant for physical activity and nutrition in ID support settings [39,40]. The framework consists of 14 environmental-asset themes relating to people, places, and preconditions for healthy living.

This draft was discussed during expert interviews. Focus points were elicited on the comprehensibility of the themes and questions of the DIHASID tool, including all possible assets relevant for healthy living in ID support settings. Firstly, the aim of the DIHASID tool and an overview of the themes were introduced. Secondly, each theme was introduced, with a description based on the HeSPID framework [39,40]. Then, for each theme, the questions were read aloud, and the participants were asked to provide feedback on how representative the questions were. In addition, further suggestions were requested. Lastly, participants were asked to reflect on the tool and share ideas on other themes that should be included.

The cognitive interviewing (CI) technique was used to check the clarity of the questions for the users. CI is a method to evaluate the quality of transferring knowledge in questionnaires and has been used successfully among people with ID [41,42]. In CI, the interviewer reads the questions aloud and asks the interviewee to think aloud when answering the question. Probing questions are used to let the interviewees paraphrase questions, discuss thoughts, feelings, and ideas, and suggest alternative wording. The Question Appraisal System (QAS-99) was used to develop the interview protocol, including probing questions related to possible problems identified by the research team [41]. The interviews started with an explanation of the aim of the interview and the tool. Then, each question was read aloud by the interviewer, and the interviewee expressed what he/she thought and what he/she would answer. If applicable, probing questions related to the question were asked. After one hour, the interview stopped, unless the interviewee explicitly wanted to continue. Interviews were audiotaped and conducted by K.V.v.A. in a place that was convenient for the interviewee.

To improve the usability of the DIHASID tool in practice, people with ID and care professionals at the three pilot locations (1) completed the DIHASID tool; (2) completed the After-Scenario Questionnaire (ASQ), a 3-item questionnaire about user satisfaction [43]; and (3) participated in a group discussion in which task usability, user satisfaction, functional usefulness, and ideas for improvements of the DIHASID tool were discussed. The group discussion topics were based on usability domains [44].

2.2. Procedures

For the expert interviews, experts were sought on physical activity, nutrition, and health promotion for people with ID. For the cognitive interviews, end-users were recruited: adults with mild/moderate ID who are able to communicate verbally, proxy respondents for persons with severe/profound ID, and a care professional. Diversity was sought in type of location (living or day-activity location). For the pilot, living or day-activity locations for people with moderate to profound ID were sought. In each pilot location, between two and four care professionals and between two and four adults with mild/moderate ID who were able to communicate verbally or between two and four proxy respondents for adults with severe/profound ID were recruited. Participants were recruited through purposive sampling. For the expert interviews, the research team's network was used to recruit participants by inviting them through email. For the cognitive interviews and pilot, the contact persons of eight ID support providers helped to recruit participants. They sent the information leaflet to team leaders and care professionals and asked them to identify potential participants.

The care professionals identified potential participants who were interested and able to participate and provide consent. Care professionals provided them with an information leaflet on the content and procedure of the study. If needed, the care professionals assisted in reading and understanding the information. Those who were interested to participate were asked to read or listen to the consent form. It was possible to contact the researcher by phone or email to ask questions. Those who agreed to participate were asked to sign the form themselves. After consent was obtained, the contact information was shared with the researcher, who contacted them or their care professional to schedule the meeting(s). For the expert interviews, informed consent was obtained when the appointment was being made.

The study was conducted according to the principles of the Declaration of Helsinki and the EU General Data Protection Regulation. The Medical Research Ethics Committee of Radboud University and Medical Center approved this study (registration number: 2018-4408).

2.3. Inclusive Approach

This study actively involved people with ID as co-researchers to deploy experiential and scientific knowledge and contribute to appropriate data collection, data quality, and relevant outcomes [45,46]. The inclusive research team consisted of researchers with ID (co-researchers) and without ID, all employed by the university, and followed Frankena's [46] guidelines in the consensus statement for inclusive health research. K.V.v.A., A.v.d.C., and H.J. developed the procedure and the data collection method and incorporated feedback from other team members and the project's advisory group, which included people with ID, care professionals, health professionals, and a manager. Data collection and analysis was conducted by K.V.v.A. The co-researchers assisted when interpretation questions arose regarding the analysis of the cognitive interviews and group discussions of the pilot. Then, they listened to the audiotapes and discussed the meaning of what participants said. After each phase, K.V.v.A., A.v.d.C., H.J., and J.N. discussed how to adjust the tool in light of the problems and possible solutions identified during data collection. Given the important contribution of the co-researchers to this study, they are also recognized as co-authors on this paper.

Collaboration between the researchers with and without ID was supported by (1) the research clock, a clock on which steps of the study were visualized to prompt memory; (2) audio recordings rather than transcripts for data analysis; (3) verbal explanation of this manuscript to obtain feedback; and (4) a training on working as a team of researchers with and without ID. In addition to this scientific paper, an easy-read abstract was written.

2.4. Analysis

Data analysis was performed using Atlas.ti software 8.2.29 and SPSS (version 25, SPSS Inc., Chicago, IL, USA. The suggestions from the expert interviews were collected and grouped based on type of problem and suggested improvements for the DIHASID tool. The audio recordings of the cognitive interviews were analyzed using Atlas.ti. The identified problems were selected and categorized according to the eight QAS-99 categories [41]. Then, the categories were thematically analyzed, and suggestions for improvements were logged.

The pilot data on the DIHASID tool and the ASQ were analyzed using descriptive statistics in SPSS. The audio recordings of the group discussions were thematically analyzed using Atlas.ti. Relevant fragments were structured in the categories of the TURF framework on usability, where TURF stands for Task, User, Representation and Function [44], and then thematically analyzed. The gathered information was discussed among the research team to finalize the DIHASID tool.

3. Results

3.1. Participants

Thirty persons participated in the development of the DIHASID tool. Seven female experts in lifestyle and health promotion participated in interviews on the comprehensibility of the DIHASID tool: three experts on physical activity for people with ID, two experts on nutrition for people with ID, and two experts on health promotion. The following end-users participated in cognitive interviews on the clarity of the DIHASID tool: people with ID, aged 18–55 (two male, three females, three filled it out for living location and two for day-activity location), a female proxy respondent (parent), and a female care professional. The tool was piloted on usability among 16 persons from three different living and/or day-activity locations for people with moderate to profound ID, i.e., six persons with ID (five males, 1 female), two female proxy respondents, seven female care professionals, and one male manager.

3.2. Comprehensive DIHASID Tool

The analysis of the expert interviews resulted in six points for improving the comprehensibility of the DIHASID tool: (i) add a theme, (ii) add answer options, (iii) clarify or divide broad or vague questions, (iv) find better matching response categories for which respondents have the knowledge to answer, (v) use reminders for what is viewed as healthy living and a healthy living environment, and (vi) personalize questions. The input was used to change the tool regarding (i) adding or changing questions and answer options, (ii) providing more instructions, and (iii) personalization of the questions. Table 2 provides a full list of the points for improvements and changes made to the DIHASID tool.

Table 2. Points for improvement suggested in expert interviews and changes to the DIHASID tool.

Point for Improvement	Changes to the DIHASID Tool
Add theme: Include communication about healthy living within an organization in questions about health-promoting organizational policies.	The question: "How do you perceive the attention on healthy living in communications by this organization?" was added.

Table 2. Cont.

Add answer options for the questions: (1) Type of disabilities: type of wheelchair, I am not allowed on the road by myself, epilepsy (2) Type of support persons: friends, occupational therapist, speech therapist (3) Type of support: others buy food/devices: bicycle for the wheelchair, book with ideas about exercise activities, games in which you need to move, meal service, and meal-in-a-box (4) Type of autonomy-supported decision making: clients choose themselves, they do not receive help.	The suggested answer options were added to the questions.
Clarify or divide broad or vague questions: (1) The answer options for the question on types of advice from types of health professionals are not complete. Many health professionals can give several types of advice. (2) How participants experience the help of others for healthy living is very broad. It might be better to split 'others' into categories such as family and friends, health professionals, care professionals, volunteers, and clients. (3) The question, "What do you think of the opportunities for healthy living in the neighborhood?" was found to be vague. This could be interpreted as places for healthy living or activities for healthy living.	(1) The question was split into two questions: "At this location, there is enough opportunity for care professionals to get tips about...?" <answer options include types of advice> and "Who is available to provide this advice?" <answer options include types of health professionals>. (2) The answer option for the question, "How well do others help with healthy living?" was split into three categories: (a) care professionals, clients, and volunteers, (b) family and friends, and (c) health professionals. (3) The question was split into: "Are there enough places for healthy eating, healthy drinking, physical activity, and sports in the neighborhood?" and "Are there enough activities for healthy living in which you/the client can participate?"
Matching response categories: (1) The answer type for the question on talking about healthy living was perceived as difficult and not appropriate. The answer type on how often talks about healthy living were held was perceived as less important than how talking is experienced. (2) The answer option for the questions, "How much time do care professionals have for activating clients?" and "How much time and attention and do care professionals have for providing food and drinks?" were perceived as too difficult. It was perceived as too difficult for participants to express this in days per week, as this largely varies between weeks.	(1) The answer options were changed to a 5-point smiley answer. (2) The answer options were changed to never/sometimes/often/always.
Use reminders: The experts stated that clients would need reminders of what is viewed as healthy living and a healthy living environment.	The explanation of healthy living was repeated at several places in the questionnaire. The subthemes of People, Places, and Preconditions were repeated above the open questions to stimulate the participants to think about all the questions that they answered about the overarching theme and formulate wishes.
Personalized questions: The participants perceived referrals in questions as too general. Personalization of the questions was perceived as helpful for clients (e.g., "Who supports you with healthy living?" instead of "Who at this location supports healthy living?").	Separate questions were devised for clients, proxies, and care professionals.

Analysis also resulted in points that did not match the aim of the DIHASID tool and therefore did not result in changes to the tool. Examples include suggestions on the knowledge or professional attitude of clients and care professionals, relaxation, and negative environmental factors. The stability of the social network of people with ID was not included in the DIHASID tool, as this was perceived as too difficult to ascertain via a questionnaire. Details on accessibility (e.g., does the swimming pool have a hoist) were not included, as this would make the list too detailed and too long.

3.3. Clarity of the DIHASID Tool

Analysis of the cognitive interviews identified 152 problems with clarity, resulting in 119 adjustments to the DIHASID tool. The problems and their adjustments are described below using the eight QAS-99 categories, see Table 3.

In the Clarity category ($n = 64$), problems related to the wording of the questions, technical terms, such as health professionals and epilepsy, and vague questions. Regarding Response categories ($n = 38$), problems related to technical terms and vague, overlapping, and missing answer options. For example, the differences between the five smileys were vague according to the participants. Problems with Instructions ($n = 23$) included lack of clarity on what to consider when answering the questions, information missing on how many answers could be chosen, and surplus information. A few problems related to Knowledge or Memory ($n = 10$), including difficulty in knowing the boundaries and facilities of—and distances from—facilities within the neighborhood and care professionals' knowledge on organizational policy and budgets. For Sensitivity or Bias ($n = 7$), problems related to questions on the nature of a person's disabilities and use of the word 'client'. Only one problem related to the Assumptions category: it was perceived as difficult to choose one smiley for how a person perceives help from all health professionals. Other problems ($n = 9$) related to the size and unclear meaning of pictures.

Table 3. Problems identified in cognitive interviews and changes to improve the clarity of the DIHASID tool.

QAS-99 Category	Description of Problems	Changes to the DIHASID Tool
1. Reading Difficulty reading the question (what and how to read)	n.a.	n.a.
2. Instructions Problems with instructions or explanations (conflicting, inaccurate, or complicated)	-unclear for participants what to consider when answering the questions -unclear instruction on the number of answers that can be chosen -unclear what to write or where to write an answer -difficult explanations: pictograms with words under them would help them understand the question better -some information was perceived as surplus -including that a support person is allowed to help was perceived as helpful for getting answers to the open questions	-shorten the questionnaire instruction -specify the instruction -explain how many answers may be chosen -specify that help from a support person is allowed -explain where to fill in the answer -include pictures and words beneath them
3. Clarity Problems related to communicating the intent of the question (wording, technical terms, vague, reference points)	-participants had difficulty understanding the sentence for some questions -technical terms, such as health professionals, aids, patient lift, masseur, epilepsy, spasm, residential and daytime support center -vague questions, for example what a neighborhood is	-change word order in sentences -give explanation or examples for unclear words -replace technical terms with easy words
4. Assumptions Problems with assumptions made or underlying logic (inappropriate, assumes constant behavior, double-barreled)	-it was perceived as difficult to choose one smiley for how a person perceives help from all health professionals	n.a.
5. Knowledge/Memory Whether respondents are likely to know or remember information (knowledge, attitude, recall failure, computation problems)	-difficulty in knowing the boundaries and facilities of, and distances from, facilities within the neighborhood -for care professionals: to know about the policy and financial budget of their organization	-make the distance from facilities broader (within 15-min walking distance, within 15-min biking distance, you need a car/cab/bus to get there) -insert "I don't know" options for questions for care professionals about budget and policy
6. Sensitivity/Bias Sensitive nature, wording, or bias of questions (sensitive content or wording and social acceptability)	-the nature of a person's disabilities -use of the word client	-include the response option "I don't want to say" for the question about disabilities -change client into resident or participant at daytime activities
7. Response categories Adequacy of range of responses (difficulty of open-ended questions, mismatch, technical terms, vague, overlapping, missing, illogical order)	-unclear technical terms: fitness center, hydrotherapy bath -vague answer options: smiley response categories because differences between the five smileys were unclear for participants -overlapping answer options: kitchen and adjusted kitchen -missing answer options: vegetable garden for the question about aids for healthy nutrition	-replace technical terms with easier words -change words or add examples for vague answer options -remove answer options (use of three instead of five smileys) -remove overlapping answer options -add open answer options for incomplete response categories
8. Other problems	-size of pictures -unclear meaning of pictures	-size of all pictures was increased -unclear pictures were changed into pictures that were perceived to be clearer

The identified problems and suggestions were used to improve the clarity of the DIHASID tool by shortening and specifying instructions, explaining how many answer options to choose and where to fill in the answer, including or changing pictograms, changing word order, replacing technical terms with easy words, explaining unclear words, removing/inserting answer options, and changing sensitive words.

3.4. Usable DIHASID Tool

The analysis of the DIHASID tool pilot provided information on (1) how the task was performed and experienced, (2) final points for improvements on usability, and (3) what the DIHASID tool can yield in practice.

It took the 16 participants on average 34 min (38 for participants with ID, 35 for proxy respondents, and 30 for care professionals) to complete the task, and only a few answers were missing. Seven participants, of which six people with ID, chose to fill the DIHASID tool out on paper, and nine used the online questionnaire; both were perceived as clear and easy to navigate. Most participants perceived the explanation and clarity of the task ($n = 13$ out of 16), the ease of the task ($n = 12$ out of 16), and the length of the task ($n = 13$ out of 16) as good. All participants viewed themselves as the right person to answers the questions, except those on financial aspects and health-promoting organizational policies, which care professionals perceived as difficult because they were not familiar with these issues. Regarding financial and policy aspects, participants identified a team leader as the right person to be involved in filling out the DIHASID tool. Participants with ID perceived the help from a care professional as pleasant, needed, and not influencing their answers.

Final points for improving the DIHASID tool included: (1) page numbering, larger answer fields, and larger fonts for the paper version, (2) allowing participants to choose more than one answer option for multiple choice questions, (3) instructing proxies that they can tick 'not applicable' for questions that are irrelevant for the person they represent, e.g., a question about talking when the person they represent cannot speak, and (4) final changes to questions and explanations to improve clarity, for example changing the description of clients 'resident or participant at daytime activities' back to 'client'.

In the group discussions, participants reflected that the DIHASID tool can help to (1) raise awareness and put healthy living in the spotlight, (2) create an overview on what is available to support healthy living, and (3) use the overview to create changes in the organization. Participants identified a summary of the outcomes as needed for generating actionable knowledge. For example, teams of care professionals can discuss this summary and devise action steps together. Participants identified the following stakeholders with whom to share this summary: clients, clients' families, care professionals, team leaders, personal support coordinators, policymakers, and quality assurance officers of the organization.

3.5. Final Version of the DIHASID Tool

The final DIHASID tool (see Supplementary Materials) consists of 37 questions divided into four parts: (1) participant and setting characteristics, (2) how people support healthy living including their social network, types of support, and values regarding healthy living, (3) how places support healthy living including tools, facilities, accessibility, and person–environment fit, and (4) the preconditions for healthy living that are available, including financial aspects and health-promoting organizational policies. Regarding the type of questions, part one includes multiple choice questions. Parts two, three, and four include the following type of questions: (1) tick boxes on presence of assets, (2) multiple choice questions (3-point smiley scale, but 5-point Likert scale for questions that are aimed only at care professionals and proxies) on how respondents experience a theme, and (3) an open question on wishes and dreams regarding the theme. The tool can be completed by people in a living or day-activity location, e.g., people with mild to moderate ID, proxy respondents for people with severe/profound ID, care professionals, and team leaders.

4. Discussion

This study aimed to develop an inclusive and functional tool for mapping assets for physical activity and healthy nutrition in ID support settings. An iterative process of applying feedback from expert interviews, cognitive interviews, and pilot testing was used to develop a comprehensive, clear, usable tool. The tool, named DIscovering Health-promoting Assets in Settings for people with Intellectual Disabilities (DIHASID), can be completed in approximately 30 min by people with mild to moderate ID who are assisted by a support person, proxy respondents for people with severe/profound ID, care professionals, and team leaders.

The DIHASID tool is an inclusive tool for people with ID and care professionals that can be used to facilitate bottom–up engagement to improve the health-promoting capacities of ID support settings. This approach is empowering and aligns with the 'Nothing about us, without us' movement that advocates for the involvement of people with ID in matters that affect them [47]. Furthermore, this bottom–up approach can create awareness among policymakers of what supports people with ID and their care professionals in facilitating healthy lifestyles. The DIHASID tool helps to implement inclusive and healthy environments and thereby facilitates policymakers in the trend toward a greater focus on environmental impacts on health. For example, the Dutch Environment Act and Green Deal provide good opportunities to include attention on health promotion in spatial planning and sustainable innovations, including a healthy living environment in the care sector [48,49].

Participants perceived the DIHASID tool as helpful for providing an overview of user-experienced assets and wishes regarding a healthy living environment for physical activity and healthy nutrition of people with ID, thereby aligning with the goals of asset mapping [24]. From an asset-based community development perspective, the next steps for building healthy ID support settings include (1) finding connectors and engaging them in (re)building relationships between people to link assets and create a health-promoting infrastructure, (2) creating a joint vision and action plan, and (3) embedding this plan and vision in the settings' organizational structure [50,51]. These steps are important but also challenging to implement in ID support settings because currently there is a lack of clarity among stakeholders on roles and responsibilities regarding health promotion. Care professionals who are involved in everyday support are often not trained on this topic. Allied health professionals often focus mostly on curative care rather than prevention and may not know how to facilitate care professionals [19,52]. Furthermore, it might be challenging to involve people with ID in developing a joint vision and action plan. Future studies could design and pilot how this bottom–up process can be tailored to their needs.

A major strength of this study is the co-design of the DIHASID tool by the inclusive research team together with experts in practice, experts in research, and experts by experience. This ensured that tailored methods were used to enable people with ID to meaningfully engage as participants and led to a better match between research and practice. In addition, the insights of the researchers with ID helped in interpreting user perspectives and in deciding on appropriate changes to improve the usability of the tool.

The number of interviews to improve the comprehensibility, clarity, and usability of the tool was limited. However, an iterative process was used, and after the pilot, hardly any changes were required. Although the DIHASID tool gives prompts about a wide range of assets in the physical, social, and organizational environment, the results depend on the participants' familiarity with local assets. Therefore, it is preferable that multiple persons in a setting fill out the DIHASID tool to gain an overview that is as complete as possible. Lastly, some caution should be exercised about implementing this tool in other countries. The type of questioning and general themes are expected to be relevant in other countries, as the tool was built on the basis of an existing international concept mapping study [39]. However, the clarity of the questions was tested in Dutch, and the tool's comprehensibility and usability were tested in the support organization in the Netherlands. Therefore, we advise anyone who wants to apply the DIHASID tool in another country to conduct a pilot to see whether adaptations are needed for that context.

Future studies could use the DIHASID tool to (1) provide insight into how people with ID are currently supported by ID support organizations to live healthily, (2) enhance intervention effectiveness in specific settings by identifying assets that can support the intervention in that particular setting and/or interweave the intervention in the setting [53], and (3) gain insight into contextual factors that might influence the outcomes and successes of health promotion interventions applied in that particular setting [54].

5. Conclusions

The DIHASID tool is a comprehensive, clear, and usable tool to map health-promoting assets in ID support settings. Using the tool provides insight into perceived environmental assets and into points for improvements regarding support for healthy nutrition and physical activity of people with moderate to profound ID in settings where they engage. The bottom–up development of this tool for co-learning ensures that the DIHASID tool asks about assets that may be relevant for users of ID support settings. The tool empowers people with ID and care professionals to pinpoint assets that they find helpful and to identify future directions for creating healthy environments for physical activity and healthy nutrition. The tool can be used together with stakeholders who are responsible for health promotion and organizational policy, and the overview of assets can be used to mobilize and build on assets to inclusively improve the health-promoting capacity of ID support settings.

Supplementary Materials: The following are available online at http://www.mdpi.com/1660-4601/17/3/794/s1, The Appendix includes the English version of the DIHASID tool. The tool was professionally translated from Dutch to English.

Author Contributions: Conceptualization and methodology, K.V.v.A., T.H., J.N., A.v.d.C., and H.J.; investigation, K.V.v.A.; analysis, K.V.v.A., A.v.d.C., and H.J.; writing—original draft preparation, K.V.v.A.; writing—review and editing, K.V.v.A., T.H., G.L., J.N., K.v.d.V., A.v.d.C., and H.J. All authors approved the submitted version. All authors have read and agreed to the published version of the manuscript.

Funding: ZonMw (Nationaal Programma Gehandicapten, grant number: 80-84500-98-118) and the Academic collaborative Stronger on Your Own Feet.

Acknowledgments: The authors would like to acknowledge ZonMw and the Academic collaborative Stronger on Your Own Feet for funding this study. Furthermore, they are very grateful for the contribution of the study participants.

Conflicts of Interest: The authors declare no conflict of interest.

Ethics Approval: The study is conducted according to the principles of the Declaration of Helsinki (October 2013, 64th WMA General Assembly) and in accordance with the EU General Data Protection Regulation. Written informed consent was obtained from all participants prior to data collection. The accredited Medical Research Ethics Committee of the Radboud University and Medical Center approved the study (registration number: 2018-4408).

References

1. Havercamp, S.M.; Scandlin, D.; Roth, M. Health disparities among adults with developmental disabilities, adults with other disabilities, and adults not reporting disability in North Carolina. *Public Health Rep.* **2004**, *119*, 418. [CrossRef] [PubMed]
2. Emerson, E. Underweight, obesity and exercise among adults with intellectual disabilities in supported accommodation in Northern England. *J. Intellect. Disabil. Res.* **2005**, *49*, 134–143. [CrossRef] [PubMed]
3. Humphries, K.; Traci, M.A.; Seekins, T. Nutrition and Adults with Intellectual or Developmental Disabilities: Systematic Literature Review Results. *Intellect. Dev. Disabil.* **2009**, *47*, 163–185. [CrossRef] [PubMed]
4. Hilgenkamp, T.I.; Reis, D.; van Wijck, R.; Evenhuis, H.M. Physical activity levels in older adults with intellectual disabilities are extremely low. *Res. Dev. Disabil.* **2012**, *33*, 477–483. [CrossRef]
5. Schrojenstein Lantman-de Valk, H.M.J. Health in People with Intellectual Disabilities: Current Knowledge and Gaps in Knowledge. *J. Appl. Res. Intellect. Disabil.* **2005**, *18*, 325–333. [CrossRef]
6. Kuijken, N.; Naaldenberg, J.; Nijhuis-van der Sanden, M.; Schrojenstein-Lantman de Valk, H. Healthy living according to adults with intellectual disabilities: Towards tailoring health promotion initiatives. *J. Intellect. Disabil. Res.* **2016**, *60*, 228–241. [CrossRef]

7. Humpel, N.; Owen, N.; Leslie, E. Environmental factors associated with adults' participation in physical activity: A review. *Am. J. Prev. Med.* **2002**, *22*, 188–199. [CrossRef]
8. Botchwey, N.D.; Falkenstein, R.; Levin, J.; Fisher, T.; Trowbridge, M. The Built Environment and Actual Causes of Death Promoting an Ecological Approach to Planning and Public Health. *J. Plan. Lit.* **2015**, *30*, 261–281. [CrossRef]
9. Popkin, B.M.; Duffey, K.; Gordon-Larsen, P. Environmental influences on food choice, physical activity and energy balance. *Physiol. Behav.* **2005**, *86*, 603–613. [CrossRef]
10. Sallis, J.F.; Floyd, M.F.; Rodríguez, D.A.; Saelens, B.E. Role of built environments in physical activity, obesity, and cardiovascular disease. *Circulation* **2012**, *125*, 729–737. [CrossRef]
11. Schalock, R.L.; Borthwick-Duffy, S.A.; Bradley, V.J.; Buntinx, W.H.E.; Coulter, D.L.; Craig, E.M.; Gomez, S.C.; Lachapelle, Y.; Luckasson, R.; Reeve, A.; et al. *Intellectual Disability: Definition, Classification, and Systems of Supports*, 11th ed.; American Association on Intellectual and Developmental Disabilities: Washington, DC, USA, 2010; ISBN -978-1-9353-0404-3.
12. Zorginstituut Nederland. *Screeningsrapport Gehandicaptenzorg Zinnige Zorg*; Zorginstituut Nederland: Diemen, The Netherlands, 2019.
13. Van Staalduinen, W.; ten Voorde, F. *Trendanalyse Verstandelijk Gehandicaptenzorg*; TNO: Amsterdam, The Netherlands, 2011.
14. Heutmekers, M.; Naaldenberg, J.; Frankena, T.K.; Smits, M.; Leusink, G.L.; Assendelft, W.J.; van Schrojenstein Lantman-de, H.M. After-hours primary care for people with intellectual disabilities in The Netherlands—current arrangements and challenges. *Res. Dev. Disabil.* **2016**, *59*, 1–7. [CrossRef] [PubMed]
15. Naaldenberg, J.; Kuijken, N.; van Dooren, K.; van Schrojenstein Lantman de Valk, H. Topics, methods and challenges in health promotion for people with intellectual disabilities: A structured review of literature. *Res. Dev. Disabil.* **2013**, *34*, 4534–4545. [CrossRef] [PubMed]
16. Bartlo, P.; Klein, P.J. Physical activity benefits and needs in adults with intellectual disabilities: Systematic review of the literature. *Am. J. Intellect. Dev. Disabil.* **2011**, *116*, 220–232. [CrossRef]
17. Steenbergen, H.A.; Van der Schans, C.P.; Van Wijck, R.; De Jong, J.; Waninge, A. Lifestyle Approaches for People with Intellectual Disabilities: A Systematic Multiple Case Analysis. *J. Am. Med. Direct. Assoc.* **2017**, *18*, 980–987. [CrossRef]
18. Kuijken, N.M.J.; Naaldenberg, J.; Vlot-van Anrooij, K.; Nijhuis-van der Sanden, M.W.; Van Schrojenstein Lantman-de Valk, H.M.J.; Leusink, G.L. Integrating health promotion in everyday life of people with ID—Extent to which current initiatives take context into account. *Intellect. Dev. Disabil.*. (accepted).
19. Kuijken, N.M.J.; Vlot-van Anrooij, K.; van Schrojenstein Lantman-de Valk, H.M.J.; Leusink, G.; Naaldenberg, J.; Nijhuis-van der Sanden, M.W. Stakeholder expectations, roles and responsibilities in Dutch health promotion for people with intellectual disabilities. *Health Promot. Int.* **2018**. [CrossRef]
20. Whitelaw, S.; Baxendale, A.; Bryce, C.; MacHardy, L.; Young, I.; Witney, E. 'Settings' based health promotion: A review. *Health Promot. Int.* **2001**, *16*, 339–353. [CrossRef]
21. Dooris, M. Expert voices for change: Bridging the silos—Towards healthy and sustainable settings for the 21st century. *Health Place* **2013**, *20*, 39–50. [CrossRef]
22. Mŭkoma, W.; Flisher, A.J. Evaluations of health promoting schools: A review of nine studies. *Health Promot. Int.* **2004**, *19*, 357–368.
23. World Health Organization. The International Network of Health Promoting Hospitals and Health Services: Integrating Health Promotion into Hospitals and Health Services: Concept, Framework and Organization. Available online: https://apps.who.int/iris/handle/10665/107859 (accessed on 13 December 2019).
24. Morgan, A.; Ziglio, E. Revitalising the evidence base for public health: An assets model. *Promot. Edu.* **2007**, *14*, 17–22. [CrossRef]
25. Alvarez-Dardet, C.; Morgan, A.; Cantero, M.T.R.; Hernán, M. Improving the evidence base on public health assets—The way ahead: A proposed research agenda. *J. Epidemiol. Community Health* **2015**, *69*, 721–723. [CrossRef] [PubMed]
26. Saelens, B.E.; Glanz, K.; Sallis, J.F.; Frank, L.D. Nutrition Environment Measures Study in Restaurants (NEMS-R): Development and Evaluation. *Am. J. Prev. Med.* **2007**, *32*, 273–281. [CrossRef]
27. Wong, F.; Stevens, D.; Connor-Duffany, K.; Siegel, K.; Gao, Y. Community Health Environment Scan Survey (CHESS): A novel tool that captures the impact of the built environment on lifestyle factors. *Glob. Health Act.* **2011**, *4*. [CrossRef] [PubMed]

28. Oldenburg, B.; Sallis, J.F.; Harris, D.; Owen, N. Checklist of Health Promotion Environments at Worksites (CHEW): Development and measurement characteristics. *Am. J. Health Promot.* **2002**, *16*, 288–299. [CrossRef] [PubMed]
29. Nederlands Instituut voor Sport en Bewegen. De Beweegvriendelijke Omgeving Scan (BVO Scan) Hoe Beweegvriendelijk is uw Buurt of Wijk? Available online: https://www.kenniscentrumsport.nl/publicatie/?de-beweegvriendelijke-omgeving-scan-bvo-scan&kb_id=16655 (accessed on 13 December 2019).
30. Gezond in. De Leefplekmeter. Wat Vind je van je leefplek? Available online: https://www.kenniscentrumsport.nl/publicatie/?de-leefplekmeter&kb_id=23868 (accessed on 13 December 2019).
31. Rijksinstituut voor Veiligheid en Milieu. Gezonde Omgeving Utrecht (Go! Utrecht). Handelingsperspectieven voor een Gezonde Leefomgeving. Available online: https://www.rivm.nl/publicaties/gezonde-omgeving-utrecht-go-utrecht-handelingsperspectieven-voor-gezonde-leefomgeving (accessed on 13 December 2019).
32. National Center for Chronic Disease Prevention and Health Promotion. Built Environment Assessment Tool. Available online: https://www.cdc.gov/nccdphp/dnpao/state-local-programs/built-environment-assessment/index.htm (accessed on 13 December 2019).
33. Green, S.H.; Glanz, K. Development of the perceived nutrition environment measures survey. *Am. J. Prev. Med.* **2015**, *49*, 50–61. [CrossRef]
34. Chow, C.K.; Lock, K.; Madhavan, M.; Corsi, D.J.; Gilmore, A.B.; Subramanian, S.V.; Li, W.; Swaminathan, S.; Lopez-Jaramillo, P.; Avezum, A.; et al. Environmental Profile of a Community's Health (EPOCH): An Instrument to Measure Environmental Determinants of Cardiovascular Health in Five Countries. *PLoS ONE* **2010**, *5*, e14294. [CrossRef]
35. DeJoy, D.M.; Wilson, M.G.; Goetzel, R.Z.; Ozminkowski, R.J.; Wang, S.; Baker, K.M.; Bowen, H.M.; Tully, K.J. Development of the Environmental Assessment Tool (EAT) to measure organizational physical and social support for worksite obesity prevention programs. *J. Occup. Environ. Med.* **2008**, *50*, 126–137. [CrossRef]
36. Shimotsu, S.T.; French, S.A.; Gerlach, A.F.; Hannan, P.J. Worksite environment physical activity and healthy food choices: Measurement of the worksite food and physical activity environment at four metropolitan bus garages. *Int. J. Behav. Nutr. Phys. Act.* **2007**, *4*, 17. [CrossRef]
37. Springer, A.E.; Evans, A.E. Assessing environmental assets for health promotion program planning: A practical framework for health promotion practitioners. *Health Promot. Perspect.* **2016**, *6*, 111–118. [CrossRef]
38. Van Bortel, T.; Wickramasinghe, N.D.; Morgan, A.; Martin, S. Health assets in a global context: A systematic review of the literature. *BMJ Open* **2019**, *9*. [CrossRef]
39. Vlot-van Anrooij, K.; Naaldenberg, J.; Hilgenkamp, T.I.M.; Vaandrager, L.; van der Velden, K.; Leusink, G.L. Towards healthy settings for people with intellectual disabilities. *Health Promot. Int.* **2019**. [CrossRef]
40. Vlot-van Anrooij, K. Perspectives of people with intellectual disabilities on people, places, and preconditions supporting healthy living. (Submitted).
41. Willis, G.B. *Cognitive Interviewing: A Tool for Improving Questionnaire Design*; Sage Publications: Thousand Oaks, CA, USA, 2004; ISBN 9780761928041.
42. Bakker-van Gijssel, E.J.; Lucassen, P.L.; olde Hartman, T.C.; Assendelft, W.J.; van Schrojenstein Lantman-de, H.M. Constructing a health assessment questionnaire for people with intellectual disabilities: A cognitive interview study. *J. Appl. Res. Intellect. Disabil.* **2019**. [CrossRef]
43. Lewis, J.R. IBM computer usability satisfaction questionnaires: Psychometric evaluation and instructions for use. *Int. J. Hum. Comput. Interact.* **1995**, *7*, 57–78. [CrossRef]
44. Zhang, J.; Walji, M.F. TURF: Toward a unified framework of EHR usability. *J. Biomed. Informatics* **2011**, *44*, 1056–1067. [CrossRef]
45. Johnson, K.; Minogue, G.; Hopklins, R. Inclusive research: Making a difference to policy and legislation. *J. Appl. Res. Intellect. Disabil.* **2014**, *27*, 76–84. [CrossRef]
46. Frankena, T.; Naaldenberg, J.; Cardol, M.; Garcia Iriarte, E.; Buchner, T.; Brooker, K.; Embregts, P.; Joosa, E.; Crowther, F.; Fudge Schormans, A.; et al. A consensus statement on how to conduct inclusive health research. *J. Intell. Disabil. Res.* **2018**, *63*, 1–11. [CrossRef]
47. United Nations. International Day of Disabled Persons, 2004—Nothing about Us, Without Us. Available online: https://www.un.org/development/desa/disabilities/international-day-of-persons-with-disabilities-3-december/international-day-of-disabled-persons-2004-nothing-about-us-without-us.html (accessed on 10 April 2019).

48. Gezondheidsraad. Meewegen van Gezondheid in Omgevingsbeleid. Evenwichtig en Rechtvaardig Omgaan Met Risico's en Kansen. Available online: http://www.omgevingsweb.nl/cms/files/2016-08/201612-meewegen-van-gezondheid-in-omgevingsbeleid.pdf (accessed on 13 December 2019).
49. Milieuplatform zorg. Concept Grean Deal Duurzame Zorg 2.0 Routekaart Cure. Available online: https://milieuplatformzorg.nl/green-deal/ (accessed on 12 November 2019).
50. McKnight, J.; Kretzmann, J. *Building Communities from the Inside out: A Path toward Finding and Mobilizing a Community's Assets*; ACTA Publications: Chicago, IL, USA, 1993; ISBN 087946108X.
51. Rasberry, C.N.; Slade, S.; Lohrmann, D.K.; Valois, R.F. Lessons Learned from the Whole Child and Coordinated School Health Approaches. *J. School Health* **2015**, *85*, 759–765. [CrossRef]
52. O'Leary, L.; Taggart, L.; Cousins, W. Healthy lifestyle behaviours for people with intellectual disabilities: An exploration of organizational barriers and enablers. *J. Appl. Res. Intellect. Disabil.* **2018**, *31*, 122–135. [CrossRef]
53. Springer, A.E.; Evans, A.E.; Ortuño, J.; Salvo, D.; Varela Arevalo, M.T. Health by design: Interweaving health promotion into environments and settings. *Front. Public Health* **2017**, *5*, 268. [CrossRef]
54. Pfadenhauer, L.M.; Gerhardus, A.; Mozygemba, K.; Lysdahl, K.B.; Booth, A.; Hofmann, B.; Wahlster, P.; Polus, S.; Burns, J.; Brereton, L.; et al. Making sense of complexity in context and implementation: The Context and Implementation of Complex Interventions (CICI) framework. *Implement. Sci.* **2017**, *12*, 21. [CrossRef] [PubMed]

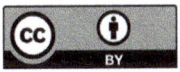

© 2020 by the authors. Licensee MDPI, Basel, Switzerland. This article is an open access article distributed under the terms and conditions of the Creative Commons Attribution (CC BY) license (http://creativecommons.org/licenses/by/4.0/).

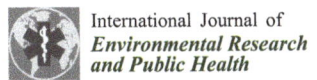

Article

Attitudes of Mainstream and Special-Education Teachers toward Intellectual Disability in Italy: The Relevance of Being Teachers

Laura Arcangeli, Alice Bacherini, Cristina Gaggioli, Moira Sannipoli and Giulia Balboni *

Department of Philosophy, Social and Human Sciences, and Education, Università degli Studi di Perugia, Piazza G. Ermini, 1, 06123 Perugia, Italy; laura.arcangeli@unipg.it (L.A.); alice.bacherini@studenti.unipg.it (A.B.); cristina.gaggioli@gmail.com (C.G.); moira.sannipoli@unipg.it (M.S.)
* Correspondence: giulia.balboni@unipg.it

Received: 29 August 2020; Accepted: 5 October 2020; Published: 7 October 2020

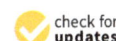

Abstract: The attitudes of teachers toward intellectual disability (ID) contribute to an effective school inclusion of students with ID, thereby enhancing their quality of life. The present study was aimed at investigating the attitude differences toward ID of mainstream and special-education teachers in Italy and the general and specific teachers' characteristics most related to these attitudes. An online version of the Attitudes toward Intellectual Disability (ATTID) questionnaire was filled by 307 mainstream teachers and 237 special-education teachers. The findings show that special-education teachers held more positive attitudes. Specific ATTID dimensions were positively affected for both types of teachers by previous training in special education/ID, perceived support, and promotion of positive attitudes toward ID, in addition to the quality of relationships with individuals with ID, while they were positively affected for special-education teachers by perceived efficacy of ID knowledge. No or very limited effects were observed for previous experience in teaching students with typical development or ID (even with severe/profound ID). Fostering resources to provide teachers with high-quality training, support, and resources and strategies to promote positive attitudes toward ID seems a relevant approach leading to favorable attitudes, thereby improving the quality of life of students with ID.

Keywords: attitudes toward ID; intellectual disability; mainstream teachers; special-education teachers; ATTID; training; support

1. Introduction

Intellectual disability (ID) is a disorder characterized by significant limitations in both intellectual functioning and adaptive behavior, as expressed in conceptual, social, and practical skills, with onset before 18 years of age or during the developmental period [1–3]. Interventions for individuals with ID should be implemented to enhance their quality of life. Based on Schalock and Verdugo's [4] model, quality of life is a multidimensional construct made up of eight core domains: personal development, self-determination, interpersonal relationships, social inclusion, rights, emotional well-being, physical well-being, and material well-being. Inclusive environments are environments that provide access to resources, information, and relationships and encourage growth and development, in addition to supporting people, accommodating psychological needs related to autonomy, competence, and relatedness [5]. These factors may improve all the dimensions of quality of life of individuals with ID.

Educational inclusion is an example of an inclusive environment. Educational inclusion implies not only the complete integration of children with ID or other special needs into programs and activities with peers [6], but also the planning of individualized projects for all students in order to promote the best opportunities for the personal growth of everyone [7–9]. Inclusion is an unending process of increasing learning, participation, and quality of life for all students, with or without ID or other special educational needs [10–12]. Social participation and school inclusion are rights for students with ID, as stated by several international documents, such as the World Declaration on Education for All [13], the Salamanca Statement [14], the No Child Left Behind American Law [15], or the Convention on the Rights of Persons with Disabilities [16]. They represent essential components for a life of quality and equality [17]. In Italy, since the end of the 1970s, Law 517 [18], Law 104 [19], and Law 96 [20] have established that students with ID, as all other students, have the right to attend mainstream education classes, supported by a special-education teacher for a number of hours per week [8,21].

An environmental factor that plays a central role in the effective social inclusion of students with ID is represented by the attitudes of teachers toward ID. Attitude is a personal evaluation toward people, objects, or events which generates either positive or negative judgments, consequently predisposing individual behavior [22]. The most used models of attitudes toward ID are based on the three-factor model of attitudes [23], which defines an attitude as a multidimensional construct represented by three dimensions: (a) cognitive (beliefs or knowledge of ID), (b) emotional (feelings created by ID), and (c) behavioral (predisposition to act toward individuals with ID).

Some studies found that teachers show more negative attitudes toward students with ID than toward those with other kinds of disabilities (e.g., physical or sensory), because students with ID need a greater level of support and adaptation for classroom activities [24–26]. Hence, studying the attitudes toward ID of teachers, as well as factors related to those attitudes, seems to be relevant; nevertheless, very few investigations were conducted on this topic [27–30]. In more detail, these studies investigated, in different countries and cultural contexts (i.e., Egypt, Turkey, Canada, and Scotland), the attitudes toward ID of elementary-school mainstream teachers or of middle-school physical education teachers. Moreover, factors related to teachers' attitudes toward ID, particularly those concerning specific teacher characteristics, were investigated (e.g., self-efficacy, training in special education or ID, years of teaching experience). A higher level of teacher self-efficacy was found to be associated with more positive attitudes toward individuals with ID [30]. Furthermore, training in ID was found to be associated with more positive attitudes [28], especially concerning knowledge of the capacity and rights of individuals with ID, as well as the willingness to interact with persons with ID [29]. However, no relationship was found between having attended special-education classes and the attitudes toward ID of teachers [30]. Similarly, Sermier Dessemontet et al. [29], but not Ozer et al. [28], revealed an association between previous experience teaching pupils with ID and higher levels of willingness to interact with persons with ID, along with less discomfort. Moreover, Ozer et al. [28] found that teachers with fewer years of teaching experience showed more positive attitudes, while Wilson et al. [30] found the opposite result.

With respect to general characteristics contributing to teachers' attitudes toward ID, it was found that prior contact with persons with ID [27], particularly, the quality rather than the quantity of prior contacts [29], is related to the attitudes of teachers. Indeed, Sermier Dessemontet et al. [29] found no associations between the frequency of contact and any dimension of the attitudes of teachers toward ID, while a higher quality of contact was found to be related to less discomfort toward individuals with ID and a higher willingness to interact with them. Finally, a younger chronological age of teachers was found to be associated with more positive attitudes toward ID [28].

More studies were realized on the attitudes of teachers toward school inclusion of students with ID or other disabilities. For example, it was found that teachers teaching at a lower school level and those with higher levels of perceived school support showed more positive attitudes toward the inclusion of pupils with ID or other disabilities [31–33]. However, other investigations did not find any association between school level and attitudes toward inclusion [34,35].

Given the Italian history with regard to the inclusion of individuals with ID and, therefore, the experience and contact of teachers with students with ID in Italy, it would be interesting to study teachers' attitudes toward ID in Italy, as well as any factors related to those attitudes. To date, in Italy, studies were only realized highlighting teachers' attitudes toward the inclusion of students with ID in mainstream classes [32,36]. It was found that special-education teachers have a better attitude than mainstream teachers, while mainstream teachers with experience in teaching pupils with ID had a better attitude and were not negatively affected by age and years of service. Moreover, mainstream high-school teachers and teachers older than 40 asked for more training [32].

The present study aimed to investigate the attitudes toward ID of mainstream teachers and special-education teachers in Italy, as well as the characteristics related to these attitudes. Firstly, we investigated the quality of the attitudes of mainstream and special-education teachers toward ID (positive, neutral, or negative) and if there were any differences between the attitudes of these two groups of teachers. Secondly, separately for mainstream teachers and special-education teachers, we investigated the relationships of attitudes toward ID with (a) the teacher's personal characteristics (general characteristics, i.e., age, prior quantity, closeness, and quality of contact with individuals with ID) and (b) characteristics specific to being teachers (teacher-specific characteristics, i.e., school level taught, previous training in special education or ID, years of teaching experience, years of experience teaching pupils with ID, experience teaching pupils with severe/profound ID, perceived efficacy of ID knowledge, perceived support, and promotion of positive attitudes toward ID). Toward this aim, separately for mainstream and special-education teachers, we first investigated the relationship between each dimension of attitude toward ID (cognitive, emotional, and behavioral) and each individual's general and teacher-specific characteristic; then, we investigated the degree to which an individual's teacher-specific characteristics affected each dimension of attitude toward ID, in addition to the individual's general characteristics. In this way, it was possible to identify the factors positively related to teachers' attitudes toward ID, which need to be taken into account when planning interventions to create an inclusive environment for students with ID.

2. Materials and Methods

This study was conducted following the ethical standards laid down in the 2013 Fortaleza version of the Declaration of Helsinki, it was a voluntary survey for adults that were not in a vulnerable condition, written informed consent was obtained from each participant, and their anonymity was guaranteed. The participants did not receive any form of incentive to participate in this study. Given that, being not a clinical study and being the participants not in a vulnerable condition, the present study is not subject to the prior ethical approval of the Ethical Committee in accordance with the Regulation of the European Parliament n. 536/2014.

2.1. Instruments

2.1.1. Attitudes toward Intellectual Disability

The Attitudes Toward Intellectual Disability Questionnaire (ATTID) [37] was used to measure attitudes toward ID. It is composed of 67 items structured in 5 dimensions that map the three-factor model of attitudes [22,23]: (a) two dimensions related to a cognitive factor measured by the knowledge of capacity and rights (20 items) and the knowledge of causes of ID (seven items); (b) two dimensions related to an affective factor measured by discomfort (17 items) and sensitivity/tenderness (6 items); (c) a dimension related to a behavioral factor measured by interaction (17 items). The discomfort dimension assesses the feelings of stress, fear, embarrassment, anxiety, or inadequacy toward persons with ID. The knowledge of capacity and rights dimension measures myths and beliefs related to ID and the rights of individuals with ID, such as the right to attend school, to work, to have a romantic partner, to be integrated into the community. It also concerns these individuals' ability and potential. The interaction dimension investigates willingness to interact with people with ID. The sensitivity/tenderness dimension evaluates the presence of feelings of pity, sadness or compassion toward persons with ID. Finally, the knowledge of causes dimension measures the knowledge of the etiology of ID. Respondents were asked to express their level of agreement/disagreement with each statement, according to a 5-point Likert scale ranging from 1 = totally agree to 5 = totally disagree. Higher scores indicate more negative attitudes toward individuals with ID.

We developed an Italian translation and adaptation of the ATTID (available upon request) in agreement with the International Test Commission Guidelines for Translating and Adapting Tests [38]. In the interaction dimension, one item was split into two items, and two more items were added in order to better evaluate the Italian school-level context (see Supplementary Materials, Note S1). As a result, the Italian ATTID consists of 70 items.

Psychometric properties of the Italian ATTID were investigated using the data collected in the present study. The factorial structure was preliminarily studied via Confirmatory Factor Analyses (CFA), using data from 485 of the 544 teachers of the present investigation (59 participants were excluded because they presented multivariate outliers for this analysis). The robust maximum likelihood estimator (MLR) was used, given that the items' score distributions were far from being multivariate normal (based on Mardia's test) [39]. A first CFA was carried out using the normalized score obtained for the 70 items of the ATTID. The latent variables were the five ATTID dimensions, and the observed variables were the 70 items; each of them loaded only the corresponding latent variable. However, two of the added items of the interaction dimension—those regarding the teachers' opinion about whether individuals with ID should attend regular preschool or middle school—had the same answers as the original items regarding attending primary school. Therefore, the two added items were deleted. Moreover, two items of the sensitivity/tenderness dimension—those regarding if individuals felt empathy or sympathy for an individual with ID that they met on the street—had no correlation with the other items of the dimension and did not load the corresponding dimension. Therefore, these two items were eliminated. A second CFA was run with the 66 remaining items loading the corresponding dimension. We found that all factor loadings of each item on the corresponding dimension were statistically significant and ranged from 0.323 to 0.879 (mean = 0.605; median = 0.602). The ATTID dimensions were correlated, with inter-correlation coefficients ranging from 0.18 to 0.69 for the discomfort, knowledge of capacity and rights, interaction, and sensitivity/tenderness dimensions; the inter-correlation coefficients ranged from -0.08 to 0.18 for the knowledge of causes of ID and the other four dimensions. The goodness-of-fit indexes were acceptable concerning the root-mean-square error of approximation (RMSEA = 0.069) and the standardized root-mean-square residual (SRMR = 0.092), but poor concerning the comparative fit index (CFI = 0.749), and the Tucker–Lewis index (TLI = 0.737) [39,40]. Data collection is in progress to increase the number of participants and make the sample less homogeneous.

Internal consistency was found to be adequate to excellent [41], with Cronbach's alpha coefficients of 0.93 for the discomfort dimension, of 0.91 for both the knowledge of rights and the interaction dimensions, of 0.86 and 0.75 for the sensitivity/tenderness and the knowledge of causes dimensions, respectively, and of 0.94 for the total scale. The construct validity was also investigated by computing the inter-correlation coefficients for the five ATTID dimensions, which produced results very similar to those reported for the original version [37]. The magnitude of the correlation coefficients was evaluated as trivial (<0.10), small (0.10–0.29), medium (0.30–0.49), large (0.50–0.69), or very large (≥0.70) [42]. The correlation coefficients for discomfort, knowledge of capacity and rights, interaction, and sensitivity/tenderness dimensions were small to large, ranging from Pearson's $r = 0.17$ to $r = 0.69$. The correlations coefficients of knowledge of causes of ID with the other four ATTID dimensions were trivial or small, ranging from Pearson's $r = -0.09$ to $r = 0.12$.

2.1.2. Individuals' General Characteristics

Questions were adapted from the ATTID or developed for investigating the following individuals' general characteristics that are generally investigated in studies regarding attitudes toward ID (see Supplementary Materials, Table S1): age (range: 1–5); quantity of contact with individuals with ID, split into (a) the number of known individuals with ID and (b) the frequency of contact with individuals with ID, which were collapsed into a unique variable called the quantity of contact with individuals with ID (range: 1–7; Cronbach's alpha = 0.63); closeness of relationships with individuals with ID (range: 1–4); quality of relationships with individuals with ID (range: 1–3). Higher scores indicated higher levels of the measured characteristic.

2.1.3. Individuals' Teacher-Specific Characteristics

Questions were developed for investigating the following individuals' teacher-specific characteristics (see Supplementary Materials, Table S2): school level taught (range: 1–4); past training in special education or ID, split into (a) type of specialization for special-education activities, based on which we classified the years of training in special education, and (b) hours of courses attended on ID, which we then collapsed into a unique variable called training in special education or ID (range: 1–7; Cronbach's alpha = 0.52); years of teaching experience (range: 1–4); years of experience teaching pupils with ID (range: 1–4); experience teaching pupils with severe or profound ID (score: 0, 1). Higher scores represented higher levels of the measured characteristic.

Moreover, we developed an additional pool of 20 items (see Supplementary Materials, Table S2) to thoroughly investigate aspects related to teachers' perceived efficacy of their own knowledge of ID or in handling pupils with ID, teachers' perceived support received from the school and community context for teaching pupils with ID, and efficacy of strategies applied in the classroom to promote positive attitudes toward ID and inclusion of students with ID by the school. The rating scale of the items was the same 5-point Likert scale as for the ATTID; however, for the analyses of the present study, the scoring system was reversed, such that higher scores represented higher levels of the measured constructs.

A principal component analysis (PCA) with a Promax rotation was carried out using the normalized score obtained for these 20 items, using data from 515 of the 544 teachers of the present investigation (29 participants were excluded because they presented multivariate outliers for this analysis) [43]. The Kaiser–Meyer–Olkin (KMO) test of sampling adequacy was meritorious, corresponding to a score of 0.87 [44], while Bartlett's test of sphericity indicated that the variables were sufficiently related to one other ($\chi^2 = 5079.61$; $p < 0.001$). The number of components to be extracted was identified considering (a) the Kaiser–Guttman criterion, (b) the scree test, and (c) the results of a parallel analysis. Both the Kaiser–Guttman criterion and the parallel analysis suggested five components to be extracted. However, the inspection of the scree plot showed a curve inflection point after the third component, thereby justifying a three-component solution. A PCA with five components showed only two items loading on the fifth component, while a PCA with four components presented an item overlapping two different components. On the contrary, the three-component solution seemed most adequate (accounting for 53.67% of the variance), with at least three items loading on each of the three components, along with no bifactor items and item factor loadings ranging from 0.42 to 0.92. The components were labeled as (a) perceived efficacy of ID knowledge (eight items), (b) perceived support (seven items), and (c) promotion of positive attitudes toward ID (five items). Internal consistency was investigated by computing Cronbach's alpha, resulting in coefficients of 0.94, 0.80, and 0.53, respectively. Given the small number of items for the third component, its Cronbach's alpha coefficient may be considered acceptable [45].

2.1.4. Social Desirability

The Balanced Inventory of Desirable Responding, Short Form (BIDR-6) [46,47] was used to detect attempts at simulation. This measure comprises 16 items with a 6-point Likert scale, ranging from 1 = strongly disagree to 6 = strongly agree, which evaluate the unconscious tendency to provide honest but positively biased responses, as well as the habitual and conscious presentation of a favorable public image. Individuals with a total score exceeding the 95th centile of the normative sample were identified as simulators. An Italian adaptation was used with adequate reliability and validity [46].

2.2. Participants

Participants were 544 Italian teachers (87% females, 11% males, and 2% who did not answer), of which 307 were mainstream teachers (90% females, 9% males, and 1% who did not answer) and 237 were special-education teachers (83% females, 14% males, and 3% who did not answer). Overall, they were recruited from 19 out of 20 Italian regions, representing 73 out of 107 Italian provinces. The schools in which they worked were located in cities with the following numbers of inhabitants (in thousands): <5 (16%), 5–20 (29%), 20–50 (19%), 50–100 (10%), 100–250 (15%), 250–500 (3%), or >500 (8%). The majority of teachers reported that their school had regular contact with local medical services (91%) and that psychologists, pedagogists, or other professionals, such as social workers or speech therapists, were available at their school (77%). Sixty-one percent of the teachers had previously attended classes on issues related to ID (e.g., inclusive education).

Originally, 691 participants were recruited; they were mainstream teachers and special-education teachers, as well as other professionals who worked in the school (e.g., school heads, administrative or technical clerks, janitors, social workers, and aides). However, 43 individuals were excluded because they did not complete the entire questionnaire ($n = 14$), because they were retired teachers ($n = 8$), trainee teachers ($n = 13$), or teachers in a foreign country ($n = 3$), or because they were not working consistently at school ($n = 5$). Then, of the remaining 648 individuals, 49 were excluded as potential simulators because they exceeded the cut-off score for social desirability, as measured by the BIDR-6. As a consequence, 599 participants remained: 307 mainstream teachers, 237 special-education teachers, and 55 other school professionals. Due to its small size, we decided to exclude the latter group, focusing our study only on the 307 mainstream and 237 special-education teachers; their characteristics are reported in Table 1.

Table 1. Characteristics of the mainstream and special-education teachers.

	Mainstream Teachers ($n = 307$)	Special-Education Teachers ($n = 237$)
Age (%)		
18–29	4	4
30–39	14	32
40–49	35	42
50–59	38	17
60+	9	5
Quantity of contact with individuals with ID (Score range: 1–7)		
Mean (SD)	4.01 (1.69)	4.66 (1.58)
Range	1–7	1–7
Closeness of relationships with individuals with ID [1] (%)		
Neighbors, offspring's schoolmates, individuals met in leisure activities or sports	3	1
Individuals met for volunteer or work activities	73	79
Relatives	12	11
Family members	12	9
Quality of relationships with individuals with ID [1] (%)		
Neutral	8	3
Good	70	60
Excellent	22	36
School level taught (%)		
Preschool	12	10
Elementary school	34	28
Middle school	23	30

Table 1. Cont.

	Mainstream Teachers ($n = 307$)	Special-Education Teachers ($n = 237$)
High school	31	32
Training in special education or ID (Score range: 1–7)		
Mean (SD)	2.99 (1.81)	4.56 (1.82)
Range	1–7	1–7
Years of teaching experience (%)		
<5	11	28
5–10	11	27
10–20	38	32
20+	40	13
Years of experience teaching pupils with ID (%)		
<5	36	41
5–10	24	28
10–20	25	22
20+	15	8
Experience teaching pupils with severe/profound ID (%)		
Yes	60	72
No	40	28
Perceived efficacy of ID knowledge (Score range: 8–40)		
Mean (SD)	28.12 (5.64)	31.81 (4.30)
Range	8–40	8–40
Perceived support (Score range: 7–35)		
Mean (SD)	24.15 (4.33)	24.30 (4.58)
Range	8–35	10–35
Promotion of positive attitudes toward ID (Score range: 5–25)		
Mean (SD)	18.70 (2.42)	18.49 (2.43)
Range	11–25	10–25

[1] The number of mainstream teachers and special-education teachers was 293 and 232, respectively, because 14 and 5 of them, respectively, reported not having had any experience with individuals with intellectual disability (ID).

Concerning the study population, based on a description of Italian classroom teachers and academic staff investigated in 2018 by the Eurostat [48], i.e., the statistical office of the European Union, the study population was mostly female (81%), relatively mature (2% aged 18–29; 11% aged 30–39; 28% aged 40–49; 40% aged 50–59; and 19% aged 60 or more), teaching at preschool (12%), elementary school (31%), middle school (22%), or high school (35%). The participants of this study were not selected randomly but based on voluntary responses. However, there was no difference between them and the study population in terms of gender ($\chi^2_{(1)} = 2.06$, $p = 0.15$), age ($\chi^2_{(4)} = 0.01$, $p = 0.99$), and school level taught ($\chi^2_{(3)} = 0.92$, $p = 0.82$).

2.3. Procedure

An online questionnaire, including the items of the ATTID Italian version, the questions we adapted or developed for measuring the individuals' general and teacher-specific characteristics, and the items of the BIDR-6, was arranged with Google Forms. Data collection took place between May 2018 and April 2019. The online questionnaire was disseminated via the most popular Facebook groups and an online magazine of mainstream and special-education teachers (i.e., Orizzonte Scuola).

Moreover, it was spread by teachers who attended the one-year post-lauream master's program in special education provided by the University of Perugia in 2018 and by university professors affiliated with the Italian Association of Special Education (SIPeS).

2.4. Data Analysis

As a prerequisite for all analyses, the score distribution in each ATTID dimension and the metric variables that measured individual characteristics (see Table 1) were checked for mainstream teachers and special-education teachers, considering the following factors: (a) the presence of univariate outliers, i.e., participants with a z-value higher than |3.29|, and multivariate outliers, i.e., participants for which the probability associated with the Mahalanobis distance was lower than 0.001; (b) univariate normality, i.e., skewness and kurtosis between −1.00 and 1.00, and multivariate normality, i.e., Mardia's test being negative.

To investigate the quality of the attitudes of mainstream and special-education teachers toward ID, descriptive statistics were computed for each of the five ATTID dimensions, with scores expressed on a 5-point Likert scale (i.e., raw score relative to the number of the corresponding items). Given that higher scores indicated more negative attitudes toward individuals with ID, as suggested by the ATTID's authors [37], scores of 1 (totally agree) and 2 (agree) were evaluated as positive attitudes, a score of 3 (neither agree nor disagree) indicated neutral attitudes, and scores of 4 (disagree) and 5 (totally disagree) represented negative attitudes.

To study if there were any differences in the five ATTID dimensions between mainstream and special-education teachers, a one-way multivariate analysis of covariance (MANCOVA) was performed. The type of teacher, i.e., mainstream or special-education teacher, was taken as the independent variable, while the five ATTID dimensions were introduced simultaneously as dependent variables. Years of teaching experience was introduced as a covariate variable to properly take into account differences in this variable between mainstream and special-education teachers (see Section 3). In the case of statistically significant differences, Cohen's d effect size was computed and evaluated as negligible (<0.19), small (0.20–0.49), medium (0.50–0.79), or large (≥0.80) [49].

Before running the MANCOVA analysis, we checked for the following: (a) adequacy of the number of participants, verifying that the ratio between the size of the two groups did not exceed 10:1; (b) homogeneity of variance–covariance matrices trough Box's M test; (c) homogeneity of the variance of each dependent variable through the Levene's test; (d) linearity of the relationships of each dependent variable with the covariate variable; (e) homogeneity of the regression slopes [41]. Moreover, we investigated whether the two groups of teachers were paired for gender, performing a χ^2 test, as well as for age and years of teaching experience, performing Mann–Whitney tests. In the case of statistically significant differences, phi and rank-biserial correlation rg effect sizes were computed for χ^2 and Mann–Whitney tests, respectively; they were both evaluated as negligible (<0.10), small (0.10–0.29), medium (0.30–0.49), or large (≥0.50) [49,50].

To study the relationship between each individual's general and teacher-specific characteristics and each ATTID dimension, correlation coefficients were computed for each group of teachers. The type of correlation coefficient depended on the measurement level of the individual's characteristics. We computed Pearson's correlation coefficient for the metric variables (i.e., age, quantity of contact with individuals with ID, training in special education or ID, perceived efficacy of ID knowledge, perceived support, and promotion of positive attitudes toward ID), Spearman's correlation coefficients for the ordinal variables (i.e., closeness and quality of relationships with individuals with ID, school level taught, years of teaching experience, and years of experience teaching pupils with ID), and point-biserial correlation coefficients for the dichotomous variable (experience teaching pupils with severe/profound ID). The magnitude of the correlation coefficients was evaluated as trivial (<0.10), small (0.10–0.29), medium (0.30–0.49), large (0.50–0.69), or very large (≥0.70) [42].

Finally, to study the degree to which the individual's teacher-specific characteristics affected each ATTID dimension, in addition to the individual's general characteristics, we ran one hierarchical multiple regression for each of the five ATTID dimensions within each group of teachers. All general characteristics (i.e., age, quantity of contact, and closeness and quality of relationships with individuals with ID) and teacher-specific characteristics (i.e., school level taught, training in special education or ID, years of teaching experience, years of experience teaching pupils with ID, experience teaching pupils with severe/profound ID, perceived efficacy of ID knowledge, perceived support, and promotion of positive attitudes toward ID) that were found to have a statistically or tendentially significant correlation ($p \leq 0.08$) with the considered ATTID dimension were entered as independent variables. At step 1, we introduced only an individual's general characteristics, while, at step 2, we introduced also the individual's teacher-specific characteristics. The sr^2 incremental, i.e., a modification of R^2, was examined to detect the contribution of an individual's teacher-specific characteristics affecting each ATTID dimension, in adjunct with the individual's general characteristics. A simple linear regression was performed for mainstream teachers between the promotion of positive attitudes toward ID as an independent variable and the knowledge of causes dimension as a dependent variable, because only this factor was significantly related to this ATTID dimension. As an effect size for each significant independent variable, f^2 was computed and evaluated as small (0.02–0.14), medium (0.15–0.34), or large (≥0.35) [49]. Given the high number of comparisons with the same participants, Benjamini and Hochberg's correction for multiple comparisons [51] was applied; however, the appropriate level of significance remained at $p < 0.05$.

Before running the regression analysis, assumptions were ascertained [43]. For mainstream and special-education teachers, we verified (a) the appropriateness of the number of participants, in accordance with the assumption that $n \geq 104 + m$ (where m is the number of independent variables); (b) the absence of multicollinearity among independent variables by computing the tolerance index, which should be higher than 0.05, and the variance inflation factor (VIF), which should be lower than 2; (c) the normality, linearity, and homoscedasticity of errors, by examining the shape of the residual distribution scatterplots; (d) the independence of errors, through the Durbin–Watson statistics; and (e) the absence of outliers in standardized residuals.

Only participants who reported never having had any relationship with individuals with ID were excluded from the correlation and regression analyses involving the variables related to closeness and quality of relationships with individuals with ID.

Statistical power of the hierarchical multiple regression analyses run was conducted with G*Power 3.1 software (Heinrich Heine Universität, Düsseldorf, Germany) [52]. With more detail, we ran post-hoc power analyses [49] for linear multiple regression fixed model with R^2 increase [53].

3. Results

For both mainstream and special-education teachers, neither univariate nor multivariate outliers were found, and the normality of the univariate and multivariate distributions of the scores for each ATTID dimension and for each metric characteristic were generally satisfied. Only the variables perceived efficacy of ID knowledge for both mainstream and special-education teachers and training in special education or ID and promotion of positive attitudes toward ID for special-education teachers presented a slight kurtosis. Therefore, correlation and regression analyses were performed with normalized scores of each metric variable.

3.1. Attitudes toward ID of Mainstream Teachers and Special-Education Teachers

3.1.1. Quality of Attitudes toward ID

Table 2 presents the means (SD) of the raw scores and the 5-point Likert scale scores (i.e., raw score relative to the number of the corresponding items) obtained for mainstream and special-education teachers for each ATTID dimension. A higher score for an ATTID dimension indicates a more negative attitude. Considering the Likert scale, given that 1 and 2 represented positive attitudes,

3 represented neutral attitudes, and 4 and 5 represented negative attitudes, both mainstream teachers and special-education teachers had positive attitudes for all ATTID dimensions.

Table 2. Means and standard deviations of raw score and 5-point Likert scale score obtained by mainstream teachers and special-education teachers for each dimension of the Attitudes Toward Intellectual Disability (ATTID) questionnaire.

	Mainstream Teachers				Special-Education Teachers			
	Raw Score		5-Point Likert Scale Score		Raw Score		5-Point Likert Scale Score	
ATTID Dimension	Mean	SD	Mean	SD	Mean	SD	Mean	SD
Discomfort	32.83	9.78	1.93	0.58	30.04	8.13	1.77	0.48
Knowledge of capacity and rights	45.61	9.23	2.28	0.46	43.77	9.63	2.19	0.48
Interaction	36.71	9.21	2.04	0.51	33.92	8.26	1.88	0.46
Sensitivity/Tenderness	10.02	3.85	2.50	0.96	9.47	3.56	2.37	0.89
Knowledge of causes of ID	16.49	4.11	2.36	0.59	16.11	3.67	2.30	0.52

3.1.2. Differences in Attitudes toward ID between Mainstream Teachers and Special-Education Teachers

The results of non-parametric statistics showed that special-education teachers, compared with mainstream teachers, were more often male ($\chi^2_{(1)}$ = 3.94, $p < 0.05$; phi = 0.09) and younger (U = 25.724, $z = -6.14$, $p < 0.001$; rg = 0.29), with fewer years of teaching experience (U = 21.510, $z = -8.519$, $p < 0.001$; rg = 0.41).

MANCOVA assumptions were satisfied, except for the homogeneity of variance–covariance matrices, given that Box's M test showed statistically significant results ($F_{(15,1031317)}$ = 1.68, $p < 0.05$). However, Box's M test is so sensitive that some authors proposed setting the level of significance at $p < 0.005$ [54]. Levene's test for homoscedasticity showed a significant result only for the dependent variable discomfort ($F_{(1,542)}$ = 7.11, $p < 0.01$). Given the results of the Box's M and Levene's tests, we used Pillai's trace criterion to report the multivariate test results, which is robust to these violations [55].

MANCOVA showed a multivariate statistically significant effect of the type of teacher on the attitude toward ID, controlled for years of teaching experience (Pillai's trace = 0.023, $F_{(5,537)}$ = 2.48, $p < 0.05$). The subsequent univariate tests showed that special-education teachers, compared with mainstream teachers, obtained statistically significant lower scores, i.e., more positive attitudes, for the ATTID dimensions discomfort ($F_{(1,541)}$ = 10.80, $p < 0.01$), interaction ($F_{(1,541)}$ = 7.13, $p < 0.01$), and sensitivity/tenderness ($F_{(1,541)}$ = 5.56, $p < 0.05$). The effect size was small in all cases, with Cohen's d equal to 0.29, 0.25, and 0.21, respectively. No statistically significant differences were found for the ATTID dimensions knowledge of capacity and rights and knowledge of causes of ID.

3.2. Relationships between General and Teacher-Specific Characteristics and Each Attitudes toward ID Dimension for Mainstream Teachers and Special-Education Teachers

3.2.1. Correlation between Characteristics and Attitudes toward ID Dimensions

Table 3 reports the correlation coefficients between the scores for variables measuring an individual's general and teacher-specific characteristics and each ATTID dimension. As can be seen, regarding an individual's general characteristics, younger age was significantly related to a greater knowledge of capacity and rights for both types of teachers and to more interactions for special-education teachers only. A higher quantity of contact and a better quality of relationship with individuals with ID were significantly correlated with less discomfort and sensitivity/tenderness and more interactions for both types of teachers and with a greater knowledge of causes of ID for special-education teachers only. A closer relationship with individuals with ID was associated with more interactions for mainstream teachers and with a greater knowledge of causes of ID for special-education teacher.

Regarding an individual's teacher-specific characteristics, teaching at a higher school level was related to a greater knowledge of capacity and rights for mainstream teachers only. More training in special education or ID was associated with less discomfort and sensitivity/tenderness for both types of teachers and with more interactions for mainstream teachers only. More years of teaching experience was related to a lesser knowledge of capacity and rights for both types of teachers and to few interactions for mainstream teachers only. More years of experience teaching pupils with ID and of experience teaching pupils with severe/profound ID was related to a lesser knowledge of capacity and rights for special-education teachers and to less sensitivity/tenderness for mainstream teachers. For mainstream teachers only, experience teaching pupils with severe/profound ID was related to less discomfort.

Higher levels of perceived efficacy of ID knowledge, perceived support, and promotion of positive attitudes were associated with more interactions for both types of teachers and with less discomfort for special-education teachers only. A higher perceived efficacy of ID knowledge was related to less sensitivity/tenderness for both types of teachers and to less discomfort for mainstream teachers only. Higher perceived support was related to a greater knowledge of capacity and rights for special-education teachers only. Finally, a higher promotion of positive attitudes was related to a greater knowledge of capacity and rights and of causes of ID for both types of teachers.

All these significant correlation coefficients had a small magnitude, except for some obtained for the quantity of contact and the quality of relationships with individuals with ID, as well as for the perceived efficacy of ID knowledge, which had a medium magnitude.

3.2.2. Regressions of Characteristics on Attitudes toward ID Dimensions

To study the degree to which an individual's teacher-specific characteristics affected each ATTID dimension, in addition to the individual's general characteristics, we ran one hierarchical multiple regression for each of the five ATTID dimensions within each group of teachers. All the individual's general and teacher-specific characteristics that were found to have a statistically or tendentially significant correlation ($p \leq 0.08$) with the considered ATTID dimension were entered as independent variables. Each ATTID dimension was taken as the dependent variable.

With regard to the regression assumptions, particularly, the appropriateness of the number of participants, a maximum of eight and seven characteristics was entered as independent variables for mainstream teachers and special-education teachers, respectively. The minimum required numbers of 112 (i.e., 104 + number of independent variables = 104 + 8 = 112) and 111 (i.e., 104 + number of independent variables = 104 + 7 = 111) participants for mainstream and special-education teachers, respectively, were lower than the actual numbers of participants in each group (equal to 307 and 237, respectively); therefore, the assumption of adequacy of the number of participants was satisfied. Moreover, within each teacher group, the absence of multicollinearity among the independent variables was ascertained, because the tolerance and the VIF index values were higher than 0.50 and lower than 2, respectively. For each independent variable taken separately, as well as within the set of predictors, the normality, linearity, and homoscedasticity of the residuals were ascertained. Indeed, an examination of the shape of the residual distribution scatterplots revealed that, in all cases, the residuals were normally distributed around each and every dependent variables' predicted score; residuals had a horizontal line relationship with the predicted dependent variables' scores—hence, the shape of the scatterplots appeared rectangular—and the variance of residual scores was approximately equal for all predicted dependent variables' scores [43]. The independence of errors in the regression solutions was satisfied too, because the Durbin-Watson values ranged from 1.75 to 2.13 and therefore fell within the suggested range of 1.5–2.2 [43]. Finally, no outliers in the standardized residuals were detected, given that no standardized residuals exceeded SD = 3.29 [43].

Table 3. Correlation coefficients between general and teacher-specific characteristics and each dimension of the ATTID questionnaire for mainstream teachers and special-education teachers.

Individual's Characteristics	ATTID Dimensions									
	Discomfort		Knowledge of Capacity and Rights		Interaction		Sensitivity/Tenderness		Knowledge of Causes of ID	
	Mainstream Teachers	Special-Education Teachers	Mainstream Teachers	Special-Education Teachers	Mainstream Teachers	Special-Education Teachers	Mainstream Teachers	Special-Education Teachers	Mainstream Teachers	Special-Education Teachers
General										
Age	0.03	0.02	0.26 **	0.16 *	0.10	0.14 *	−0.04	−0.05	0.07	0.05
Quantity of contact with individuals with ID	−0.43 **	−0.24 **	0.00	0.11	−0.27 **	−0.17 *	−0.29 **	−0.18 **	−0.04	−0.15 *
Closeness of relationships with individuals with ID [1]	−0.10 °	0.08	0.04	−0.02	−0.11 *	−0.02	−0.07	0.09	−0.03	−0.16 *
Quality of relationships with individuals with ID [1]	−0.47 **	−0.30 **	−0.08	−0.11	−0.38 **	−0.37 **	−0.33 **	−0.17 **	−0.02	−0.19 **
Teacher-specific										
School level taught	0.02	−0.04	−0.13 *	0.03	−0.03	0.09	0.04	−0.04	0.09	−0.05
Training in special education or ID	−0.23 **	−0.23 **	−0.04	0.08	−0.19 **	−0.12 °	−0.25 **	−0.25 **	−0.05	0.03
Years of teaching experience	0.06	−0.07	0.20 **	0.20 **	0.14 *	0.05	−0.07	−0.12 °°	0.09	−0.01
Years of experience teaching pupils with ID	−0.08	−0.10	0.08	0.23 **	−0.03	0.08	−0.16 **	−0.12 °°	−0.03	−0.05
Experience teaching pupils with severe/profound ID	−0.18 **	−0.09	0.02	0.15 *	−0.10	−0.02	−0.14 *	−0.12 °°	0.01	0.04
Perceived efficacy of ID knowledge	−0.37 **	−0.38 **	−0.11 °°	−0.06	−0.31 **	−0.29 **	−0.27 **	−0.17 **	−0.10	−0.02
Perceived support	−0.09	−0.14 *	−0.11 °	−0.18 **	−0.26 **	−0.25 **	0.02	0.05	−0.07	0.04
Promotion of positive attitudes toward ID	−0.07	−0.16 *	−0.11 *	−0.14 **	−0.13 *	−0.19 **	0.08	0.01	−0.24 **	−0.19 **

[1] The number of mainstream teachers and special-education teachers was 293 and 232, respectively, because 14 and 5 of them, respectively, reported not having had any experience with individuals with ID. ** $p \leq 0.01$; * $p \leq 0.05$; °°° $p \leq 0.06$; °° $p \leq 0.07$; ° $p \leq 0.08$.

Table 4 represents the results of the regression analyses, and β (i.e., standardized beta regression coefficients), adjusted R^2 (i.e., explained variance), F (i.e. ANOVA F value of the overall significance of the regression), and sr^2 incremental are reported. Step 1 shows which of the individual's general characteristics affected each ATTID dimension for mainstream and special-education teachers. Step 2 shows which of these individual's general characteristics persisted in affecting the ATTID dimensions when considered simultaneously with the individual's teacher-specific characteristics, which of the individual's teacher-specific characteristics affected each ATTID dimension, and the degree to which the individual's teacher-specific characteristics affected each ATTID dimension, in addition to the individual's general characteristics (i.e., sr^2 incremental).

Step 2 shows that an individual's teacher-specific characteristics improved the precision of score prediction for the majority of ATTID dimensions for both types of teachers. Specifically, for special-education teachers only, a higher perceived efficacy of ID knowledge positively affected the discomfort ($f^2 = 0.12$, power = 0.99) and interaction ($f^2 = 0.06$, power = 0.86) dimensions. For both mainstream teachers and special-education teachers, higher perceived support positively affected the interaction dimension ($f^2 = 0.05$, power = 0.87, for mainstream teachers; $f^2 = 0.06$, power = 0.86, for special-education teachers), higher promotion of positive attitudes positively affected the knowledge of causes of ID dimension ($f^2 = 0.06$, power = 0.99, for mainstream teachers; $f^2 = 0.04$, power = 0.73, for special-education teachers), and higher training in special education or ID positively affected the sensitivity/tenderness dimension ($f^2 = 0.04$, power = 0.81, for mainstream teachers; $f^2 = 0.06$, power = 0.83, for special-education teacher). Lastly, for mainstream teachers only, a higher school level taught positively affected the knowledge of capacity and rights dimension ($f^2 = 0.02$, power = 0.43), and more years of teaching experiences negatively affected the interaction dimension ($f^2 = 0.02$, power = 0.43).

Finally, regarding the individual's general characteristics affecting attitudes when considered simultaneously with an individual's teacher-specific characteristics, a higher age was found to negatively affect the knowledge of capacity and rights dimension ($f^2 = 0.07$, power = 0.96) for mainstream teachers and the interaction dimension ($f^2 = 0.04$, power = 0.68) for special-education teachers. A higher quantity of contact positively affected the discomfort ($f^2 = 0.13$, power = 1.00) and sensitivity/tenderness ($f^2 = 0.04$, power = 0.81) dimensions for mainstream teachers only. Closer relationships with individuals with ID positively affected the knowledge of causes of ID dimension ($f^2 = 0.02$, power = 0.41) for special-education teachers. Finally, for both types of teachers, a better quality of relationships with individuals with ID positively affected the discomfort dimension ($f^2 = 0.22$, power = 1.00, for mainstream teachers; $f^2 = 0.05$, power = 0.79, for special-education teachers) and the interaction dimension ($f^2 = 0.12$, power = 1.00, for mainstream teachers; $f^2 = 0.13$, power = 1.00, for special-education teachers), while it positively affected the sensitivity/tenderness dimension ($f^2 = 0.09$, power = 0.99) for mainstream teachers only.

The values of f^2 showed a small effect size for all predictors in both groups of teachers, except for the contribution of the quality of relationships with individuals with ID to the discomfort dimension for mainstream teachers, for which the effect size was medium. The explained variance by the factors inserted at Step 2 ranged from 27% (discomfort dimension of mainstream teachers) to 5% (sensitivity/tenderness and knowledge of causes of ID dimensions of special-education and mainstream teachers, respectively), confirming that the explanation power of the independent variables over the dependent variable was very limited.

Table 4. Hierarchical multiple regression analyses of general and teacher-specific characteristics for each dimension of the ATTID questionnaire for mainstream teachers and special-education teachers.

	ATTID Dimensions									
	Discomfort [1]		Knowledge of Capacity and Rights		Interaction [1]		Sensitivity/Tenderness [1]		Knowledge of Causes of ID	
	Mainstream Teachers	Special-Education Teachers	Mainstream Teachers	Special-Education Teachers	Mainstream Teachers	Special-Education Teachers	Mainstream Teachers	Special-Education Teachers	Mainstream Teachers [2]	Special-Education Teachers [1]
Individual's Characteristics	β	β	β	β	β	β	β	β	β	β
Step 1										
General										
Age	-	-	0.26 ***	0.16 *	-	0.21 **	-	-	-	-
Quantity of contact with individuals with ID	−0.28 ***	−0.17 *	-	-	−0.13 *	−0.10	−0.17 **	−0.13	-	−0.12
Closeness of relationships with individuals with ID	0.04	-	-	-	−0.01	-	-	-	-	−0.13 *
Quality of relationships with individuals with ID	−0.37 ***	−0.25 ***	-	-	−0.33 ***	−0.36 ***	−0.26 *	−0.12	-	−0.13
Adjusted R^2	0.27 ***	0.10 ***	0.06 ***	0.02 *	0.15 ***	0.17 ***	0.13 ***	0.03 *	-	0.05 **
ANOVA F	36.83 ***	14.31 ***	21.29 ***	6.08 *	17.77 ***	16.25 ***	22.19 ***	4.69 *	-	5.25 **
Step 2										
General										
Age	-	-	0.23 **	0.08	-	0.23 **	-	-	-	-
Quantity of contact with individuals with ID	−0.24 ***	−0.06	-	-	−0.11	−0.03	−0.14 †	0.07	-	0.10
Closeness of relationships with individuals with ID	0.03	-	-	-	−0.05	-	-	-	-	−0.12 *
Quality of relationships with individuals with ID	−0.33 ***	−0.14 *	-	-	−0.25 ***	−0.28 ***	−0.24 ***	−0.09	-	−0.09
Teacher-specific										
School level taught	-	-	−0.14 *	-	-	-	-	-	-	-

Table 4. Cont.

	ATTID Dimensions									
	Discomfort [1]		Knowledge of Capacity and Rights		Interaction [1]		Sensitivity/Tenderness [1]		Knowledge of Causes of ID	
	Mainstream Teachers	Special-Education Teachers	Mainstream Teachers	Special-Education Teachers	Mainstream Teachers	Special-Education Teachers	Mainstream Teachers	Special-Education Teachers	Mainstream Teachers [2]	Special-Education Teachers [1]
Training in special education or ID	−0.04	−0.08	-	-	−0.03	-0.09	−0.15 *	−0.24 **	-	-
Years of teaching experience	-	-	0.02	−0.02	0.12 *	-	-	0.01	-	-
Years of experience teaching pupils with ID	-	-	-	0.14	-	-	−0.06	0.07	-	-
Experience teaching pupils with severe/profound ID	−0.01	-	-	0.09	-	-	0.01	-0.01	-	-
Perceived efficacy of ID knowledge	−0.10	−0.26***	−0.07	-	−0.09	−0.15 *	−0.01	−0.04	-	-
Perceived support	-	−0.09	−0.07	−0.13	−0.17 **	−0.19 **	-	-	-	-
Promotion of positive attitudes toward ID	-	−0.02	−0.11	−0.12	−0.06	−0.04	-	-	−0.24 ***	−0.16 *
Adjusted R^2	0.27 ***	0.17 ***	0.09 ***	0.07 *	0.21 ***	0.22 ***	0.14 ***	0.05 **	0.05 ***	0.07 ***
ANOVA F	19.37 ***	8.68 ***	5.94 ***	3.92 **	10.46 ***	10.24 ***	8.82 ***	2.80 **	18.20 ***	5.55 ***
sr^2 incremental	0.01	0.08 ***	0.04 *	0.07 **	0.07 ***	0.07 **	0.03	0.04	-	0.02*

[1] The number of mainstream teachers and special education teachers was 293 and 232, respectively, because 14 and 5 of them, respectively, reported not having had any experience with individuals with ID. [2] Simple linear regression. *** $p \leq 0.001$; ** $p \leq 0.01$; * $p \leq 0.05$.

4. Discussion

The present study was aimed at investigating the attitudes toward ID of Italian mainstream teachers and special-education teachers and verifying if there were any differences between them. In agreement with a previous study [29], both mainstream and special-education teachers reported positive attitudes; however, special-education teachers were found to be more willing to interact with individuals with ID, feeling less pity and discomfort. This outcome may be due to the higher preparation in teaching students with ID and the closer relationships with individuals with ID exhibited by special-education teachers compared to mainstream teachers [26,32]. The two teacher groups were matched for years of teaching experience but not for chronological age, leading to statistically significant differences, albeit with a small effect size. Therefore, the better attitude of the special-education teachers could also be due to their lower age, given that studies found a better attitude of younger teachers [28]. The two teacher groups were also different for gender, but previous studies did not reveal any effect of gender on teachers' attitudes toward ID [28].

We also found that an individual's teacher-specific characteristics overall affected the attitude toward ID, in addition to the individual's general characteristics. Specifically, for both mainstream teachers and special-education teachers, we found that teachers with a higher level of training in special education or ID showed less pity, sadness, or compassion toward persons with ID, in agreement with previous investigations [28,29], while teachers with higher levels of promotion of positive attitudes toward ID had a better knowledge of causes of ID, in line with a previous study [30]. Furthermore, teachers with higher perceived support from the school and community contexts had greater willingness to interact with persons with ID, in line with a previous study about the inclusion of students with disabilities [31]. The magnitude of the effect sizes was similar for mainstream and special-education teachers, indicating that these characteristics were equally important for both types of teachers. Only special-education teachers with higher levels of perceived efficacy of ID knowledge showed less discomfort and were more willing to interact with individuals with ID. These findings might indicate that they feel confident in their competence and skills with regard to managing students with ID, and this security has positive effects on their attitudes toward ID [29,30]. Only mainstream teachers teaching at higher school levels showed a greater knowledge of capacity and rights of individuals with ID. Teachers at a higher school level, compared to those at a lower school level, might have had experience with students with a defined support system, who would, thus, be included in the classroom and in the community and be able to express their needs and show their strengths.

On the contrary, in spite of the relationships found with the correlation analyses among years of teaching experience, years teaching students with ID, and experience teaching pupils with severe/profound ID and the specific dimensions of attitudes, the regression analyses showed that, when considered simultaneously with all other characteristics, these factors were not associated with any attitude dimension for both type of teachers. The only exception was for mainstream teachers with fewer years of teaching experience, who showed more willingness to interact with individuals with ID. Our findings are in agreement with Ozer et al. [28], who found the same kind of relationships between attitudes and teaching experience but not with experience teaching pupils with ID, while they disagree with Sermier Dessemontet et al. [29], who found an association between attitudes of teachers toward ID and experience teaching students with ID.

Among all the individual's general characteristics that affected attitude toward ID, when taken into account simultaneously with teacher-specific characteristics, the quality of relationships with individuals with ID affected a greater number of dimensions, along with having a higher effect size. Indeed, both types of teachers with a better quality of contacts felt less discomfort toward persons with ID and less reluctance when interacting with them, and only mainstream teachers had fewer feelings of sadness and pity. The magnitude of effect sizes was similar for both types of teachers, except for the higher effect size found with regard to discomfort for mainstream teachers, indicating that, particularly for this type of teacher, the quality of the relationships with students with ID is relevant to better interact with them without discomfort. On the contrary, the quantity of contact with individuals with ID positively affected discomfort and sensitivity/tenderness for mainstream teachers only, supporting previous findings indicating that the quality of contact with individuals with ID is more relevant than the frequency of contact [29].

Only special-education teachers with a closer relationship with persons with ID had a better knowledge of causes of ID. This result may be explained by the previous training in ID of special-education teachers, which allows them to know better the literature on ID and the possible causes of this disorder.

Finally, in agreement with a previous study [28], we found that younger mainstream teachers and special-education teachers had a better knowledge of the capacity and rights of persons with ID or were more willing to interact with them, respectively. These findings might be due to the better quality of training in special education or ID for younger mainstream teachers and to the greater motivation and willingness of younger special-education teachers.

The uniqueness of the present study consists of having studied the individual characteristics related to attitudes toward ID of both mainstream and special-education teachers, while simultaneously considering general characteristics, such as previous contact with individuals with ID and teacher's age, as well as characteristics strictly connected with being teachers, such as previous training, experience in teaching, and perceived support. In summary, we found that, for both types of teachers, previous training in special education or ID, perceived support, and promotion of positive attitudes toward ID, in addition to the quality of the relationships with individuals with ID, are the factors that most affect the attitude toward ID. For special-education teachers only, the perceived efficacy of knowledge was also related to the attitude toward ID. On the contrary, previous experience teaching students plays a very limited role in affecting attitudes of mainstream teachers toward ID, and previous experience in teaching pupils with ID, even with severe/profound ID, was not found to be related to the attitude toward ID.

These findings highlight how the school and community context may promote the development of positive attitudes of teachers toward ID. Indeed, a school or community which can provide their teachers with high-quality training in disability, which is supportive in terms of social and material resources, and which allows the teachers to promote positive attitudes toward ID can foster favorable attitudes toward ID. Previous positive relationships of teachers with individuals with ID may reinforce these positive effects. A favorable disposition toward ID of the teachers may, in turn, stimulate the development of a positive attitude toward ID in their peers, as well as in other professionals working at the school. This would drastically increase the acceptance and the participation of students with ID in classrooms and social activities, in addition to their school and community inclusion, thereby improving their quality of life.

Limitations and Future Directions

The participants of the present study were not selected randomly but based on their voluntary responses. Nevertheless, the participants were selected from 19 out of 20 Italian regions, represented 73 out of 107 Italian provinces, and were non statistically different from the study population in terms of gender, age, and school level taught. However, the method of selection based on voluntary response might have disproportionately selected teachers who were interested in the topic investigated. Indeed, most of the teachers who participated in this study reported having had positive prior contact with persons with ID, while none reported having had negative prior contact. This might have reduced the score variance in the ATTID questionnaire, thereby limiting the generalizability of the present results to teachers with a good predisposition toward ID. This indicates the need for further research of randomly selected individuals. However, this method of selection would require mandatory response to the questionnaire by all teachers; this is not feasible and would likely return answers that are not thoroughly sincere.

In accordance with previous studies in the narrow field of teachers' attitudes toward the school inclusion of students with disabilities [31,34,56], the variance in attitude scores as explained by individual characteristics was quite low. Therefore, other variables might significantly affect teachers' attitudes toward ID. Examples of possible variables are teachers' assumptions or prejudice toward individuals with ID. Also, dimensions of teachers' personality should be taken into account and, in particular, the openness to experience Big Five personality traits, which was found to have the greatest effect on social attitudes [57], such as those toward individuals with mental disorders [58] or autism spectrum disorder [59]. Identifying these factors is fundamental to implementing interventions aimed at changing negative attitudes toward ID.

5. Conclusions

Despite these limitations, the current study provides a detailed overview of attitudes toward ID, as well as of the related factors, for mainstream and special-education teachers who teach at different school levels in a country such as Italy, with a long history of school inclusion (approximately 50 years). This study shows how school and community contexts are relevant in promoting favorable attitudes toward ID, which are essential for the development of an inclusive environment for students with ID and, therefore, for the improvement of their quality of life.

Supplementary Materials: The following are available online at http://www.mdpi.com/1660-4601/17/19/7325/s1, Note S1: Description of the item modifications for the Italian adaptation of the Attitudes toward Intellectual Disability Questionnaire (ATTID); Table S1: Questions to investigate general characteristics; Table S2: Questions to investigate teachers-specific characteristics.

Author Contributions: Conceptualization, L.A., A.B., C.G., M.S., and G.B.; Data curation, A.B. and G.B.; Formal analysis, A.B. and G.B.; Funding acquisition, L.A., M.S., and G.B.; Investigation, L.A., A.B., C.G., M.S., and G.B.; Methodology, L.A., A.B., C.G., M.S., and G.B.; Project administration, G.B.; Resources, L.A., C.G., M.S., and G.B.; Supervision, G.B.; Validation, A.B. and G.B.; Writing—original draft, A.B. and G.B.; Writing—review & editing, L.A., A.B., C.G., M.S., and G.B. All authors have read and agreed to the published version of the manuscript.

Funding: This study was partially funded by the research grant "Progetto Atteggiamenti del personale scolastico verso individui con disabilità intellettiva: Effetto dell'esperienza, Finanziato con il Fondo Ricerca di Base, Anno 2018 dell'Università degli Studi di Perugia" (Attitudes of school teachers and staff towards individuals with intellectual disabilities: Effect of experience, Fondo Ricerca di Base, Year 2018, University of Perugia).

Acknowledgments: The authors thank Silvia Di Falco for her help in the Italian translation and adaptation and the development of the online version of the Attitudes Toward Intellectual Disability Questionnaire.

Conflicts of Interest: The authors declare no conflict of interest. The funders had no role in the design of the study; in the collection, analyses, or interpretation of data; in the writing of the manuscript, or in the decision to publish the results.

References

1. American Psychiatric Association. *Diagnostic and Statistical Manual of Mental Disorders*, 5th ed.; American Psychiatric Association: Washington, DC, USA, 2013.
2. Schalock, R.L.; Borthwick-Duffy, S.A.; Bradley, V.J.; Buntinx, W.H.E.; Coulter, D.L.; Craig, E.M.; Gomez, S.C.; Lachapelle, Y.; Luckasson, R.; Reeve, A.; et al. *Intellectual Disability: Diagnosis, Classification, and Systems of Supports*, 11th ed.; American Association on Intellectual and Developmental Disabilities: Washington, DC, USA, 2010.
3. World Health Organization. ICD-11 for Mortality and Morbidity Statistics. Available online: https://icd.who.int/browse11/l-m/en#/ (accessed on 19 August 2020).
4. Schalock, R.L.; Verdugo, M.A. *Handbook on Quality of Life for Human Service Practitioners*; American Association on Mental Retardation: Washington, DC, USA, 2002.
5. Schalock, R.L.; Luckasson, R.; Tassé, M.J. The contemporary view of intellectual and developmental disabilities: Implications for psychologists. *Psicothema* **2019**, *31*, 223–228.
6. Cagran, B.; Schmidt, M. Attitudes of Slovene teachers towards the inclusion of pupils with different types of special needs in primary school. *Educ. Stud.* **2011**, *37*, 171–195. [CrossRef]
7. Ainscow, M.; César, M. Inclusive education ten years after Salamanca: Setting the agenda. *Eur. J. Psychol. Educ.* **2006**, *21*, 231–238. [CrossRef]

8. European Agency for Special Needs and Inclusive Education. *Five Key Messages for Inclusive Education: Putting Theory into Practice*; European Agency for Special Needs and Inclusive Education: Odense, Denmark, 2014. Available online: https://www.european-agency.org/sites/default/files/Five%20Key%20Messages%20for%20Inclusive%20Education.pdf (accessed on 19 August 2020).
9. Srivastava, M.; De Boer, A.; Pijl, S.J. Inclusive education in developing countries: A closer look at its implementation in the last 10 years. *Educ. Rev.* **2013**, *67*, 179–195. [CrossRef]
10. UNESCO. *Policy Guidelines on Inclusion in Education*; UNESCO: Paris, France, 2009. Available online: https://unesdoc.unesco.org/ark:/48223/pf0000177849 (accessed on 19 August 2020).
11. Avramidis, E.; Kalyva, E. The influence of teaching experience and professional development on Greek teachers' attitudes towards inclusion. *Eur. J. Spéc. Needs Educ.* **2007**, *22*, 367–389. [CrossRef]
12. Dessemontet, R.S.; Bless, G. The impact of including children with intellectual disability in general education classrooms on the academic achievement of their low-, average-, and high-achieving peers. *J. Intellect. Dev. Disabil.* **2013**, *38*, 23–30. [CrossRef] [PubMed]
13. UNESCO. *World Declaration on Education for All*; UNESCO: New York, NY, USA, 1990. Available online: https://www.right-to-education.org/sites/right-to-education.org/files/resource-attachments/UNESCO_World_Declaration_For_All_1990_En.pdf (accessed on 19 August 2020).
14. UNESCO. *The Salamanca Statement and Framework for Action on Special Needs Education*; UNESCO: Salamanca, Spain, 1994. Available online: https://www.right-to-education.org/sites/right-to-education.org/files/resource-attachments/Salamanca_Statement_1994.pdf (accessed on 19 August 2020).
15. No Child Left Behind. 2001. Available online: https://www.congress.gov/bill/107th-congress/house-bill/1/text (accessed on 7 August 2020).
16. United Nations. *Convention on the Rights of Persons with Disabilities*; United Nations: New York, NY, USA, 2006.
17. Verdugo, M.A.; Navas, P.; Gómez, L.E.; Schalock, R.L. The concept of quality of life and its role in enhancing human rights in the field of intellectual disability. *J. Intellect. Disabil. Res.* **2012**, *56*, 1036–1045. [CrossRef]
18. Law 517. 1977. Available online: https://www.gazzettaufficiale.it/eli/id/1977/08/18/077U0517/sg (accessed on 7 August 2020).
19. Law 104. 1992. Available online: https://www.gazzettaufficiale.it/eli/id/1992/02/17/092G0108/sg (accessed on 7 August 2020).
20. Law 96. 2019. Available online: https://www.gazzettaufficiale.it/eli/id/2019/08/28/19G00107/SG (accessed on 7 August 2020).
21. Lauchlan, F.; Fadda, R. The "Italian model" of full inclusion: Origins and current directions. In *What Works in Inclusion?* Boyle, C., Topping, K.J., Eds.; Open University Press: Maidenhead, UK, 2012; pp. 31–40.
22. Eagly, A.H.; Chaiken, S. *The Psychology of Attitudes*; Harcourt Brace Jovanovich: Fort Worth, TX, USA, 1993.
23. Rosenberg, M.J.; Hovland, C.I. Cognitive, affective, and behavioral components of attitude. In *Attitude Organization and Change*; Rosenberg, M., Hovland, C., McGuire, W., Abelson, R., Brehm, J., Eds.; Yale University Press: New Haven, CN, USA, 1960; pp. 1–14.
24. Avramidis, E.; Norwich, B. Teachers' attitudes towards integration/inclusion: A review of the literature. *Eur. J. Spéc. Needs Educ.* **2002**, *17*, 129–147. [CrossRef]
25. De Boer, A.; Pijl, S.J.; Minnaert, A. Regular primary schoolteachers' attitudes towards inclusive education: A review of the literature. *Int. J. Incl. Educ.* **2011**, *15*, 331–353. [CrossRef]
26. Scruggs, T.E.; Mastropieri, M.A. Teacher Perceptions of Mainstreaming/Inclusion, 1958–1995: A Research Synthesis. *Except. Child.* **1996**, *63*, 59–74. [CrossRef]
27. Hassanein, E.E.A. Changing Teachers' Negative Attitudes Toward Persons With Intellectual Disabilities. *Behav. Modif.* **2014**, *39*, 367–389. [CrossRef] [PubMed]
28. Özer, D.; Nalbant, S.; Ağlamış, E.; Baran, F.; Samut, P.K.; Aktop, A.; Hutzler, Y. Physical education teachers' attitudes towards children with intellectual disability: The impact of time in service, gender, and previous acquaintance. *J. Intellect. Disabil. Res.* **2012**, *57*, 1001–1013. [CrossRef] [PubMed]
29. Dessemontet, R.S.; Morin, D.; Crocker, A.G. Exploring the Relations between In-service Training, Prior Contacts and Teachers' Attitudes towards Persons with Intellectual Disability. *Int. J. Disabil. Dev. Educ.* **2014**, *61*, 16–26. [CrossRef]
30. Wilson, C.; Woolfson, L.M.; Durkin, K. The impact of explicit and implicit teacher beliefs on reports of inclusive teaching practices in Scotland. *Int. J. Incl. Educ.* **2019**, *23*, 1–19. [CrossRef]

31. Ahmmed, M.; Sharma, U.; Deppeler, J. Variables affecting teachers' attitudes towards inclusive education in Bangladesh. *J. Res. Spéc. Educ. Needs* **2012**, *12*, 132–140. [CrossRef]
32. Balboni, G.; Pedrabissi, L. Attitudes of Italian teachers and parents toward school inclusion of students with mental retardation: The role of experience. *Educ. Train. Ment. Retard. Dev. Disabil.* **2000**, *35*, 148–159.
33. Memisevic, H.; Hodzic, S. Teachers' attitudes towards inclusion of students with intellectual disability in Bosnia and Herzegovina. *Int. J. Incl. Educ.* **2011**, *15*, 699–710. [CrossRef]
34. Malinen, O.-P.; Savolainen, H.; Xu, J. Beijing in-service teachers' self-efficacy and attitudes towards inclusive education. *Teach. Teach. Educ.* **2012**, *28*, 526–534. [CrossRef]
35. Ojok, P.; Wormnæs, S. Inclusion of pupils with intellectual disabilities: Primary school teachers' attitudes and willingness in a rural area in Uganda. *Int. J. Incl. Educ.* **2013**, *17*, 1003–1021. [CrossRef]
36. Cornoldi, C.; Terreni, A.; Scruggs, T.E.; Mastropieri, M.A. Teacher Attitudes in Italy After Twenty Years of Inclusion. *Remedial Spéc. Educ.* **1998**, *19*, 350–356. [CrossRef]
37. Morin, D.; Crocker, A.G.; Beaulieu-Bergeron, R.; Caron, J. Validation of the attitudes toward intellectual disability - ATTID questionnaire. *J. Intellect. Disabil. Res.* **2012**, *57*, 268–278. [CrossRef] [PubMed]
38. International Test Commission. International Test Commission Guidelines for Translating and Adapting Tests, 2nd ed. 2017. Available online: https://www.intestcom.org/files/guideline_test_adaptation_2ed.pdf (accessed on 19 August 2020).
39. Schermelleh-Engel, K.; Moosbrugger, H.; Müller, H. Evaluating the fit of structural equation models: Tests of significance and descriptive goodness-of-fit measures. *Methods Psychol. Res.* **2003**, *8*, 23–74.
40. Jackson, D.L.; Gillaspy, J.A.; Purc-Stephenson, R. Reporting practices in confirmatory factor analysis: An overview and some recommendations. *Psychol. Methods* **2009**, *14*, 6–23. [CrossRef] [PubMed]
41. Evers, A.; Hagemeister, C.; Høstmælingen, A.; Lindley, P.; Muñiz, J.; Sjöberg, A. EFPA Review Model for the Description and Evaluation of Psychological and Educational Tests. Test Review Form and Notes for Reviewers, Version 4.2.6. 2013. Available online: http://www.efpa.eu/download/650d0d4ecd407a51139ca44ee704fda4 (accessed on 19 August 2020).
42. Cicchetti, D.; Koenig, K.; Klin, A.; Volkmar, F.R.; Paul, R.; Sparrow, S. From Bayes Through Marginal Utility to Effect Sizes: A Guide to Understanding the Clinical and Statistical Significance of the Results of Autism Research Findings. *J. Autism Dev. Disord.* **2010**, *41*, 168–174. [CrossRef]
43. Tabachnick, B.G.; Fidell, L.S. *Using Multivariate Statistics*, 6th ed.; Pearson: New York, NY, USA, 2013.
44. Kaiser, H.F.; Rice, J. Little Jiffy, Mark Iv. *Educ. Psychol. Meas.* **1974**, *34*, 111–117. [CrossRef]
45. Cortina, J.M. What is coefficient alpha? An examination of theory and applications. *J. Appl. Psychol.* **1993**, *78*, 98–104. [CrossRef]
46. Bobbio, A.; Manganelli, A.M. Measuring social desirability responding. A short version of Paulhus' BIDR 6. *Test. Psychom. Methodol. Appl. Psychol.* **2011**, *18*, 117–135.
47. Paulhus, D.L. Measurement and Control of Response Bias. In *Measures of Personality and Social Psychological Attitudes*; Robinson, J.P., Shaver, P.R., Wrightsman, L.S., Eds.; Academic Press: New York, NY, USA, 1991; pp. 17–59.
48. European Commission Eurostat. *Classroom Teachers and Academic Staff by Education Level, Programme Orientation, Sex and Age Groups*; European Commission Eurostat: Kirchberg, Luxembourg, 2020. Available online: https://ec.europa.eu/eurostat/web/products-datasets/-/educ_uoe_perp01 (accessed on 16 September 2020).
49. Cohen, J. *Statistical Power Analysis for the Behavioral Sciences*, 2nd ed.; L. Erlbaum Associates: Hillsdale, NJ, USA, 1988.
50. King, B.M.; Minium, E.W. *Statistical Reasoning in Psychology and Education*, 4th ed.; Wiley and Sons: New York, NY, USA, 2003.
51. Benjamini, Y.; Hochberg, Y. Controlling the False Discovery Rate: A Practical and Powerful Approach to Multiple Testing. *J. R. Stat. Soc. Ser. B Stat. Methodol.* **1995**, *57*, 289–300. [CrossRef]
52. Faul, F.; Erdfelder, E.; Lang, A.-G.; Buchner, A. G*Power 3: A flexible statistical power analysis program for the social, behavioral, and biomedical sciences. *Behav. Res. Methods* **2007**, *39*, 175–191. [CrossRef]
53. Faul, F.; Erdfelder, E.; Buchner, A.; Lang, A.-G. Statistical power analyses using G*Power 3.1: Tests for correlation and regression analyses. *Behav. Res. Methods* **2009**, *41*, 1149–1160. [CrossRef]
54. Huberty, C.J.; Petoskey, M.D. Multivariate Analysis of Variance and Covariance. In *Handbook of Applied Multivariate Statistics and Mathematical Modeling*; Tinsley, H.E.A., Brown, S.D., Eds.; Academic Press: New York, NY, USA, 2000; pp. 183–208.

55. Olson, C.L. Practical considerations in choosing a MANOVA test statistic: A rejoinder to Stevens. *Psychol. Bull.* **1979**, *86*, 1350–1352. [CrossRef]
56. Savolainen, H.; Engelbrecht, P.; Nel, M.; Malinen, O.-P. Understanding teachers' attitudes and self-efficacy in inclusive education: Implications for pre-service and in-service teacher education. *Eur. J. Spéc. Needs Educ.* **2011**, *27*, 51–68. [CrossRef]
57. McCrae, R.R. Social consequences of experiential openness. *Psychol. Bull.* **1996**, *120*, 323–337. [CrossRef] [PubMed]
58. Wolska, A.; Malina, A. Personality and attitudes towards people with mental disorders: Preliminary studies results. *Int. J. Soc. Psychiatry* **2020**, *66*, 270–278. [CrossRef] [PubMed]
59. Gillespie-Lynch, K.; Daou, N.; Sanchez-Ruiz, M.-J.; Kapp, S.K.; Obeid, R.; Brooks, P.J.; Someki, F.; Silton, N.; Abi-Habib, R. Factors underlying cross-cultural differences in stigma toward autism among college students in Lebanon and the United States. *Autism* **2019**, *23*, 1993–2006. [CrossRef] [PubMed]

© 2020 by the authors. Licensee MDPI, Basel, Switzerland. This article is an open access article distributed under the terms and conditions of the Creative Commons Attribution (CC BY) license (http://creativecommons.org/licenses/by/4.0/).

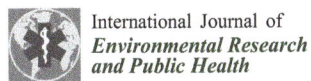

Article

Communication Support Needs in Adults with Intellectual Disabilities and Its Relation to Quality of Life

Juan Carlos García [1], Emiliano Díez [2,*], Dominika Z. Wojcik [2] and Mónica Santamaría [2,3]

1   Fundación Grupo AMÁS Social, 28914 Madrid, Spain; jc.garcia@grupoamas.org
2   Institute for Community Inclusion (INICO), University of Salamanca, 37005 Salamanca, Spain; d.z.wojcik@usal.es (D.Z.W.); msantamariado@upsa.es (M.S.)
3   Faculty of Education, Universidad Pontificia de Salamanca, 37002 Salamanca, Spain
*   Correspondence: emid@usal.es

Received: 26 August 2020; Accepted: 5 October 2020; Published: 9 October 2020

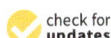

Abstract: Research suggests that individuals with intellectual disabilities (ID) experience difficulties in communication, ranging from intelligibility issues to more severe problems in the use and comprehension of spoken, written or sign language. Despite the negative effects that the inability to communicate have on quality of life (QoL), not much research has explored the relationship between communicative competence and QoL in the adult population with ID. The aim of this study was to describe the global communication profile of a sample of 281 adults with ID recruited from Grupo AMÁS Social Foundation, who differed in their level of communication support needs (CSN). The relationships between communicative competence and CSN with QoL were further examined. The results showed lower QoL indices for those participants characterized by their limited use of discourse and inability to exhibit certain communicative purposes, with the largest differences in the dimensions of self-determination, social inclusion, interpersonal relationships, emotional wellbeing and personal development. Overall, low levels of QoL were found for all participants, with even lower scores for the group identified as having CSN. A multiple regression model revealed that having speech/discourse competence is a powerful predictor of QoL, along with the level of disability and having the communicative competences to express likes and preferences or to establish new relationships. This clear relationship between communication and QoL is an important argument for disability support services when it comes to setting communication supports as a priority and as an important preventive step towards the protection of those at risk of exclusion.

Keywords: intellectual disability; communication support needs; quality of life

1. Introduction

The growing presence and visibility of persons with intellectual disabilities (ID) in our society is a remarkable milestone on the road to full inclusion. Although the research suggests that the improvement in areas such as communication skills has a direct impact on quality of life [1–3], hitherto, communication support needs (CSN) in adults with ID have still not been properly addressed.

Communication support needs are very frequent in people with ID. Typically, people with CSN may need support with understanding and/or expressing themselves. For example, in a recent study, Smith et al. [4] identified communication skills in a sample of 601 adults with ID, finding that 57.9% experienced communication difficulties and, in 23.5% of cases, the difficulties were of a severe nature. This high prevalence of communication difficulties in this study was related to factors such as level of ID, low social participation, challenging behaviors or a diagnosis of Down syndrome.

The difficulties with communication that people with ID may experience are diverse, ranging from the intelligibility or fluency of speech [5], through to the understanding and comprehension of spoken, written or sign language [6], to the transmission of messages or the pragmatic use of language [7]. These three aspects, i.e., receptive, expressive and pragmatic language functioning, form an important part in a person's communicative competence that can be assessed and measured across different situations [8]. Given that the communicative competence allows us to express desires, ideas, needs, or enables us to ask questions, etc., people who have difficulties within this area are at a direct risk of exclusion. This exclusion is understood as physical, legal, financial, and attitudinal barriers that prevent individuals from being an active participant in their community [1]. Indeed, despite the rapid advances in our understanding of the challenges that people with complex communication needs have, many of these individuals continue to experience significant challenges when it comes to inclusion into different environments, such as educational, vocational, community, healthcare, etc. [9,10]. Moreover, a growing amount of empirical work, such as the one by Snowling et al. [11], demonstrated an association between children's language delay and an increased risk of emotional and educational problems. What is more, Clegg and Ginsborg [12], further showed that these problems continue into adulthood. Studies have also shown a heightened risk of social exclusion in adults with ID, because of a reduced amount of opportunities to establish meaningful social connections and to participate in fulfilling social activities [13,14].

The degree of impact that living with a disability can have on everyday life may be explained using the idea of quality of life (QoL). Quality of life is considered a multi-layered construct [15–17] which entails several distinct dimensions at both individual (micro) and environmental (macro) levels [18] that interact with each other, and reflect both objective and subjective aspects. Despite the fact that there is no universally agreed definition of QoL [2,19] and despite the existence of different definitions [20,21], there is a wide consensus that QoL provides us with a robust tool that measures individuals' health and wellbeing and is often taken into account in clinical decision making and research [22]. There also seems to be a consensus among experts (i.e., the National Joint Committee for the Communication Needs of Persons With Severe Disabilities) that any QoL consideration must include the degree to which people can communicate effectively with members of their community, with communication being regarded as both a basic need and a human right [1].

Many studies have explored QoL in different types of conditions. An important finding from these studies suggests that individuals' level of functioning is highly correlated with their QoL [23–25], whereby individuals who are high functioning also show better QoL. More importantly, for this paper, in some studies, a direct relationship has been found between aspects related to communication and QoL. For example, Biggs and Carter [26] examined the subjective health and wellbeing of 389 transition-age young people with autism or intellectual disability. They found that speech, as the primary mode of communication, along with challenging behaviors, being diagnosed with autism, and age were predictive of lower ratings of wellbeing. Similarly, Davis et al. [27] found that 11 life domains were important for the QoL of children with cerebral palsy and intellectual disability, communication being one of them.

Although communicative competence has been related to QoL in children and adolescents, the literature on adults is relatively sparse. What is more, to the best of our knowledge, little research has directly explored how QoL is related to communicative competence in adults with ID who display communication needs. There are, however, indications in the literature on cognitive communication disorders that suggest that diverse difficulties in communicative competence have an impact on different aspects of QoL [28]. For example, with regard to the inability to communicate orally, Cruice et al. [29] found that aphasic people's functional communication ability and language functioning predicted their psychological wellbeing and social health. In fact, in a review of the topic, Hilari et al. [30] concluded that communication disability, along with other factors such emotional distress/depression, extent of aphasic impairment, the presence of other medical problems and activity level, were predictors of health-related quality of life (HRQL). Additionally, Hilari and Byng [31] found that the HRQL of individuals with severe aphasia is far more compromised than in individuals with mild aphasia. This study shows that not all people with aphasia will have the same needs and that, depending on the severity of communication and language impairment, these patients' QoL will be differentially affected.

In the literature about people with intellectual and developmental disabilities, we can also find some studies that relate communicative competence to the family quality of life (FQoL). Schertz et al. [32], for example, looked at FQoL in children with severe neurodevelopmental disabilities and significant communication needs. The results showed that the degree of communication support offered to the family was related to the overall FQoL score and individual domains of health and family relationships. In the same vein, a research review done by Saito [3] revealed that the implementation of augmentative and alternative communication from a family perspective rather thnt from an individual point of view has a direct impact on all domains of FQoL.

Finally, there is also a widespread idea among support staff for people with ID that working on improving communicative competence can be also a good way to improve QoL. For example, when Dalton and Sweeney [33] asked 138 support staff about ways to provide help in the area of communication difficulties for people with ID in residential services, 87% of them answered that setting appropriate communication goals could improve their QoL.

Given the importance of communicative competence for QoL and the lack of literature in the area, the aim of our study is to explore the consequences that living with communication needs have in different dimensions of QoL in adults with ID. Although there are various perspectives from which to measure the QoL construct, in this paper, we focus on the quality of life model proposed by Schalock and Verdugo [34]. The model is composed of eight quality of life dimensions: self-determination, rights, emotional wellbeing, social inclusion, personal development, interpersonal relations, material wellbeing, and physical wellbeing and has proven to be useful mainly because it considers quality of life not only from the perspective of health, but also because it allows for a better understanding of how to provide the necessary support to improve QoL. Thus, it considers QoL as a dynamic and multidimensional concept, with both universal and culture-tied properties, with objective and subjective components influenced by the characteristics of the person as well as contextual factors [35]. This broad perspective outlines a set of possible areas where support can be provided, which, in turn, can have a direct impact on the QoL. In fact, in Spain, Schalock and Verdugo's model has been shown to be a useful tool in planning support for people with ID, as well as having the capacity for encouraging institutions and organizations towards the use of QoL as the outcome measurement [36,37]. Furthermore, as stated by Navas et al. [38], there is a clear alignment between the dimensions of the Schalock and Verdugo's QoL model and the articles of the Convention on the Rights of Persons with Disabilities [39].

In summary, in this research, we first intend to describe the global communication profile of a large sample of adults with ID that differ in their needs in relation to support for communication and, second, to explore in detail the relationships between communicative competence and communication support needs in all the QoL dimensions outlined by the Schalock and Verdugo's model. In our study, we use the term 'communication profile' to reflect the communicative competence that captures the classification of communication mode and communication purpose. This preliminary diagnosis would be the first step to initiate a medium-term program to improve the support in the area of communication for users of disability support services belonging to Fundación Grupo AMÁS Social.

2. Method

2.1. Participants

The sample consisted of 281 individuals (134 women and 147 men) with complex needs. Both younger and older adults with communication needs were recruited from five live-in disability support services, four occupational disability support services, and four day disability support services, all belonging to Fundación Grupo AMÁS Social in Madrid. Most of the participants ($n = 235$) resided in disability support service establishments. To ascertain whether participants had complex and communication needs, the existing assessment files of each service user were consulted. Likewise, disability percentage, coexisting conditions (for $n = 213$), dependency levels (for $n = 276$) and intensity of support (for $n = 217$), were obtained from previous cognitive, social and health assessments carried out by professionals from each disability support service. The participants' characteristics are depicted in Table 1.

Table 1. Participants' characteristics.

Variable Description	Value
Mean (SD) age	42.3 (13.7)
Age range	19–71
Mean (SD) % disability	79.8 (9.7)
% disability range	37–99
Conditions associated with ID:	
Physical disability	116
Sensorial disability	70
Behavioral problems	69
Cerebral palsy	60
Dependency assessment:	
Moderate level	32
High level	112
Unknown	5
Intensity of support:	
Extensive support	133
Generalized support	84
Unknown	64

2.2. Instruments

2.2.1. Quality of Life—San Martín Scale

To measure the QoL, we used the field test version of the San Martín Scale [40], designed specifically for individuals who cannot participate in self-report due to profound I/DD and/or barriers to communication. It is composed of eight subscales that correspond to the eight quality of life domains by Schalock and Verdugo's model [34], and consists of a total of 95 items. The scale is a self-administered questionnaire in which a third-party respondent who knows the service user well answers questions about their QoL. Given the communicative problems of many of the participants, completing the scale based on their opinions was not possible. Thus, all items are formulated as third person declarative statements and are randomly organized by domains. The respondents are asked to give their answers on a frequency scale with four options (never, sometimes, often, and always). The scale has shown to have an adequate reliability and validity [40] and has been used across different studies that evaluate QoL in adults with ID [41,42].

2.2.2. Communication Profile Questionnaire

To explore the communication profile of participants, a custom-made checklist adapted from the Communication Device Use Checklist [43] was built with twelve yes/no questions about how the person communicates (communication modes checklist). Eleven questions were about the communication purpose and how the person communicates it (communication purpose checklist); one yes/no question asked if the person had communication support needs (a binary variable that was used in the analysis); another question checked previous participation in augmentative and alternative communication (AAC) interventions; and two final, broad questions assessed in detail the perception of professionals as to whether or not their disability support services were implementing good practice on cognitive accessibility and AAC training. The checklists and the two final questions can be consulted in the Supplementary Materials.

2.3. Procedure

The evaluation was carried out by a group of ninety-six professional supporting staff, working in the participating disability support services. Of these, 77.1% were women ($n = 74$) and 22.9% were men ($n = 22$) and their age ranged between 22 and 56 years ($M = 34$). As for the qualifications, almost half ($n = 49$) were direct care professionals with a degree related to social healthcare (51%): 27 were social integration technicians (28.1%), 11 were psychologists (11.45%) and 9 were managers (9.4%). The staff's experience in providing support for people with intellectual disabilities ranged from 2 to 21 years.

The type of relationship between the healthcare workers and the person with an intellectual disability was, in all cases, professional in nature and, in all cases, the person with an intellectual disability was someone who the participating professionals knew well and they had provided support for the person for at least six months.

The evaluation was completed by the professionals within a period of 4 months, during the months from February to May 2015, using a custom-made Microsoft Excel template to record the data for each participant.

This study was approved and regulated by a collaboration agreement between the Fundación Grupo AMÁS and the first author, and all the procedures performed in this research were in accordance with the ethical standards as laid down in the 1964 Declaration of Helsinki and its later amendments or comparable ethical standards.

2.4. Data Analysis

Data were analyzed using R [44]. The significance level set by the researchers to conduct the statistical analyses was = 0.05.

Participant communication profiles were analyzed using chi-squared tests with the number of participants as dependent variables and the CSN group to which they belonged as the independent variable. Standardized differences were calculated according to Austin [45].

In the analysis of communication needs and QoL, the global index of QoL as well as the QoL scores of each dimension was used as dependent variables and CSN group belonging as an independent variable. For MANOVA (multivariate analysis of variance) analysis we used R package MANOVA.RM to calculate a modified ANOVA-type statistic (MATS) for multivariate designs [46] as it is applicable for non-normal error terms, different sample sizes and/or heteroscedastic variances, and p-values were calculated based on a parametric bootstrap approach with 10,000 iterations.

The Quality of Life Index (QLI) was used as a dependent variable in all the regression models. The selection of variables that were due to be included in the regression models was done with the glmulti function of the glmulti package. This function performs an exhaustive search for the best subsets of the variables in 'x' for predicting 'y' in linear regression. We used a branch-and-bound algorithm (the leaps function from the leaps package). Due to violations of assumptions of heteroscedasticity, normal distribution of residuals and the presence of outliers, we calculated bivariate and multiple linear regression coefficients with robust statistical methods using the R package robustbase (function lmrob), which provides different robust regression techniques (e.g., MM estimation) as well as robust univariate and multivariate methods. The function bootcoefs from the package complmrob was used to bootstrap the regression coefficients of robust linear regression models.

3. Results

3.1. Participant Communication Profile

First, we were interested in exploring the participants' communication profiles, especially of those who were identified by the professionals as having communication support needs. It is noteworthy that direct care professionals identified as many as 182 people (64.8% of the total sample) as individuals with communication support needs (CSN group). This group included individuals who were supported, although not sufficiently, and those who did not receive support at all.

Table 2 shows the communication modes used by the participants according to their communication needs.

Table 2. Participants who use different communication modes as a percentage of each communication support needs (CSN) group.

Communication Modes	CSN No (n = 98)	CSN Yes (n = 182)	χ^2 p-Value	SMD
Speech/Discourse	93.8	9.3	**	3.2
Single words	82.7	41.2	**	0.9
Writing/Drawing	37.8	7.7	**	0.8
Gestures	53.1	75.8	**	0.5
Pictograms	19.4	19.2	n.s.	0.0
Manual Signs/Sign Language	6.1	8.8	n.s.	0.1
Communication Board/book	3.1	3.9	n.s.	0.0
Simple communication device	6.1	5.0	n.s.	0.1
Complex communication device	4.1	1.7	n.s.	0.1
Communication software on a device	1.0	2.8	n.s.	0.1
Phone	61.2	14.9	**	1.1
E-mail	4.1	0.6	n.s.	0.2

n.s. = non-significant difference; ** $p < 0.001$; SMD = Standardized Mean Difference; CSN = communication support needs.

As can be seen in Table 2, participants in the CSN group were mostly people who did not use speech or writing and used mainly single words and gestures. Pictograms were used equally in both groups and communication devices of different complexities and emails had a rather low usage rate in both groups (<10% in all cases). Finally, there was also a notable difference in the use of the telephone in favor of the non-CSN group.

It was also interesting to explore the communicative purposes of the participants. Table 3 shows the percentage of participants in each group that exhibit a certain communicative purpose.

Table 3. Percentage of participants who are able to communicate for different purposes as a function of communication support needs.

Communicative Purposes	CSN No (n = 98)	CSN Yes (n = 182)	χ^2 p-Value	SMD
Express needs and desires	99.0	80.8	<0.001	0.6
Ask for help	99.0	74.7	<0.001	0.8
Show likes and preferences	99.0	80.8	<0.001	0.6
Express opinions	93.9	46.7	<0.001	1.2
Exchange information	92.9	39.6	<0.001	1.4
Discuss ailments	98.0	70.3	<0.001	0.8
Express feelings	98.0	66.5	<0.001	0.9
Talk to family and friends	96.9	52.7	<0.001	1.2
Storytelling	90.8	25.8	<0.001	1.8
Talk to people around them	93.9	36.8	<0.001	1.5
Have new relationships	92.9	43.3	<0.001	1.3

SMD = Standardized Mean Difference (Austin, 2008); CSN = communication support needs.

Here, we can observe that, in the CSN group, the percentage of participants exhibiting communication purposes was generally lower than in the non-CSN group. In a way, this is a logical result and indicates the validity of the classification made by professionals when determining whether or not a participant needs support in communication. However, for communication purposes, such as expressing needs and desires, asking for help, or showing likes and preferences, the standardized differences were low. Therefore, it could be said that people who should be supported in communication are largely successful in expressing these fundamental communication purposes. Nevertheless, for other communication purposes, such as expressing opinions, exchanging information, expressing feelings, talking to family and friends, chatting with people in their environment and being able to have new relationships, the differences between the groups were larger.

Globally, the CSN group was, therefore, characterized by a limited use of discourse and reliance on gestures and, although these limited modes of communication may serve certain basic communicative purposes, the limited communication profile could probably directly influence some dimensions of QoL such as interpersonal relationships, inclusion, rights, or emotional wellbeing.

3.2. Communication Needs and Quality of Life Index

Once the profile of the group with needs had been identified, it was important to explore the impact of the communication difficulties on their QoL.

The mean QLI, a standard score (with an average of 100 and a standard deviation of 15) of the total sample reached an average value of 92.1 (SD = 16.1; mean percentile = 36.9). Therefore, the QoL profile of the participants is considered slightly low. Indeed, as can be seen in Table 4, the scores for each of the QoL dimensions did not exceed the standard score of 10 (the standard scores on the San Martín Scale have a mean of 10 and a standard deviation of three) with the dimensions of physical wellbeing, material wellbeing and interpersonal relationships scoring the lowest (<9).

Table 4. Mean (SD) standard quality of life scores by dimension and group.

Quality of Life Dimension	All Sample	CSN		CSN versus Non-CSN	
		No (n = 98)	Yes (n = 182)	Welsch's t p-Value	Cohen's d [95% CI]
Self-determination	9.4 (3.8)	12.9 (2.1)	7.6 (3.2)	<0.001	1.8 [1.5, 2.2]
Emotional wellbeing	9.2 (2.78)	10.9 (2.2)	8.3 (2.7)	<0.001	1.0 [0.7, 1.3]
Physical wellbeing	8.5 (3.4)	10.1 (2.8)	7.6 (3.4)	<0.001	0.8 [0.5, 1.0]
Material wellbeing	7.6 (3.2)	8.94 (3.0)	6.9 (3.1)	<0.001	0.7 [0.4, 0.9]
Rights	8.7 (3.3)	10.1 (2.7)	7.9 (3.4)	<0.001	0.7 [0.5, 1.0]
Personal Development	8.9 (2.9)	10.6 (2.1)	8.0 (2.8)	<0.001	1.0 [0.7, 1.3]
Social inclusion	9.1 (3.2)	11.7 (2.0)	7.7 (2.8)	<0.001	1.5 [1.3, 1.9]
Interpersonal relationships	8.2 (3.3)	10.7 (2.2)	6.9 (3.1)	<0.001	1.4 [1.0, 1.7]
Global QLI	92.1 (16.1)	104.29 (11)	85.48 (15.57)	<0.001	1.4 [1.1, 1.7]

CSN = communication support needs.

To further explore the differences in QoL as a function of CSN, a one-factor MANOVA analysis was conducted, showing that there were significant differences in QoL scores across the different dimensions (MATS = 871.2; $p < 0.001$). As presented in Table 4, post-hoc mean difference Welsch's t tests showed significant differences in QLI and all QoL dimensions between groups with and without CSN. Large differences ($d > 0.80$) were found for self-determination, social inclusion, interpersonal relationships, emotional wellbeing and personal development. The QLI of the participants of the CSN group was rather low and significantly lower than that of the non-CSN group.

Additional MANOVAs showed a significant interaction of CSN with the level of disability (MATS = 45.65; $p = 0.003$) and a non-significant interaction with age (MATS = 3.09; $p = 0.819$).

3.3. Quality of Life Relative to Communicative Profiles

In order to further explore the relationship of QoL with the communicative profiles of the sample, point-biserial correlations were carried out between the items of the communicative profile (modes and purposes) and the standard scores in the different dimensions of quality of life. Figure 1 shows two correlograms representing the correlations of communication modes and purposes with the eight quality of life dimensions.

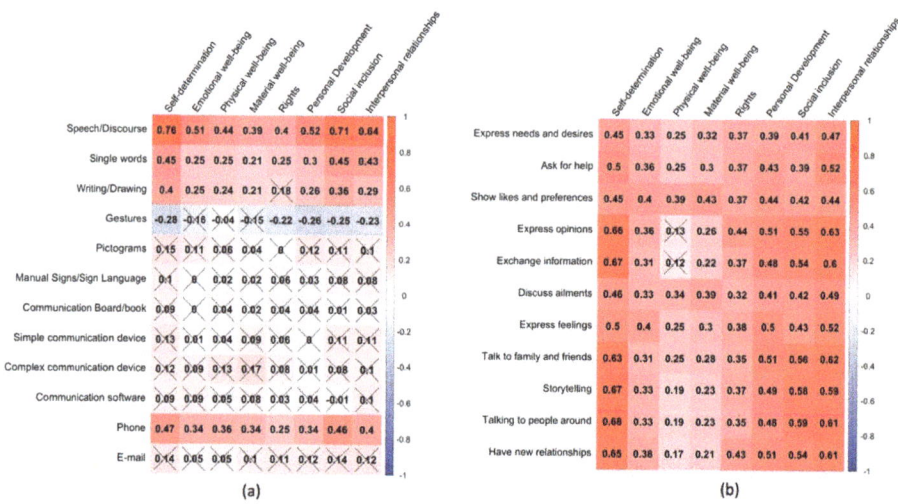

Figure 1. Correlograms representing point-biserial correlations among (**a**) modes of communication and (**b**) purposes of communication and quality of life dimension standard scores. The intensity and color of squares represent the magnitude and sign (red = positive and blue = negative) of the correlation, respectively. A crossed value indicates a non-significant correlation ($p > 0.05$; Bonferroni–Holm correction).

With regard to the modes of communication (Figure 1, panel a), it can be seen that the dimensions of self-determination, social inclusion and interpersonal relationships showed significant and greater correlations with the most complex modes of communication, with values greater than 0.64 for speech/discourse, and ranging from 0.29 to 0.47 for single words, writing/drawing and the use of a phone. The rest of the QoL dimensions showed correlations from 0.21 to 0.52 with that set of communication modes. Noteworthily, there was a moderate, though significant, negative correlation between the use of gestures and all QoL dimensions except physical and material wellbeing.

In the case of communication purposes, a very similar pattern was obtained, but with stronger correlations (Figure 1, panel b) and with almost all correlations being significant. Again, self-determination was the dimension that showed the highest correlations, followed by interpersonal relations, social inclusion and personal development dimensions.

Overall, this pattern of results points to the importance of having the ability to use some modes of communication (e.g., speech/discourse) and the need for work towards promoting certain communication purposes as a possible route towards improving QoL. This is particularly the case for the dimensions of self-determination, interpersonal relations and social inclusion that seem quite dependent on an adequate communication profile.

3.4. Personal and Communicative Factors as Predictors of Quality of Life

The second objective of this work was to explore how personal and communication factors impact the QoL of the participants with and without CSN. For this purpose, we carried out a multiple regression analysis with the QLI as a dependent variable and the demographic variables (age, sex, level of disability, number of disabilities, and dependency level) and communication modes (the twelve modes are displayed in Panel b of Figure 1) as independent variables.

In order to find meaningful predictors for QoL, we first tested our set of independent variables in each group by bivariate robust regressions using the function lmrob within the R package robustbase. We obtained the coefficient of determination (R^2) as a measure of the explained variance by each independent variable. Table 5 shows the results of this analysis.

Table 5. Results of bivariate robust regression analyses and correlation coefficients with Quality of Life Index by group.

	Communication Support Needs			
	No		Yes	
Predictors	R^2	r	R^2	r
Personal characteristics				
Age	0.10 **	0.31 *	0.05 **	0.22 *
Sex	0.001	−0.005	0.01	−0.08
Level of disability	0.04	−0.06	0.12 ***	−0.32 ***
Number of additional conditions	0.04	−0.11	0.08 ***	−0.25 ***
Additional conditions				
Physical disability	0.01	−0.07	0.11 ***	−0.33 ***
Sensory—hearing	0.02	−0.15	0.01	−0.09
Sensory—visual	0.004	0.09	0.04 *	−0.18 *
Cerebral palsy	0.07	−0.25 *	0.04 *	−0.18 *
Epilepsy	0.02	−0.14	0.03 *	−0.18 *
Mental health	0.02	−0.20 *	0.02	−0.13
Down syndrome	0.05	−0.21 *	0.001	−0.01
Serious health problems	0.05	−0.20	0.01	−0.08
Behavior problems	0.11 *	−0.33 ***	0.01	−0.07
Modes of communication				
Speech/discourse	0.33	0.24 *	0.22 ***	0.43 ***
Single words	0.08 **	−0.16	0.10 ***	0.32 ***
Writing/drawing	0.05	0.08	0.05 ***	0.22 **
Gestures	0.14 ***	−0.32 **	0.03	−0.15 *
Pictograms	0.04	−0.05	0.06 ***	0.26 **
Manual signs/sign language	0.000	0.03	0.02 *	0.14
Communication board/book	0.06	−0.20 *	0.02 *	0.15 *
Simple communication device	0.01	−0.08	0.02	0.13
Complex communication device	0.000	0.03	0.03 ***	0.15 *
Communication software on a device	0.03 ***	−0.14	0.04 ***	0.18 *
Phone	0.01	0.14	0.10 ***	0.28 ***
E-mail	0.003	0.05	0.01 ***	0.09
Purposes of communication				
Express needs and desires	0.23 ***	0.17	0.19 ***	0.40 ***
Ask for help	0.23 ***	0.17	0.18 ***	0.39 ***
Show likes and preferences	0.23 ***	0.17	0.27 ***	0.46 ***
Express opinions	0.000	0.14	0.15 ***	0.39 ***
Exchange information	0.01	0.15	0.11 ***	0.34 ***
Discuss ailments	0.01 ***	0.18	0.25 ***	0.42 ***
Express feelings	—	0.21 *	0.16 ***	0.39 ***
Talk to family and friends	0.02	0.13	0.17 ***	0.42 ***
Storytelling	0.01	0.11	0.09 ***	0.30 ***
Talk to people around	0.01	0.13	0.12 ***	0.36 ***
Have new relationships	0.02	0.20*	0.14 ***	0.37 ***

— not converged; *** $p < 0.001$; ** $p < 0.01$; * $p < 0.05$.

We then selected the predictors that had a $R^2 \geq 0.04$, which is the recommended minimum effect size representing a "practically" significant effect for social science data [47]. With those predictors, the best subset regression procedure [48] was used to find out the best-fit model from all possible subset models according to goodness-of-fit criteria. Specifically, both the Bayesian information criterion (BIC) and Akaike information criterion (AIC) were evaluated for models selected with a branch-and-bound algorithm and no interactions were considered, in order to build a parsimonious (simple) and a complex model, respectively. The complex model retained 10 variables, while the simple retained only five (see Table 6).

Table 6. Variables included in the two best models (simple and complex) selected with best subset regression procedure.

Predictor	Simple Model (BIC)	Complex Model (AIC)
Age		YES
Level of disability	YES	YES
Physical disability		YES
Speech/discourse	YES	YES
Pictograms		YES
Communication software	YES	YES
Express needs and desires		YES
Show likes and preferences	YES	YES
Storytelling		YES
Have new relationships (yes)	YES	YES

The two models were fitted with robust regression techniques, verifying the reduction in robust deviance achieved in comparison with an intercept-only model for both. Moreover, a significant reduction in robust deviance for the simple model with respect to the complex model was found (deviance-type test (5268) = 30.56; $p < 0.001$); thus, we will report the results of the most parsimonious model only.

In Table 7, bootstrapped regression coefficients are shown for the simple model fitted with the whole sample. Multiple R^2 showed that the model explained 66% of the variance, denoting a large effect. All predictor variables except communication software use were significant for predicting QLI. Having competences for speech/discourse and for showing likes and preferences showed a large effect with increments of one for the standard deviation of QoL. Similarly, the use of communication to initiate new relationships showed a significant effect, although of a more moderate size. The level of disability showed a small negative effect on QoL.

Table 7. Bootstrapped robust multiple regression coefficients (whole sample).

	B (95 % CI)	Bias	SE (Standard Error)	p
(Intercept)	82.2 (69.0,96.6)	0.1	7.0	0.001 ***
Speech/discourse (yes)	17.7 (14.5,20.8)	−0.0	1.6	0.001 ***
Communication software (yes)	16.7 (−14.9,40.6)	−1.4	13.5	0.111
Show likes and preferences (yes)	15.5 (10.8,20.0)	0.1	2.4	0.002 ***
Have new relationships (yes)	4.3 (−0.02,7.7)	−0.1	1.9	0.026 *
Level of disability	−0.2 (−0.3,−0.0)	−0.0	0.1	0.009 **

*** $p < 0.001$; ** $p < 0.01$; * $p < 0.05$.

In Table 8, bootstrapped regression coefficients are shown for the simple model fitted with the CSN group data. Multiple R^2 showed that the model explained 54% of the variance, denoting, again, a large effect. In this case, all the predictors were significant, with similar values as the model with the total sample. The use of communication software was significant, with a large effect, although it also had a wide confidence interval.

Table 8. Bootstrapped robust multiple regression coefficients (CSN group).

	B (95 % CI)	Bias	SE	p
(Intercept)	90.6 (71.3,114.8)	1.4	11.2	0.001 ***
Speech/discourse (yes)	18.8 (14.1,23.6)	−0.1	2.3	0.001 ***
Communication software (yes)	19.7 (−1.7,34.7)	−0.2	8.4	0.034 *
Show likes and preferences (yes)	15.0 (9.8,19.3)	−0.2	2.6	0.005 **
Have new relationships (yes)	3.8 (−0.5,7.8)	−0.2	2.1	0.039 *
Level of disability	−0.3 (−0.5,−0.1)	−0.0	0.1	0.005 **

*** $p < 0.001$; ** $p < 0.01$; * $p < 0.05$.

3.5. Professionals' Perceptions: ACC Use and Training

Finally, we looked at the opinions of the professionals on the situation of cognitive accessibility and support in the environment for communication and training on the AAC necessary to support people with CSN. The results are shown in Table 9.

Table 9. Percentage of yes responses as a function of communication support needs.

Supports Provided	CSN			
	No ($n = 98$)	Yes ($n = 182$)	χ^2 p-Value	SMD
Have the disability support services ever worked with the user using AAC (Augmentative/Alternative Communication)?	8.4	21.8	<0.01	0.38
Are the disability support services adapted from the point of view of cognitive accessibility for the user?	68.0	51.1	<0.01	0.35
Is the training received to provide communication support (e.g., AAC) adequate, taking into account the person's profile?	35.4	14.1	<0.001	0.51

In general, it was verified that a low percentage of people in the CSN group had received some kind of intervention by way of AAC. The supporting staff reported that the disability support services were adapted from the point of view of cognitive accessibility for a little more than half of the persons in the CSN group (51.1%) and in a significantly higher percentage (68%) in the group without CSN. Finally, with regard to the question on the training received in relation to the profile of the person, it was verified that the professionals consider the training received to be much less adequate in the case of the group of persons with CSN.

4. Discussion

This research aimed to describe the communication profile in adults with intellectual disabilities who differ in their degree of required communication support needs, as well as to explore the relationship between their communication profile and their quality of life.

On the one hand, it was possible to verify that the great majority of people in the CSN group (90.7%) do not use speech or discourse and depend greatly on the use of gestures to communicate. This restricted mode of communication allows them, however, to exhibit communicative purposes related to basic needs, although in a significantly lower percentage than in the group without support needs. However, there is also a notable difficulty in the ability to communicate with a more complex social function, such as expressing opinions or exchanging information, and talking with people in their surroundings or initiating new relationships.

On the other hand, a clear relationship between the communication profile and QoL has been verified, with lower QoL levels on all the dimensions of Schalock and Verdugo's model for people in the CSN group. We also found evidence showing that the dimensions of self-determination, social inclusion, interpersonal relationships and personal development are the ones that have the strongest relationship to the communication profile. That is, the greater the ability to communicate in ID, the higher the score in the abovementioned QoL dimensions.

In general, the results are convergent with those of other studies that relate high levels of functioning to high levels of QoL, especially those studies which consider that communication skills contribute to increased self-determination [49–51]. With regard to this relationship, a pattern of strong positive correlations between communication purposes and self-determination have also been found, clearly showing the importance of promoting certain communication purposes that can also be considered as rights as far as the UN Convention [39] and the Communication Bill of Rights [1] are concerned. These entail rights such as the freedom and security of the person or the right to live independently and be included in the community, and communication purposes such as the right to express personal preferences and feelings, to interact socially, to maintain social closeness, to build relationships or to make comments and share opinions, to name a few.

Our results, therefore, extend the findings of previous investigations [26] into the adult population with ID, in verifying that having speech/discourse competence is a powerful predictor of QoL. Moreover, in the current work, it has been observed that the relationship between speech/discourse competence and QoL is of the greatest magnitude in the case of the dimensions of self-determination, social inclusion and interpersonal relations. In addition, other general factors related to QoL have been identified, such as having a communication profile that enables one to show likes and preferences or to establish new relationships. These findings stress, therefore, the need to intervene explicitly in the improvement of communication profiles to allow for the boosting of those QoL dimensions in ID. In the case of the CSN group, the use of AAC communication software was also a significant predictor of QoL, showing the importance of AAC systems for people with complex communication needs. Overall, our finding of a set of significant predictors has the potential to be implemented in practice, as it may aid the development of tools that target the identification of people at risk of low QoL. At the same time, the results point to different aspects of communication that might deserve special attention when it comes to the development of interventions.

Finally, the need for the training of professionals in the field of communication supports (e.g., knowledge of AAC systems) has been verified. This result is consistent with that obtained by Dalton and Sweeney [33], evidencing that support staff do not always have the training or resources to provide the support required by their users. This in turn, is likely to impinge on the staff's possibility to adequately plan for communication support.

This study has some limitations. The first has to do with the selection of the sample. Although it is a sample with an adequate size, it was not possible to carry out totally random sampling, so there is a danger of a selection bias occurring. Along with this, the fact that the professionals carried out the assessment of both quality of life and of the identification of which group the participants belonged to (CSN/non-CSN) could limit the scope of our results. Ideally, the individuals with ID themselves should be the ones responding to the survey; however, this was not possible due to the nature of the communication difficulties of some of the participants. In this sense, we agree with Nieuwenhuijse et al. [52] in considering that research on QoL in people who cannot express themselves is a challenge and that new ways to carry out the QoL assessment should be explored. Moreover, it can be noted that our sample was very heterogeneous in terms of age, with some individuals as young as 19 and others in their seventies. Future studies could recruit participants within different age groups and directly compare whether or not there are any age effects on communication needs and their relation to QoL. Moreover, caution should be taken when generalizing our results to adults who reside in their family homes, as their reality in terms of the level of support and subsequent QoL can be different to the one experienced by individuals who are institutionalized.

5. Conclusions

This study has explored communication profiles and their relationship to QoL in a sample of 281 adults with ID. Overall, low levels of QoL were found for the entire sample, and especially for the group of participants who were identified as having communication support needs. More specifically, another significant finding to emerge from this study is that communicative profile is related to some of the QoL dimensions, such as self-determination, social inclusion and interpersonal relationships. This is especially important given the close link between those quality of life dimensions and some fundamental rights of people with disabilities [38,39]. Moreover, the close relationship between the communication profile and QoL in adults with intellectual disabilities, in particular for those with communication support needs, makes it clear that interventions to provide communication support for improving everyday communication should be a priority for disability support services providing services to users with these profiles. We think that a good starting point for addressing these challenges is the guidance document of the National Joint Committee for the Communication Needs of People with Severe Disabilities (NJC) [1,53], which offers information derived from a recent literature review that could be used by professionals interested in implementing effective communication services and opportunities.

This study has also found that professionals perceive the need for training on how to support people with ID as well as on how to address the necessary adaptations in the environment that facilitate communication to ensure that their right to communicate is upheld. Therefore, specific training plans are needed in relation to issues such as communication assessment, goal selection, interventions to improve communication, and interventions to improve environmental supports such as cognitive accessibility, adaptations to easy-reading or signage.

The main implication of the results of this research is to highlight, with supporting evidence, the potential for communication support interventions to improve QoL. One consequence of this research is that disability support services ought to explicitly address the communication needs of their users. In the case of AMÁS Social Foundation, the participants' home disability support service, this research has led to the creation of group of interest in communication and cognitive accessibility, in which professionals from all the adult disability support services participate. These groups also participate in promoting measures to improve cognitive accessibility and support in the environment, as well as in providing specialized support for all the people who need support with communication. To this end, specific measures have been taken, such as promoting the participation of experts in AAC in all disability support services, and developing a training plan for AAC and accessibility for all professionals and volunteers. The next step will be to carry out a post-intervention evaluation, to assess the impact of these measures. If the relationship between communication and QoL is as strong as observed in this study, we hope to observe, in a future investigation, that increased measures to support communication will lead to improved QoL among people with complex support needs.

Supplementary Materials: The following are available online at http://www.mdpi.com/1660-4601/17/20/7370/s1, Document S1: Communication profile questionnaire.

Author Contributions: Conceptualization, J.C.G. and E.D.; data curation, E.D.; formal analysis, E.D.; investigation, J.C.G.; methodology, J.C.G. and E.D.; project administration, J.C.G.; resources, J.C.G.; software, E.D.; supervision, E.D.; writing—original draft, J.C.G., E.D. and D.Z.W.; writing—review and editing, J.C.G., E.D., D.Z.W. and M.S. All authors have read and agreed to the published version of the manuscript.

Funding: This research received no external funding.

Acknowledgments: The authors would like to thank professionals from Fundación Grupo AMÁS who participated in the study.

Conflicts of Interest: The authors declare no conflict of interest.

References

1. Brady, N.C.; Bruce, S.; Goldman, A.; Erickson, K.; Mineo, B.; Ogletree, B.T.; Paul, D.; Romski, M.A.; Sevcik, R.; Siegel, E.; et al. Communication Services and Supports for Individuals with Severe Disabilities: Guidance for Assessment and Intervention. *Am. J. Intellect. Dev. Disabil.* **2016**, *121*, 121–138. [CrossRef]
2. Markham, C.; van Laar, D.; Gibbard, D.; Dean, T. Children with speech, language and communication needs: Their perceptions of their quality of life. *Int. J. Lang. Commun. Disord.* **2009**, *44*, 748–768. [CrossRef]

3. Saito, Y. Augmentative and alternative communication practice in the pursuit of family quality of life: A review of the literature. *Res. Pract. Pers. Sev. Disabil.* **2007**, *32*, 50–65. [CrossRef]
4. Smith, M.; Manduchi, B.; Burke, É.; Carroll, R.; McCallion, P.; McCarron, M. Communication difficulties in adults with Intellectual Disability: Results from a national cross-sectional study. *Res. Dev. Disabil.* **2020**, *97*, 103557. [CrossRef]
5. Coppens-Hofman, M.C.; Terband, H.; Snik, A.F.M.; Maassen, B.A.M. Speech Characteristics and Intelligibility in Adults with Mild and Moderate Intellectual Disabilities. *Folia Phoniatr. Logop.* **2016**, *68*, 175–182. [CrossRef]
6. Marrus, N.; Hall, L. Intellectual disability and language disorder. *Child Adolesc. Psychiatr. Clin. N. Am.* **2017**, *26*, 539–554. [CrossRef]
7. Tuffrey-Wijne, I.; McEnhill, L. Communication difficulties and intellectual disability in end-of-life care. *Int. J. Palliat. Nurs.* **2008**, *14*, 189–194. [CrossRef]
8. Purcell, M.; Morris, I.; McConkey, R. Staff Perceptions of the Communicative Competence of Adult Persons with Intellectual Disabilities. *Br. J. Dev. Disabil.* **1999**, *45*, 16–25. [CrossRef]
9. Chew, K.L.; Iacono, T.; Tracy, J. Overcoming communication barriers - working with patients with intellectual disabilities. *Aust. Fam. Physician* **2009**, *38*, 10–14.
10. Light, J.; Mcnaughton, D. Designing AAC Research and Intervention to Improve Outcomes for Individuals with Complex Communication Needs. *Augment. Altern. Commun.* **2015**, *31*, 85–96. [CrossRef]
11. Snowling, M.J.; Adams, J.W.; Bishop, D.V.M.; Stothard, S.E. Educational attainments of school leavers with a preschool history of speech-language impairments. *Int. J. Lang. Commun. Disord.* **2001**, *36*, 173–183. [CrossRef]
12. Ball, S.J. *Language and Social Advantage: Theory into Practice*; Clegg, J., Ginsborg, J., Eds.; John Wiley and Sons, Ltd.: Chichester, UK, 2006.
13. Gilmore, L.; Cuskelly, M. Vulnerability to loneliness in people with intellectual disability: An explanatory model: Vulnerability to loneliness. *J. Policy Pract. Intellect. Disabil.* **2014**, *11*, 192–199. [CrossRef]
14. Overmars-Marx, T.; Thomése, F.; Verdonschot, M.; Meininger, H. Advancing social inclusion in the neighbourhood for people with an intellectual disability: An exploration of the literature. *Disabil. Soc.* **2014**, *29*, 255–274. [CrossRef]
15. Felce, D. Defining and applying the concept of quality of life. *J. Intellect. Disabil. Res.* **1997**, *41*, 126–135. [CrossRef] [PubMed]
16. Hughes, C.; Hwang, B.; Kim, J.H.; Eisenman, L.T.; Killian, D.J. Quality of life in applied research: A review and analysis of empirical measures. *Am. J. Ment. Retard.* **1995**, *99*, 623–641.
17. McVilly, K.R.; Rawlinson, R.B. Quality of life issues in the development and evaluation of services for people with intellectual disability. *J. Intellect. Dev. Disabil.* **1998**, *23*, 199–218. [CrossRef]
18. McIntyre, D. The difficulties of inclusive pedagogy for initial teacher education and some thoughts on the way forward. *Teach. Teach. Educ. Int. J. Res. Stud.* **2009**, *25*, 602–608. [CrossRef]
19. Rapley, M. *Quality of Life Research: A Critical Introduction*; SAGE Pubications: London, UK, 2003.
20. Rusch, F.R.; Millar, D.M. Emerging transition best practices. In *Beyond High School: Transition from School to Work*; Rusch, F.R., Chadsey, J.G., Eds.; Wadsworth Publishing Co.: Belmont, CA, USA, 1998.
21. Taylor, S.J.; Bogdan, R.C. Quality of life and the individual's perspective. In *Quality of Life: Perspectives and Issues*; American Association on Mental Retardation: Washington, DC, USA, 1990; pp. 27–40.
22. Bowling, A. *Measuring Health: A Review of Quality of Life Measurement Scales*, 2nd ed.; Open University Press: Buckingham, PA, USA, 1997.
23. Kraemer, B.R.; McIntyre, L.L.; Blacher, J. Quality of life for young adults with mental retardation during transition. *Ment. Retard.* **2003**, *41*, 250–262. [CrossRef]
24. Schalock, R.L.; Keith, K.D. *Quality of Life Questionnaire*; IDS: Worthington, OH, USA, 1993.
25. Schalock, R.L.; Lemanowicz, J.A.; Conroy, J.W.; Feinstein, C.S. A multi-variate investigative study of the correlates of quality of life. *J. Dev. Disabil.* **1994**, *3*, 59–73.
26. Biggs, E.E.; Carter, E.W. Quality of Life for Transition-Age Youth with Autism or Intellectual Disability. *J. Autism Dev. Disord.* **2016**, *46*, 190–204. [CrossRef]
27. Davis, E.; Reddihough, D.; Murphy, N.; Epstein, A.; Reid, S.M.; Whitehouse, A.; Williams, K.; Leonard, H.; Downs, J. Exploring quality of life of children with cerebral palsy and intellectual disability: What are the important domains of life? *Child. Care Health Dev.* **2017**, *43*, 854–860. [CrossRef] [PubMed]

28. Neumann, S.; Quinting, J.; Rosenkranz, A.; de Beer, C.; Jonas, K.; Stenneken, P. Quality of life in adults with neurogenic speech-language-communication difficulties: A systematic review of existing measures. *J. Commun. Disord.* **2019**, *79*, 24–45. [CrossRef] [PubMed]
29. Cruice, M.; Worrall, L.; Hickson, L.; Murison, R. Finding a focus for quality of life with aphasia: Social and emotional health, and psychological well-being. *Aphasiology* **2003**, *17*, 333–353. [CrossRef]
30. Hilari, K.; Needle, J.J.; Harrison, K.L. What are the important factors in health-related quality of life for people with aphasia? A systematic review. *Arch. Phys. Med. Rehabil.* **2012**, *93*, S86–S95. [CrossRef] [PubMed]
31. Hilari, K.; Byng, S. Health-related quality of life in people with severe aphasia. *Int. J. Lang. Commun. Disord.* **2009**, *44*, 193–205. [CrossRef]
32. Schertz, M.; Karni-Visel, Y.; Tamir, A.; Genizi, J.; Roth, D. Family quality of life among families with a child who has a severe neurodevelopmental disability: Impact of family and child socio-demographic factors. *Res. Dev. Disabil.* **2016**, *53–54*, 95–106. [CrossRef]
33. Dalton, C.; Sweeney, J. Communication supports in residential services for people with an intellectual disability. *Br. J. Learn. Disabil.* **2013**, *41*, 22–30. [CrossRef]
34. Schalock, R.L.; Verdugo, M.Á. *Handbook on Quality of Life for Human Service Practitioners*; American Association on Mental Retardation: Washington, DC, USA, 2002.
35. Van Hecke, N.; Claes, C.; Vanderplasschen, W.; De Maeyer, J.; De Witte, N.; Vandevelde, S. Conceptualisation and Measurement of Quality of Life Based on Schalock and Verdugo's Model: A Cross-Disciplinary Review of the Literature. *Soc. Indic. Res.* **2018**, *137*, 335–351. [CrossRef]
36. Schalock, R.L.; Verdugo, M.A. El concepto de calidad de vida en los servicios y apoyos para personas con discapacidad intelectual [The concept of quality of life in services and supports for people with intellectual disabilities]. *Siglo Cero Rev. Esp. Sobre Discapac. Intelect.* **2007**, *38*, 21–36.
37. Tamarit Cuadrado, J. La transformación de los servicios hacia la calidad de vida. Una iniciativa de innovación social de FEAPS. *Siglo Cero Rev. Esp. Sobre Discapac. Intelect.* **2015**, *46*, 47. [CrossRef]
38. Navas, P.; Gomez, L.E.; Verdugo, M.A.; Schalock, R.L. Derechos de las personas con discapacidad intelectual: Implicaciones de la Convención de Naciones Unidas [Rights of Persons with Intellectual Disabilities: Implications of the United Nations Convention]. *Siglo Cero Rev. Esp. Sobre Discapac. Intelect.* **2012**, *43*, 7–28.
39. United Nations. Convention on the Rights of Persons with Disabilities. Available online: http://www.ohchr.org/EN/Issues/Disability/Pages/TrainingmaterialCRPDConvention_OptionalProtocol.aspx (accessed on 1 July 2020).
40. Verdugo, M.A.; Gómez, L.E.; Arias, B.; Navas, P.; Schalock, R.L. Measuring quality of life in people with intellectual and multiple disabilities: Validation of the San Martín scale. *Res. Dev. Disabil.* **2014**, *35*, 75–86. [CrossRef] [PubMed]
41. Hierro Zorrilla, I.; Verdugo Alonso, M.Á.; Gómez Sánchez, L.E.; Fernández Ezquerra, S.; Cisneros Fernández, P. Evaluación de la calidad de vida en personas con discapacidades significativas: Aplicación de la Escala San Martín en la Fundación Obra San Martín. *Rev. Esp. Discapac.* **2015**, *3*, 93–105. [CrossRef]
42. Vega Córdova, V.; Jerano Rio, C.; Flores Robaina, N.; Cruz Ortiz, M.; Artaza, C. Calidad de vida de adultos con discapacidad intelectual institucionalizados en Chile desde la perspectiva de los proveedores de servicios. *Univ. Psychol. Ed. Electrónica* **2013**, *12*, 1–27. [CrossRef]
43. Fried-Oken, M.; Fox, L.; Rau, M.T.; Tullman, J.; Baker, G.; Hindal, M.; Wile, N.; Lou, J.-S. Purposes of AAC device use for persons with ALS as reported by caregivers. *Augment. Altern. Commun. Baltim. Md 1985* **2006**, *22*, 209–221. [CrossRef]
44. R Core Team. *R: A Language and Environment for Statistical Computing*; R Foundation for Statistical Computing: Vienna, Austria, 2020.
45. Austin, P.C. Using the standardized difference to compare the prevalence of a binary variable between two groups in observational research. *Commun. Stat. Simul. Comput.* **2009**, *38*, 1228–1234. [CrossRef]
46. Friedrich, S.; Pauly, M. MATS: Inference for potentially singular and heteroscedastic MANOVA. *J. Multivar. Anal.* **2018**, *165*, 166–179. [CrossRef]
47. Ferguson, C.J. An effect size primer: A guide for clinicians and researchers. *Prof. Psychol. Res. Pract.* **2009**, *40*, 532–538. [CrossRef]
48. Zhang, Z. Variable selection with stepwise and best subset approaches. *Ann. Transl. Med.* **2016**, *4*, 136. [CrossRef]

49. Beukelman, D.R.; Mirenda, P.; Ball, L.J. *Augmentative and Alternative Communication: Supporting Children and Adults with Complex. Communication Needs*; Paul H. Brookes Baltimore: Baltimore, MD, USA, 2012.
50. Brown, F.; Gothelf, C.R.; Guess, D.; Lehr, D.H. Self-Determination for Individuals with the Most Severe Disabilities: Moving beyond Chimera. *J. Assoc. Pers. Sev. Handicaps* **1998**, *23*, 17–26. [CrossRef]
51. Light, J. "Communication is the essence of human life": Reflections on communicative competence. *Augment. Altern. Commun.* **1997**, *13*, 61–70. [CrossRef]
52. Nieuwenhuijse, A.M.; Willems, D.L.; van Goudoever, J.B.; Echteld, M.A.; Olsman, E. Quality of life of persons with profound intellectual and multiple disabilities: A narrative literature review of concepts, assessment methods and assessors. *J. Intellect. Dev. Disabil.* **2019**, *44*, 261–271. [CrossRef]
53. National Joint Committee for the Communication Needs of Persons with Severe Disabilities. Guidelines for Meeting the Communication Needs of Persons with Severe Disabilities. Available online: https://www.asha.org/policy/GL1992-00201/ (accessed on 20 June 2020).

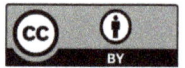

© 2020 by the authors. Licensee MDPI, Basel, Switzerland. This article is an open access article distributed under the terms and conditions of the Creative Commons Attribution (CC BY) license (http://creativecommons.org/licenses/by/4.0/).

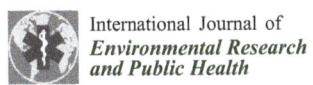

Article

Toward a Better "Person–Environment Fit" through Items Calibration of the SIS-C

Víctor B. Arias [1], Antonio M. Amor [1,*], Miguel A. Verdugo [1], María Fernández [1], Benito Arias [2] and Alba Aza [1]

1. Institute on Community Integration, Department of Personality, Assessment and Psychological Treatments, Faculty of Psychology, University of Salamanca, 37005 Salamanca, Spain; vbarias@usal.es (V.B.A.); verdugo@usal.es (M.A.V.); mariafernandez@usal.es (M.F.); azhernandez@usal.es (A.A.)
2. Institute on Community Integration, Department of Psychology, Faculty of Education and Social Work, University of Valladolid, 47011 Valladolid, Spain; barias@psi.uva.es
* Correspondence: aamor@usal.es; Tel.: +34-670576341

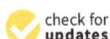

Received: 15 April 2020; Accepted: 14 May 2020; Published: 15 May 2020

Abstract: The Supports Intensity Scale–Children's Version (SIS-C) is the only available tool to assess extraordinary support needs for children and adolescents with intellectual disability. In past years, several works have proclaimed the need for its ongoing improvement as a measurement instrument. To contribute to this line of research, the goal of this work is to analyze the reliability of the SIS-C and its usefulness to distinguish between different levels of intensity of support needs. To address this, 814 children and adolescents with intellectual disability (M = 11.13 years; SD = 3.41) were assessed using the SIS-C Spanish version. Item response theory analyses were conducted to estimate latent scores and assess measurement quality along the support needs continuum. The SIS-C items showed good overall discrimination and information values, and none showed problems that required their removal or modification. However, all the scales composing the SIS-C showed problems in discerning high levels of intensity of support needs, especially for children and adolescents with severe/profound intellectual disability. This ceiling effect may be an obstacle for both research and practice involving the SIS-C. Implications for research and practice are discussed, and future lines of research for improving the SIS-C are provided.

Keywords: context-based intervention; social-ecological model of disability; person–environment fit; supports paradigm; support needs; support needs assessment; quality of life; rights; Supports intensity scale (SIS)

1. Introduction

Framed in a social-ecological approach and in a strengths-based perspective, the supports paradigm conceives intellectual disability (ID) as a state of functioning characterized by a mismatch between the persons with ID competencies and the environmental demands, defined by the contexts of participation and the age and culturally appropriate activities to develop in such contexts [1]. This mismatch originates support needs, understood as a "psychological construct referring to the pattern and intensity of supports necessary for a person to participate in activities linked with normative human functioning" [2] (p. 135).

Leaving behind the concept of ID as a deficit within the person and emphasizing the interaction person–environment is the defining characteristic of the supports paradigm [1]. From this paradigm, it is assumed that all persons have support needs because everyone experiences mismatches in certain situations or activities. Thus, through the lens of the supports paradigm, the main difference between persons with and without ID concerns the nature of their support needs. In this sense, persons with ID, given that they experience intense and ongoing mismatches, have extraordinary support needs that extend beyond what most typically functioning people need to participate in the same contexts and activities [2].

Beyond this conceptualization, the supports paradigm has also brought a renewal in professional practices in the field of ID. Contrary to approaches focused on the functional rehabilitation of persons with ID [3], the supports paradigm emphasizes the "support needs assessment and planning" process. Through this process, persons with ID define first, without restrictions, those contexts and activities in which they would like to participate following their vital expectations. These contexts and activities are the bases to determine the pattern and intensity of the extraordinary support needs that persons with ID require in order to offer them personalized supports. Supports are defined as "resources and strategies that aim to promote the development, education, interests, and personal well-being of a person and that enhance individual functioning" [2] (pp.135). Supports can be classified according to their nature and focus. Thompson et al. [2] distinguish between personal supports (i.e., those including natural or informal supports and paid or professional supports), technological supports (i.e., including high technology, like a wheelchair; medium technology, like an app; or low technology, like the use of reminders), and environmental adaptations, modifications and accommodations. According to their focus, supports can be person-directed (i.e., those whose focus is to build upon the strengths of the person) or be directed at modifying environmental demands and tasks, making them more accessible [1]. No matter their nature and focus, from this social-ecological perspective, supports are bridges that maximize the person-environment fit, and aim to meet the needs and improve the functioning and participation of persons with ID in their life project–which is critical for them to achieve personal desired outcomes that increase their quality of life (QoL) [1,3–5]. In a nutshell, the supports paradigm allows the building of bridges for persons with ID to be causal agents over their lives, consistent with the United Nation's Convention on the Rights of Persons with Disabilities [6].

The importance of the support needs construct within the supports paradigm has motivated a growing emphasis on its measurement. Although there exist different approaches to assess support needs, the current trend focuses on developing standardized measures of extraordinary support needs for persons with ID based on the supports paradigm [7,8], such as the Service Needs Assessment Profile [9]; the Instrument to Classify Support Needs for People with Disability [10]; and the Supports Intensity Scale [11], updated as the Supports Intensity Scale–Adult's Version (SIS-A) [12]. Of these, the SIS-A is the most used at the international level, translated into 13 languages and used in 16 countries according to the American Association on Intellectual and Developmental Disabilities (AAIDD) [13]. The SIS-A allows the measurement of the extraordinary support needs that adults with ID aged 16–64 require to participate in 49 activities in six contexts of daily living: Home living, Community living, Lifelong learning, Employment, Health and safety, and Social activities. To assess extraordinary support needs, each activity is rated following three measurement methods: frequency, daily support time, and type of support. Several works have reported evidence on the good psychometric properties of the scores obtained using the SIS-A (for an in-detail study, see [7]).

The proliferation of standardized measures of extraordinary support needs, such as the SIS-A [12], has facilitated the implementation of the supports paradigm. These tools have not only boosted the support needs assessment and planning process [8], but also improved the efficiency of resources allocation at organizational level, a critical resource to optimize supports planning for improving the QoL of persons with ID [14,15]. Given that support needs assessment and planning should be started as soon as possible and be offered through the lifespan of the person with ID [16], the AAIDD, given the lack of standardized measures of extraordinary support needs for children and adolescents with ID and taking as a reference the good psychometric properties reported in relation to the SIS-A, developed and validated the Supports Intensity Scale–Children's Version (SIS-C) [17], the version for children and adolescents of the SIS-A.

The SIS-C (described subsequently in the instrument section) was designed to assess extraordinary support needs in children and adolescents with ID between 5 and 16 years [17]. Starting from the hypothesis of the influence of age on support needs (i.e., the younger the children, the stronger their support needs), the standardization sample for developing norms was stratified following six age cohorts (i.e., 5–6, 7–8, 9–10, 11–12, 13–14, and 15–16). The standardized portion of the tool aims for the assessment of the extraordinary support needs that children and adolescents with ID may require to participate in 61 activities in seven contexts: Home living activities (HLA), Community and neighborhood activities (CNA), School participation activities (SPA), School learning activities (SLA), Health and safety activities (HSA), Social activities (SA), and Advocacy activities (AA). As in the SIS-A [12], each activity is rated across three measurement methods (i.e., type of support, frequency, and daily support time) and the scores obtained through the use of the SIS-C count with evidence of validity and reliability [7]. The SIS-C has been adapted and validated in different contexts (e.g., [18]) and there is an increasing interest in investigating its appropriateness and evidence of validity and reliability for children and adolescents with other disabilities [19–21].

Since its availability, the SIS-C [17] has been used by various studies for support needs assessment and planning for children and adolescents with ID. For example, Walker et al. [22], on the basis of the SIS-C use, developed personalized educational plans that, rather than focusing only on student's literacy, aimed to enhance other relevant personal outcomes such as participation in their community. Recently, Schalock, van Loon et al. [23] used the SIS-C to inform a personalized support plan for improving the QoL of a student with ID in inclusive settings in the Netherlands. However, despite these works, use of the SIS-C is still not as generalized as that of the SIS-A [24], so efforts are being made to promote its use within general education settings to enhance outcomes for students with ID [25].

Notwithstanding the evidence on the use of the SIS-C and the good psychometric properties reported for its use with children and adolescents with ID [7], a critical issue concerning the SIS-C use is its refinement as a measurement instrument—a need that has already started to be addressed by research. Specifically, one line of research that has gathered much attention is the analysis of the SIS-C properties by considering the three measurement methods used to score support needs [26,27]. Seo et al. [26] explored seven multitrait–multimethod (MTMM) models, each one including a substantive trait (i.e., the support needs domain) and three method factors matching the three measurement models used in the assessment (i.e., type of support, frequency, and daily support time). The authors found that, in general, the factorial loadings of the substantive traits were significantly higher than those of the method factors ($p < 0.01$), except for the items of the CNA and AA domains, whose average factorial loadings were significantly higher for the "daily support time" method than for the substantive trait. With these results, the authors concluded that the MTMM model used demonstrated enough evidence of convergence validity to support the use of the raw scores obtained through the three measurement models used in the SIS-C.

Although the previous study highlighted the existence of effects associated with the measurement methods, it did not yield enough information to make decisions based on the relevance of such effects. A way to facilitate the interpretation of the MTMM model used in the previous research would be through the quantification of the size of the factors in terms of explained variance and the proportion of reliable variance. With the evidence of the abovementioned study, the interpretation of the bifactor model needed the quantification of its impact on the unidimensionality of the model and of the reliability with which the substantive trait reproduces the target construct. Starting from this rationale, Verdugo et al. [27] replicated the previous work in Spain and extended it by analyzing the relevance of the method effects to determine whether these effects hindered a precise support needs assessment, and if they were relevant enough to change the way individual scores are produced or even to generate modifications to the SIS-C. To address this, the authors used a bifactor model as an approximation to analyze the MTMM and monotrait–heteromethod matrices. Essentially, the findings were similar to those reported by Seo et al. [26] regarding the location of the main sources of method variances, with the CNA and HSA domains the most affected and the method variance concentrated in the daily support time items. The implications of this work are relevant, indicating that the raw scores obtained through the daily support time measurement method are significantly contaminated by the variance unrelated to the support needs construct [27].

The cited studies have focused on investigating the construct validity of the SIS-C through the comparison of different factorial structures. One aspect that has been less studied is the reliability of the SIS-C and its utility for the purposes for which it was designed. Traditionally, the extent to which a set of items works well is judged by a single index such as the alpha coefficient [28]. Here, the standard error of measurement (SEM) of the assessed person is inversely related to the reliability coefficient so that the reliability and the standard error are constant for all the persons, no matter their score in the test of their real level in the construct. However, it is more realistic and valid to assume that a measure will present different accuracy levels at different ranges of the latent variable [29–33] so that a measurement instrument may be reliable for a certain range of the latent variable but not very reliable in others, as is usually the case, for example, in clinical screening instruments [34].

That said, the main goal of the SIS-C is to assess extraordinary support needs to provide personalized systems of supports to enhance the person's QoL [8]. Consequently, it is expected that the SIS-C assesses with reliability a wide range of intensity of support needs so that most children and adolescents with ID are evaluated with enough reliability no matter the intensity of their support needs. However, to the best of our knowledge, there are no works that have investigated the reliability of the SIS-C at different ranges of support needs. Is the SIS-C reliable enough for the assessment of support needs at all ranges of support needs? How accurately does the SIS-C capture individual differences in the continuum of support needs? Is the SIS-C useful in the case of all the children and adolescents with ID, or is it only useful for certain ranges of the intensity of support needs? Is it necessary to reformulate, remove, or add items to improve the functioning of the SIS-C? Answering these questions will generate a better knowledge of the psychometric properties and utility of the SIS-C, as well as suggest improvement actions for its refinement—all being critical issues for improving current practices regarding support needs assessment and planning for children and adolescents with ID. With the purpose of addressing these questions, this study aimed to analyze the SIS-C reliability and its usefulness in distinguishing between different levels of intensity of support needs. Specifically, we used models based on item response theory (IRT) to obtain the location and discrimination parameters of the 61 activities (i.e., items) of the SIS-C. IRT does not conceptualize the reliability as a constant property for all the assessed persons, but rather allows the measurement error to vary along the latent continuum depending on the interaction between the properties of the items and the characteristics of the persons. This, along with the possibility of estimating the amount of information provided by each item, will allow us to obtain relevant insights regarding the quality and the usefulness of the measure for its purposes.

2. Materials and Methods

2.1. Instrument

The SIS-C is the only standardized measure available to assess extraordinary support needs in children and adolescents with ID aged 5–16 years [17]. As mentioned (see Introduction), the tool is normed following age bands (i.e., 5–6, 7–8, 9–10, 11–12, 13–14, and 15–16). Regarding its structure, the SIS-C comprises two parts. The first part consists of eight items from which to make an a priori estimation of the probable extraordinary support needs that the child or adolescent with ID may have in seven daily living contexts and in general. The second part has two sections: (a) a section related to "Exceptional Medical and Behavioral Support Needs" and (b) the "Support Needs Scale." The Exceptional Medical and Behavioral Support Needs section identifies specific medical conditions (e.g., parenteral feeding) and challenging behaviors (e.g., truancy) that may require substantial levels of support, regardless of the relative intensity of support needs required by the person. These conditions are rated following a three-point Likert rating scale, where higher scores indicate greater needs (i.e., 0 = No support needed; 1 = Some support needed; 2 = Extensive support needed).

The Support Needs Scale is the standardized section of the SIS-C. It includes seven daily living contexts and is designed to assess extraordinary support needs that children and adolescents with ID require to participate in 61 activities related to such contexts. Table 1 describes each activity domain along with the three measurement methods used to rate the intensity of the extraordinary support needs for these domains.

Table 1. Supports Intensity Scale–Children's Version (SIS-C) domains' descriptions and measurement methods for the 'Support Needs Scale' section.

SIS-C activity domains
HLA includes nine household activities. Examples include "eating" and "using electronic devices."
CNA is composed of eight activities involved in being a member of the neighborhood or the community. Exemple activities include "using public services" and "shopping."
SPA incorporates nine activities linked to school participation. "Following classroom and school rules" and "participating in activities in common school areas" are examples of activities in this domain.
SLA is made up of nine activities associated with acquiring knowledge and/or skills while attending school (e.g., "learning" and "completing homework assignments").
HSA involves eight activities linked to assuring safety and health across home, school, and community. Examples are "maintaining physical fitness" and "responding in emergency situations."
SA includes nine activities related to social interactions with others. Among these activities, examples are "making and keeping friends" and "maintaining conversation."
AA are core activities relevant to being the causal agent over one's life. Exemple activities involve "making personal choices and decisions."

Measurement methods' rating scales for each SIS-C activity		
Type of support	Frequency of support	Daily support time
0 = None	0 = Negligible	0 = None
1 = Monitoring	1 = Infrequently	1 = Less than 30 minutes
2 = Verbal/gestural prompting	2 = Frequently	2 = 30 minutes to less than 2 hours
3 = Partial physical assistance	3 = Very frequently	3 = 2 hours to less than 4 hours
4 = Full physical assistance	4 = Always	4 = 4 hours or more

Note. HLA = Home living activities; CNA = Community and neighborhood activities; SPA = School participation activities; SLA = School learning activities; HSA = Health and safety activities; SA = Social activities; AA = Advocacy activities.

Each activity is scored by adding the value given to each measurement method (i.e., each activity can have a score between 0 and 12). Raw scores are transformed into standard scores for each domain. The sum of the standard scores allows calculation of the "Support Needs Index," a measure of the intensity of the extraordinary support required by the child or adolescent with ID. As the SIS-C is normed following age bands, the standard scores and the Support Needs Index give information on the percentile of each child or adolescent, making it possible to know where he/she is along the support needs continuum regarding his/her same-age peers with ID for each domain and globally. The standard scores for each domain also allow calculation of the "Support Needs Profile," which gives information on the distribution of the extraordinary support needs across the domains [17].

The SIS-C follows a semi-structured interview implemented by a qualified interviewer to at least two informants [17]. This semi-structured interview involves an interaction between the interviewer and the informants, and its adequate functioning is necessary to gather an accurate estimation of the extraordinary support needs that the child or adolescent with ID may have. There are different considerations for this semi-structured interview to be regarded as adequate [8,17]: (a) the interviewer's knowledge on the supports paradigm and in the SIS-C; (b) the establishment of a good rapport between the stakeholders; (c) the interviewer's ability to guide the conversations elicited during the interview; and (d) the characteristics and composition of the informants. First, the interviewer should be familiar with the supports paradigm, with the SIS-C goal, and he/she should have completed at least a four-year degree. Second, it is common that the informants, especially when they meet for the first time with the interviewer, feel anxious or that they have the wrong expectations about the interview or the meaning of the SIS-C assessment. Paying attention to the respondents' concerns and doubts, showing flexibility, and adjusting their expectations about the SIS-C goals are chief to establish a good rapport. Third, the interview should flow as a conversation, it being the role of the interviewer to help the respondents focus on the SIS-C purpose whenever necessary. It is the responsibility of the interviewer to gather the relevant information on the extraordinary support needs that the child or adolescent with ID may have for all the SIS-C activities and domains. To gather this information, the interviewer asks the informants about the "extra" support that the child or adolescent with an ID of a certain age band (e.g., 14–15 years) requires beyond the support that a typically developing same-age peer would need to participate in the activity. The interviewer also has to clarify the different measurement methods and the rating scale options and, if there is a disparity between the informants regarding the support needs of the assessed person, then it is necessary to discuss and reach an agreement between all those present in the interview. Finally, regarding the composition and the nature of the informants, it is better to select a dyad of informants composed by a professional and a family member to have a more complete picture of the extraordinary supports required by the child or adolescent with ID in all the SIS-C domains. To be selected as informants, they must have known the assessed child or adolescent for at least three months, and they must have had recent interactions with him/her in the contexts included in the SIS-C [35].

The standardized section of the SIS-C, specifically, its translation and validation in Spanish [18], was used to address the aim of this paper. The SIS-C Spanish follows Tassé and Craig's guidelines to adapt standardized measures to different contexts from the original [36] and the recommendations of the International Test Commission [37]. As in the original version, the SIS-C Spanish has optimal evidence of validity and reliability regarding its scores [7].

2.2. Participants

The use of the SIS-C to assess extraordinary support needs involves, beyond interviewers, the assessed children or adolescents with ID and the informants reporting on their support needs [17].

A total of 814 children and adolescents with ID were assessed (M = 11.13 years; SD = 3.41). The students who were assessed comprised a heterogeneous sample according to sociodemographic and clinical variables, as detailed in Table 2.

Table 2. Sociodemographic and clinical variables of the assessed children and adolescents.

Sociodemographic variables	N	%	Clinical variables	N	%
Gender			**Etiology of ID**		
Male	528	64.86	Non-specific	317	38.94
Female	286	35.14	Down's Syndrome	111	13.64
Total	814	100	Autism Spectrum Disorder	248	30.47
[1] **Autonomous Community**			Cerebral Palsy	101	12.42
Andalusia	113	13.88	Rare diseases	35	4.29
Aragon	23	2.83	Co-occurrence	2	0.24
Canary Islands	86	10.56	Total	814	100
Cantabria	27	3.32	[2] **Adaptive behavior limitations**		
Castile-La Mancha	101	12.41	Mild	174	21.38
Castile and Leon	154	18.92	Moderate	314	38.57
Extremadura	23	2.83	Severe	200	24.57
Galicia	50	6.14	Profound	67	8.23
Madrid	145	17.81	N/A	59	7.25
Murcia	28	3.44	Total	814	100
Valencia	64	7.86	[2] **Intellectual functioning limitations**		
Total	814	100	Mild	206	25.31
Primary language			Moderate	290	35.63
Spanish	784	96.32	Severe	195	23.96
Galician	2	0.24	Profound	65	7.98
Romanian	2	0.24	N/A	58	7.12
Arabian	3	0.36	Total	814	100
Valencian	8	0.98	**Assistive technology use**		
English	1	0.13	Yes	157	19.29
Ukrainian	1	0.13	No	657	80.71
SSL	1	0.13	Total	814	100
Missing	12	1.47	**Sensory condition associated**		
Total	814	100	Yes	91	11.18

Table 2. Cont.

Sociodemographic variables.	N	%	Clinical variables	N	%
Age cohort			No	723	88.82
5–6	110	13.51	Total	814	100
7–8	108	13.27	Physical condition associated		
9–10	100	12.28	Yes	174	21.38
11–12	148	18.18	No	640	78.62
13–14	195	23.95	Total	814	100
15–16	153	18.81	Language condition associated		
Total	814	100	Yes	389	47.79
Schooling			No	425	52.21
Special education	493	60.56	Total	814	100
General education	179	21.99			
Combined	129	15.84			
Missing data	13	6.61			
Total	814	100			
Educational stage					
Elementary	110	13.51			
Primary	356	43.73			
Secondary	348	42.76			
Total	814	100			
Living					
Family home	777	95.45			
Foster family home	9	1.11			
Small group home (< 7)	7	0.86			
Midsize group home (7–15)	9	1.11			
Large residential facility (> 15)	3	0.36			
Missing data	9	1.11			
Total	814	100			

Note. SSL = Spanish sign language. [1] Autonomous Community = Region with administrative and legislative autonomy of the Kingdom of Spain. [2] Adaptive behavior and intellectual functioning limitations are based on educational records, not actual scores on standardized assessments. N / A = Not available.

Regarding the informants, most were professionals, essentially teachers (63%), psychologists (8%), speech therapists (6%), therapeutic pedagogy teachers (5%), therapists (3%), physiotherapists (2%), Snoezelen therapists (1.6%), and caregivers (1.4%). On average, these informants had known the children or adolescents with ID for more than 3 months (M = 3.31 months). Following the SIS-C guidelines [17], we sought to have at least two informants for each assessment. This was possible for 732 interviews. For these interviews, the additional informants were family members for 460 cases (mothers in 84% of interviews).

2.3. Procedure

Participants were recruited following a non-probabilistic convenience sampling method. To recruit participants, the research team wrote a letter presenting the research project and the inclusion criteria to participate (i.e., as interviewer, informant, or student with ID). The letter was sent by e-mail to various organizations, schools, and high schools providing supports to children and adolescents with ID (who were between 5 and 16 years) in the 17 Spanish Autonomous Communities. The research team received a positive answer from 48 organizations from 10 Autonomous Communities, each one providing, on average, 15 participants (ranging from 3 to 63). Subsequently, the organizations willing to participate were contacted by telephone, and informed consent forms and all the details regarding the project were sent to them to share with the families and/or legal guardians of the children and adolescents to be assessed.

Once the consent forms were filled, the assessments of children and adolescents with ID started. Approximately one-third of the assessments were conducted by the research team. When it was not possible, the research team asked the organizations to select one person who would serve as the interviewer within the organization. Then, a twofold measure was taken to ensure consistency between the interviews conducted by the research team and those done by the interviewers selected by the organizations. First, the research team requested the organizations to select as the interviewer a person who matched the requirements stated in the SIS-C for the interview process (see Instrument section) [17]. On the other hand, the selected interviewers were trained by a research team member through face-to-face meetings or via online training sessions. Training consisted of training sessions on the supports paradigm and how to implement the SIS-C. The training sessions included both theoretical content and role-playing exercises. Once the assessments were completed, all data were introduced in a database and were treated for their subsequent analyses.

All the procedures described in this paper followed the ethical standards required by research that involves human participants. As a requisite to start the research, the research project was assessed and approved by the Bioethics Committee of the University of Salamanca (resolution available upon request to the contact author). This research also followed the standards on data protection in force in Spain, aligned with the General Regulation on Data Protection of the European Union (Regulation EU2016/679), so alphanumeric codes were assigned to all the participants to guarantee their anonymity. All procedures comply with the principles of the 1964 Declaration of Helsinki and its amendments.

2.4. Data analysis

All data were analyzed with the software IRTPRO 4.0 using the graded response model (GRM) [38]. The GRM assumes, in addition to the usual IRT assumptions, that the categories in which the child or adolescent is rated can be ordered, as is the case, for example, with the probabilistic rating scales of summative estimates or "Likert type." The model aims to obtain more information than if the response levels were only two (e.g., yes or no) and, in this sense, it is an extension of the two-parameter logistic model (2-PLM) to ordered polytomous categories.

The GRM specifies a person's probability of being rated with an *ik* category or higher as opposed to being rated with a lower category when the rating scale has at least three categories, and is expressed as:

$$P^*_{ik}(\theta_j) = \frac{e^{D\alpha_i(\theta_j - \beta_{ik})}}{1 + e^{D\alpha_i(\theta_j - \beta_{ik})}} \quad (1)$$

$$P_{ik}(\theta_j) = P^*_{ik}(\theta_j) - P^*_{ik+1}(\theta_j), \quad (2)$$

where k is the ordered response option, $P_{ik}(\theta_j)$ is the probability of answering to option k in item i with a latent trait level θ_j, $P^*_{ik}(\theta_j)$ is the probability of answering to option k or higher in item i with a latent trait level θ_j, θ_j is the person's latent trait level, β_{ik} is the location parameter of alternative k of Item i, α_i is the discrimination parameter of Item i, and D is the constant 1.702.

Prior to estimating the GRMs, it was verified that the data met the criteria of unidimensionality and local independence through optimized parallel analysis [39], the estimation of the explained variance by the first factor in exploratory factor analysis (i.e., unweighted least squares), and the indices of closeness to unidimensionality based on minimum rank factor analysis recommended by Ferrando and Lorenzo–Seva [40]: the explained common variance (ECV; values above 0.85 suggests that data can be treated essentially as unidimensional) and the mean of item residual absolute loadings (MIREAL; values below 0.30 indicate the lack of relevant sources of local dependency). Moreover, for each SIS-C domain, the strength and the replicability of the unidimensional model and the quality of the individual scores were assessed through the generalized replicability of the latent construct (H-G) [41], the factor determinacy index (FDI) [42], and the marginal reliability calculated from the estimated a posteriori scores. H-G values above 0.80 indicate that the factor is robust and stable across samples and studies. FDI values higher than 0.90 suggest that the factor scores are good proxies of the latent scores in the factor. Values of marginal reliability above .80 mean that the scores have been estimated with enough accuracy.

3. Results

3.1. Unidimensionality, Local Independency, and Quality of the Measure

Table 3 shows the results of the previous analyses for the estimations of the GRMs. For all the SIS-C scales (hereafter, the term "domain" is substituted by "scale," a term more accurate for this field of data analysis), the parallel analysis recommended retaining a single factor. The first eigenvalue of the unidimensional models retained between the 79% (SPA and SA) and the 87% (HLA) of the total variance of data. For all cases, the ECV values were above 0.90 (M = 0.94) and the MIREAL values were below 0.20 (M = 0.16). The FDI and H-G indices and the marginal reliability were above 0.95 for all cases. All these results suggest that all the scales acquired high unidimensionality, that there was no evidence on strong violations of local independency, and that data presented high quality and reliability.

Table 3. Results of dimensionality, reliability, and local independence analyses.

Scale	EV-FA	PA	ECV	MIREAL	FDI	H-G	MR
HLA	0.87	1	0.95	0.17	0.98	0.97	0.97
CAN	0.83	1	0.96	0.14	0.98	0.97	0.97
SPA	0.79	1	0.94	0.15	0.98	0.97	0.97
SLA	0.84	1	0.95	0.17	0.99	0.98	0.98
HAS	0.81	1	0.95	0.19	0.98	0.96	0.97
SA	0.79	1	0.94	0.18	0.98	0.97	0.97
AA	0.84	1	0.95	0.18	0.99	0.98	0.98

Note. HLA = Home living activities; CNA = Community and neighborhood activities; SPA = School participation activities; SLA = School learning activities; HSA = Health and safety activities; SA = Social activities; AA = Advocacy activities; EV-FA = Variance explained by the first eigenvalue; PA = Number of factors recommended by parallel analysis; ECV = Explained common variance; MIREAL = Mean of item absolute residuals; FDI = Factor determinacy index; H-G = Latent index of replicability; MR = Marginal reliability of estimated a posteriori scores.

As these results were considered adequate to guarantee the unidimensionality and quality of the data, we then proceeded to estimate the GRMs.

3.2. Estimation of Graded Response Models

Table 4 shows the estimated parameters for each scale. The alpha parameter represents the capacity of the item to discern between different levels of the latent variable (i.e., support needs). The items obtained alpha values between 2.21 ("sleeping and/or napping" in HLA) and 5.96 ("taking action and attaining goals" in AA), with a mean of 4.02. Given that α_i values of 0.01–0.24 can be considered very low, values of 0.25–0.64 low, values of 0.65–1.34 moderate, values of 1.35–1.69 high, and values ≥ 1.7 very high [43], it can be concluded that, in absolute terms, the discrimination parameters were very high for all the items of the seven scales. Likewise, the standard errors were low for all cases, indicating that the GRMs estimated the parameters accurately.

Figure 1 depicts, as an example, the characteristic response curves for Item 7 ("following classroom and school rules") of the SPA scale. The abscissa axis represents the latent variable theta (M = 0; SD = 1). Five curves are plotted per item (solid lines), each one showing the probability, represented on the left ordinate axis, of belonging to each of the response categories. Thus, in the commented item, for the most probable response to be "full physical assistance" (Category 5), the child/adolescent must present a level of support needs greater than 0.86 standard deviations above the mean. In contrast, the most probable response category for a child situated in the mean (Theta = 0) would be "verbal/gestural prompting" (Category 3). The dashed line represents the zone of the latent variable in which the item is most informative (i.e., it can discriminate between participants with different levels of extraordinary support needs). For this item, the peak of information is approximately between −1.5 and +1 theta scores, thus covering a range of 2.5 standard deviations around the mean of the latent variable.

Table 4. Model parameters.

Scale	Item	α	α s.e.	β1	β1 s.e.	β2	β2 s.e.	β3	β3 s.e.	β4	β4 s.e.
HLA	1	3.41	0.20	−1.66	0.08	−0.97	0.05	−0.14	0.04	0.61	0.05
	2	3.79	0.22	−0.79	0.05	−0.21	0.04	0.22	0.04	0.98	0.06
	3	5.84	0.39	−1.21	0.06	−0.64	0.04	−0.26	0.04	0.45	0.04
	4	5.05	0.32	−1.04	0.05	−0.52	0.04	−0.19	0.04	0.66	0.05
	5	4.88	0.30	−0.68	0.04	−0.17	0.04	0.12	0.04	0.74	0.05
	6	2.21	0.13	−0.31	0.05	0.30	0.05	0.89	0.06	1.53	0.08
	7	2.98	0.17	−0.97	0.06	−0.35	0.05	0.21	0.05	0.69	0.05
	8	2.42	0.14	−1.17	0.07	−0.45	0.05	0.20	0.05	0.98	0.07
	9	2.55	0.15	−1.21	0.07	−0.47	0.05	−0.09	0.05	0.58	0.06
CNA	1	4.11	0.25	−1.45	0.07	−0.76	0.05	−0.37	0.04	0.24	0.05
	2	3.70	0.21	−1.35	0.06	−0.75	0.05	−0.18	0.04	0.47	0.05
	3	3.62	0.21	−1.34	0.06	−0.66	0.05	0.05	0.05	0.75	0.06
	4	4.91	0.31	−1.59	0.07	−0.99	0.05	−0.45	0.04	0.13	0.05
	5	5.04	0.32	−1.37	0.06	−0.81	0.05	−0.30	0.04	0.28	0.05
	6	3.90	0.23	−1.76	0.08	−1.07	0.05	−0.42	0.04	0.22	0.05
	7	3.42	0.20	−1.47	0.07	−0.85	0.05	−0.14	0.05	0.39	0.05
	8	4.71	0.29	−1.49	0.06	−0.75	0.05	−0.24	0.04	0.39	0.05
SPA	1	3.00	0.18	−1.75	0.09	−1.19	0.06	−0.47	0.05	0.20	0.05
	2	4.63	0.28	−1.24	0.06	−0.60	0.04	0.02	0.04	0.67	0.05
	3	4.37	0.27	−1.46	0.06	−0.83	0.05	−0.23	0.04	0.45	0.05
	4	2.67	0.16	−1.48	0.08	−0.75	0.05	−0.33	0.05	0.27	0.05
	5	4.57	0.27	−0.97	0.05	−0.40	0.04	0.20	0.05	0.83	0.06
	6	2.43	0.16	−2.18	0.12	−1.40	0.07	−0.52	0.05	−0.09	0.05
	7	3.45	0.19	−1.26	0.06	−0.64	0.05	0.17	0.05	0.86	0.06
	8	3.92	0.23	−1.02	0.05	−0.51	0.04	0.09	0.05	0.60	0.05
	9	4.22	0.25	−1.06	0.05	−0.61	0.04	0.09	0.04	0.58	0.05
SLA	1	4.55	0.33	−2.04	0.13	−1.50	0.09	−0.69	0.06	−0.15	0.05
	2	5.49	0.41	−2.06	0.13	−1.51	0.09	−0.64	0.05	0.03	0.05
	3	5.28	0.41	−2.03	0.13	−1.56	0.10	−0.79	0.06	−0.26	0.05
	4	5.57	0.42	−1.88	0.11	−1.40	0.09	−0.61	0.05	0.02	0.05
	5	3.56	0.24	−1.81	0.11	−1.23	0.08	−0.50	0.05	0.37	0.05
	6	4.26	0.30	−2.02	0.13	−1.54	0.10	−0.59	0.05	0.02	0.05
	7	5.25	0.40	−1.85	0.11	−1.46	0.09	−0.67	0.05	−0.23	0.05
	8	3.76	0.26	−1.81	0.11	−1.32	0.08	−0.62	0.06	0.06	0.05
	9	3.71	0.26	−1.90	0.12	−1.23	0.08	−0.53	0.05	0.07	0.05
HSA	1	3.07	0.18	−1.11	0.06	−0.67	0.05	0.04	0.05	0.59	0.06
	2	3.36	0.20	−1.39	0.07	−1.01	0.06	−0.29	0.05	0.26	0.05
	3	3.20	0.19	−1.63	0.08	−1.09	0.06	−0.13	0.05	0.49	0.06
	4	4.53	0.29	−1.50	0.07	−0.94	0.05	−0.25	0.05	0.29	0.05
	5	4.34	0.31	−1.66	0.08	−1.21	0.06	−0.75	0.05	−0.30	0.05
	6	4.82	0.36	−1.75	0.08	−1.30	0.06	−0.78	0.05	−0.35	0.05
	7	4.04	0.27	−1.72	0.08	−1.19	0.06	−0.62	0.05	−0.19	0.05
	8	3.70	0.23	−1.52	0.07	−0.98	0.06	−0.39	0.05	0.15	0.05
SA	1	4.08	0.24	−1.32	0.06	−0.78	0.05	0.06	0.05	0.81	0.06
	2	2.90	0.17	−1.24	0.06	−0.68	0.05	0.03	0.05	0.64	0.06
	3	4.35	0.27	−1.34	0.06	−0.88	0.05	−0.11	0.04	0.31	0.05
	4	4.19	0.27	−1.75	0.08	−1.18	0.05	−0.34	0.04	0.03	0.05
	5	2.63	0.15	−1.42	0.07	−0.87	0.06	0.06	0.05	0.81	0.06
	6	4.67	0.29	−1.35	0.06	−0.88	0.05	−0.19	0.04	0.23	0.05
	7	4.48	0.27	−1.39	0.06	−0.88	0.05	−0.13	0.04	0.44	0.05
	8	2.70	0.15	−1.13	0.06	−0.49	0.05	0.09	0.05	0.66	0.06
	9	3.09	0.20	−1.67	0.08	−1.13	0.06	−0.51	0.05	−0.15	0.05
AA	1	2.85	0.17	−1.05	0.07	−0.46	0.05	0.43	0.06	1.12	0.07
	2	5.11	0.35	−1.72	0.09	−1.24	0.06	−0.48	0.05	−0.09	0.05
	3	5.96	0.43	−1.81	0.09	−1.36	0.07	−0.49	0.05	0.02	0.05
	4	3.61	0.22	−1.66	0.09	−1.11	0.06	−0.07	0.05	0.48	0.06
	5	4.13	0.27	−1.45	0.07	−0.96	0.06	−0.34	0.05	0.10	0.05
	6	5.48	0.38	−1.68	0.08	−1.25	0.06	−0.51	0.05	−0.07	0.05
	7	3.26	0.19	−1.21	0.07	−0.74	0.06	0.09	0.05	0.74	0.06
	8	4.59	0.31	−1.70	0.09	−1.26	0.07	−0.45	0.05	−0.09	0.05
	9	5.06	0.34	−1.89	0.10	−1.40	0.07	−0.57	0.05	−0.02	0.05

Note. HLA = Home living activities; CNA = Community and neighborhood activities; SPA = School participation activities; SLA = School learning activities; HSA = Health and safety activities; SA = Social activities; AA = Advocacy activities; s.e. = Standard error of estimation.

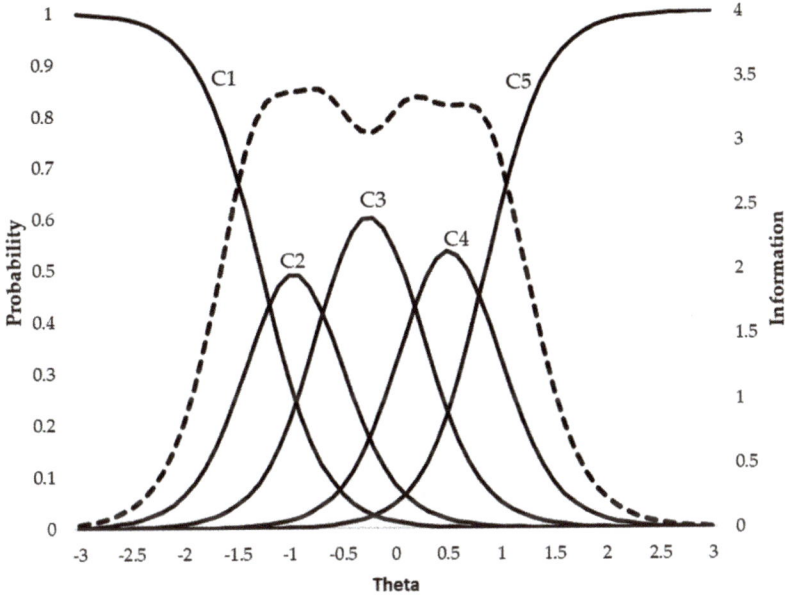

Figure 1. Rating scale categories curves and item information. Solid lines represent the probability of each rating scale category (C1, C2, etc.) conditional to the theta level. The dashed line represents the item information function.

Figure 2 shows the test information curve (TIC; panel a) and the test characteristic curve (TCC; panel b) of the CNA scale. The TIC is the result of adding the information curves of all the items of the scale, and it represents the amount of information provided by the test, conditional to the level in the latent variable (theta, depicted in the abscissa axis). The figure also includes the standard error of measurement (dashed line), which represents the reliability of the test along the theta continuum (right ordinate axis). In the CNA scale, the maximum information and reliability were observed at the peak of the TIC approximately between −1.5 and 0.25 theta scores. The effective operational range (EOR) is the area of the variable that is productive for the measure, which on this scale is between −2.1 and +0.9 theta scores. Consequently, the scale was not reliable to assess children with very low support needs (below −2.1 standard deviations) or children with moderate-high or high support needs (above +0.9 standard deviations). Panel b in Figure 2 shows the TCC, which represents the relationship predicted by the model between the raw scores in the CNA scale (ordinate axis) and the latent level of support needs (theta in the abscissa axis). The EOR can be observed clearly in this panel—above the theta score of +0.9 the scale has a strong ceiling effect, where all children obtained the same score independently of their level in the latent trait of support needs; therefore, the scale was not capable of discerning between children with intense extraordinary support needs. Results concerning the TIC, the TCC, and the EOR (as well as the ceiling effect) were similar for all the scales (data and figures for the TIC, the TCC, and the EOR of the HLA, SPA, SLA, HSA, SA, and AA scales are available upon request to the contact author).

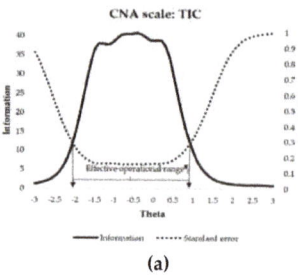
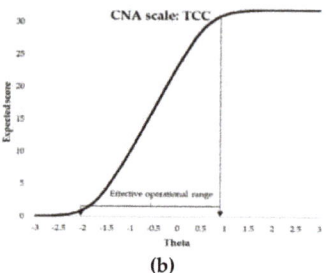

Figure 2. CNA scale: (a) test information curve and standard error; (b) Test characteristic curve. CNA = Community and neighborhood activities.

An interesting question to assess the utility of scales is how many of the assessed children obtained scores that fell out of the EOR (in other words, for which proportion of the participants the scale has been reliable and useful). Table 5 shows, for each scale, the EOR, as well as the number of children and adolescents with ID who fell out of the EOR and, consequently, were assessed with questionable reliability. The number of participants with scores below the EOR was low (between 0.3% and 4.5%, M = 1.3%). However, the proportion of participants located in the upper EOR was substantially higher (between 13% and 31%, M = 19%). It was explored whether the probability that a child was observed in the upper EOR had any relationship with grouping variables such as gender, age, and degree of disability. The degree of disability was the only variable that showed a strong and consistent relationship. Children with severe/profound ID had more probability ($p > 0.01$) of obtaining scores above the upper EOR for all the scales, with very strong size effects, between Phi = 0.44 (odds ratio = 19.4) in the SPA scale and Phi = 0.58 (odds ratio = 28.9) in the CNA scale. Table 5 also shows the proportion of children and adolescents with severe/profound ID who were observed above the upper EOR (between 74% for SLA and 93% for SA and AA).

Table 5. Effective operational ranges and scores distribution.

	HLA	CNA	SPA	SLA	HSA	SA	AA
EOR lower bound	−1.4	−2.1	−1.9	−2.5	−2.2	−2	−2.2
EOR upper bound	1.3	0.9	1.2	0.5	0.8	1.1	0.7
EOR range	2.7	3	3.1	3	3	3.1	2.9
% children below EOR	4.5	0.6	1.2	0.3	0.6	1.2	0.8
% children above EOR	13	21	13	31	22	14	21
% children with S/P ID above upper EOR	90	88	87	74	83	93	93

Note. HLA = Home living activities; CNA = Community and neighborhood activities; SPA = School participation activities; SLA = School learning activities; HSA = Health and safety activities; SA = Social activities; AA = Advocacy activities; S / P ID = Severe / Profound Intellectual disability.

4. Discussion

Using a large sample of children and adolescents with ID, the present authors applied the GRM method [38] to estimate the discrimination, location, and information functions of the 61 items of the SIS-C [17]. All the items showed high discrimination and information values, and none showed problems that required their removal or review. Considering the discrimination and location of the items together, the results of the IRT scale scores estimations showed substantial variability between individuals, with a score of approximately −2.5 to +1 standard deviations around the latent mean. This result suggests that the SIS-C scales have very good accuracy at low and medium ranges of support needs, but that they may be unreliable at high levels. Prior to drawing a discussion on the findings of this work, it is necessary to acknowledge that the training and expertise of the interviewers selected by each organization, as well as the possible relationship between the interviewer and the assessed child/adolescent with ID, may have influenced the results of this study. Notwithstanding this, although any possible disparity between the interview style followed by the interviewers selected by the organizations versus that followed by the research team may have supposed a bias source, the present authors designed and implemented a training program to make the interviews as homogeneous as possible, always following the SIS-C guidelines for the interview process [17].

The proportion of children and adolescents with extraordinary support needs located in the low reliability zone was between 13% (HLA) and 31% (SLA). To better illustrate this result, we can take as an example the SLA scale—the scores discriminated very well between participants with support needs between −2.5 and +0.5 standard deviations along the latent continuum, but remained constant in the range from +0.5 to +3 standard deviations, giving rise to a strong and extensive ceiling effect (i.e., two children with substantially different support needs would obtain the same observed scores). This ceiling effect was observed for the seven scales. It does not seem to be related to the age or gender of the participants, supporting the decision to use the same set of items for all age bands, as suggested in previous research [44–46]. The probability of being observed in the low discrimination range strongly depended on the level of ID given that, on average, 87% of the cases located in the ceiling effect area had severe/profound ID.

One central question is to what extent a ceiling effect poses a problem for the usefulness of the SIS-C [17]. The presence of wide ranges of low discrimination can only be regarded as a deficiency in a tool if it interferes with the goals for which it was developed. In clinical diagnosis scales, it is common to observe strong floor effects because the indicators must concentrate their discriminative power at high levels of the variable, which is useful for classifying persons into groups (e.g., affected and unaffected). For example, in an adaptive behavior scale whose goal is the diagnosis of ID, it is possibly not applicable to evaluate in detail medium and low deficit levels, so the items will be designed to provide maximum information in high areas of the variable—those relevant for diagnosis. However, the aim of the SIS-C is not to diagnose but to assess the pattern and intensity of needs that serve for supports planning [8,17]. Consequently, the SIS-C is expected to accurately measure a wide range of intensity of support needs so that most people are assessed accurately enough regardless of the intensity of their support needs. Under these circumstances, a strong ceiling effect may interfere with the goals of the SIS-C, which implies potentially important consequences for both research and practice.

Regarding research, the low variability in a significant proportion of the participants may bias the results of the data analyses. The support needs in the ceiling area will tend to behave as a constant rather than as a variable, inhibiting the possibility of analyzing heterogeneity in an important part of the sample and its relationship with other predictor, criterion, or grouping variables. This may bias research results in persons with high levels of support needs. An example is research that focuses on investigating the impact of support needs on QoL by using a linear or nonlinear regression model. For this, it is necessary that the criterion variable has variance—if, for a large proportion of participants the criterion behaves like a constant, the regression weights will be unable to capture part of the variability of the criterion, altering the results and making their interpretation difficult. Another example is studies analyzing the impact of supports planning—possibly, any real impact of the program would be hidden because of the problem of measurement discrimination in high areas of the variable.

As regards the applied field, support needs assessment obeys the need to understand the pattern and intensity of the extraordinary support that children and adolescents with ID require with the aim of providing personalized supports that enhance their functioning and QoL [1], such as personalized education plans that include goals beyond literacy [22] and the use of personalized support plans to improve personal outcomes in inclusive settings [23]. However, for children and adolescents with ID located in the ceiling effect area, no pattern of support needs will be obtained—rather, homogeneous scores where all or almost all the indicators acquire the maximum score. For these children, the SIS-C is not able to capture individual differences, does not allow recognition of the real pattern of support needs, and ultimately does not provide useful information for planning personalized programs or for evaluating the effectiveness of the intervention. These issues hinder efficiency in supports planning regarding children and adolescents with ID, which, in turn, may have negative effects on the efforts made to enhance their inclusion and QoL. The problem is that the main environmental demands that interact with their capacities are related to educational contexts and activities. It is precisely these contexts on which economic cuts have had the greatest impact over the last decade, which makes it especially necessary to have instruments that allow different levels of support needs to be adequately discerned to support more efficient decision-making in resources and supports implementation to enhance QoL [8].

There are solutions to the research and applied problems described above. In instruments aimed at measuring a wide spectrum of individual differences (such as the SIS-C), it is common to observe poor discrimination in extreme areas of the latent variable, as usually happens, for example, in the assessment of general intelligence [47]. In practice, this is not relevant if the tails of the distribution are short, contain few people, and the scale is capable of accurately capturing individual differences in most of those assessed. That said, the SIS-C assesses low to medium levels of support needs with good precision, but it presents significant discrimination difficulties at high levels. To solve this problem, it is necessary to change the traditional idea of fixed-length scales by the idea of personalized instruments based on pools of items calibrated using IRT models. As has been shown in this study, it is possible to know how well each item differentiates between people who are at different levels of the latent variable, so it is possible to combine different items to maximize information in different ranges of the assessed continuum. Therefore, it would be possible to develop a pool of indicators with high discrimination and with location parameters distributed over a range of the latent variable as wide as necessary. In the IRT, the true position of the assessed person in the latent variable does not depend on the specific set of items administered [31]; therefore, this calibrated pool of items would allow the development of instruments adapted to the assessment needs of each person or group (e.g., by applying only discriminatory items in the moderate-high range of support needs for persons with severe/profound ID). This would make it possible to minimize the problem of the ceiling effect, improve substantially the assessment accuracy for all the ranges of support needs (which would facilitate more efficient supports planning), and reduce the length of the test without prejudice to reliability, as well as further the development of high-quality and efficient assessment systems such as computerized adaptive tests [48]. For the case of children with severe/profound ID, developing and calibrating such set of indicators would translate into better opportunities to obtain positive outcomes regarding the different environments considered by the SIS-C. These indicators would allow to obtain personalized profiles of support needs in which to base a thoughtful provision of supports aligned with their vital expectations, something that, in turn, can help to overcome the idea of the "more is better" in supports planning and resources allocation, an idea which is especially anchored regarding persons with severe/profound ID and which has been used in (not a few) occasions to neglect the provision of opportunities with those with extensive support needs [49].

5. Conclusions

The SIS-C items showed high discrimination and information capacity; therefore, its modification does not appear necessary. However, all scales showed discrimination problems in children and adolescents with high support needs, especially people with severe/profound ID. This ceiling effect may be an important obstacle for both research and practice involving the SIS-C. A key objective for future research to improve the SIS-C is to design reliable and discriminatory indicators in areas of high intensity of support needs.

Author Contributions: Conceptualization, V.B.A., A.M.A., M.A.V., M.F., B.A. and A.A.; methodology, V.B.A., A.M.A., M.A.V. and B.A.; software, V.B.A.; validation, B.A.; formal analysis, V.B.A. and B.A.; investigation, A.M.A., M.A.V., M.F. and A.A.; resources, A.M.A. and M.A.V.; data curation, V.B.A. and A.M.A.; writing—original draft preparation, V.B.A. and A.M.A.; writing-review and editing, M.A.V., M.F., B.A. and A.A.; visualization, A.M.A; supervision, M.A.V. and B.A.; project administration, A.M.A.; funding acquisition, M.A.V. All authors have read and agreed to the published version of the manuscript.

Funding: This research was funded by The Spanish Ministry of Economy and Competitiveness, grant numbers PSI2015-65193-P and BES-2016-078252.

Acknowledgments: We are thankful to the schools, high schools, organizations, and families who participated in this research.

Conflicts of Interest: The authors declare no conflict of interest.

References

1. Schalock, R.L.; Borthwick-Duffy, S.A.; Bradley, V.J.; Buntinx, W.H.E.; Coulter, D.L.; Craig, E.M.; Gomez, S.C.; Lachapelle, Y.; Luckasson, R.; Reeve, A.; et al. *Intellectual Disability: Definition, Classification, and Systems of Supports*, 11th ed.; American Association on Intellectual and Developmental Disabilities: Washington, DC, USA, 2010.
2. Thompson, J.R.; Bradley, V.J.; Buntinx, W.H.E.; Schalock, R.L.; Shogren, K.A.; Snell, M.E.; Wehmeyer, M.L. Conceptualizing supports and the supports needs of people with intellectual disability. *Intellect. Dev. Disabil.* **2009**, *47*, 135–146. [CrossRef] [PubMed]
3. Verdugo, M.A. Conceptos clave que explican los cambios en la provisión de apoyos a las discapacidades intelectuales y del desarrollo en España. *Siglo Cero* **2018**, *49*, 35–52. [CrossRef]
4. González, J.A. Intensidad de apoyos, salud mental, empleo y su relación con resultados de calidad de vida. *Siglo Cero* **2019**, *50*, 73–88. [CrossRef]
5. Schalock, R.L. Six ideas that are changing the IDD field internationally. *Siglo Cero* **2018**, *49*, 21–33. [CrossRef]
6. United Nations. Convention on the Rights of Persons with Disabilities. 2006. Available online: https://www.un.org/development/desa/disabilities/convention-on-the-rights-of-persons-with-disabilities/convention-on-the-rights-of-persons-with-disabilities-2.html (accessed on 15 April 2020).
7. American Association on Intellectual and Developmental Disabilities. Evidence for the reliability and validity of the Supports Intensity Scales. Available online: https://www.aaidd.org/docs/default-source/sis-docs/evidence-for-the-reliabilityandvalidity-of-the-sis.pdf?sfvrsn=7ed3021_0 (accessed on 15 April 2020).
8. Verdugo, M.A.; Amor, A.M.; Arias, V.B.; Guillén, V.M.; Fernández, M.; Arias, B. Examining measurement invariance and differences across groups in the support needs of children with and without intellectual disability. *J. Appl. Res. Intellect. Disabil.* **2019**, *32*, 1535–1548. [CrossRef] [PubMed]
9. Gould, A. *The Service Needs Assessment Profile*, 1st ed.; ATG and Associates Pty Ltd.: Sydney, Australia, 1998.
10. Llewellyn, G.; Parmenter, T.; Chan, J.; Riches, V.; Hindmarsh, G. *I-CAN: Instrument to Classify Support Needs for People with Disability*; University of Sydney: Sydney, Australia, 2005.
11. Thompson, J.R.; Bryant, B.R.; Campbell, E.M.; Craig, E.M.; Hughes, C.M.; Rotholz, D.A.; Schalock, R.L.; Silverman, W.; Tassé, M.J.; Wehmeyer, M.L. *Supports Intensity Scale: User's Manual*; American Association on Mental Retardation: Washington, DC, USA, 2004.
12. Thompson, J.R.; Bryant, B.R.; Schalock, R.L.; Shogren, K.A.; Tassé, M.J.; Wehmeyer, M.L.; Campbell, E.M.; Craig, E.M.; Hughes, C.; Rotholz, D.A. *Supports Intensity Scale-Adult Version (SIS-A): User's Manual*; American Association on Intellectual and Developmental Disabilities: Washington, DC, USA, 2015.
13. American Association on Intellectual and Developmental Disabilities. International SIS use. Available online: https://www.aaidd.org/sis/international (accessed on 15 April 2020).
14. Chou, Y.C.; Lee, Y.C.; Chang, S.C.; Yu, A.P. Evaluating the Supports Intensity Scale as a potential assessment instrument for resources allocation for persons with intellectual disability. *Res. Dev. Disabil.* **2013**, *34*, 2056–2063. [CrossRef]
15. Giné, C.; Font, J.; Guàrdia-Olmos, J.; Balcells-Balcells, A.; Valls, J.; Carbó-Carreté, M. Using the SIS to better align the funding of residential services to assessed support needs. *Res. Dev. Disabil.* **2014**, *35*, 1144–1151. [CrossRef]
16. Seo, H.; Wehmeyer, M.L.; Shogren, K.A.; Hughes, C.; Thompson, J.R.; Little, T.D.; Palmer, S.B. Examining underlying relationships between the Supports Intensity Scale-Adult version and the Supports Intensity Scale-Children's version. *Assess. Eff. Interv.* **2017**, *42*, 237–247. [CrossRef]
17. Thompson, J.R.; Wehmeyer, M.L.; Hughes, C.M.; Shogren, K.A.; Seo, H.; Little, T.D.; Schalock, R.L.; Realon, R.E.; Copeland, S.R.; Patton, J.R.; et al. *The Supports Intensity Scale-Children's Version (SIS-C): User's Manual*; American Association on Intellectual and Developmental Disabilities: Washington, DC, USA, 2016.

18. Guillén, V.M.; Adam, A.L.; Verdugo, M.A.; Giné, C. Comparison between the Spanish and Catalan versions of the Supports Intensity Scale for Children (SIS-C). *Psicothema* **2017**, *29*, 126–132. [CrossRef]
19. Aguayo, V.; Arias, V.B.; Verdugo, M.A.; Amor, A.M. Measuring support needs in children with motor disability: Validity and utility of the Supports Intensity Scale (SIS-C). *Res. Dev. Disabil.* **2019**, *95*, 103509. [CrossRef]
20. Aguayo, V.; Verdugo, M.A.; Arias, V.B.; Guillén, V.M.; Amor, A.M. Assessing support needs in children with intellectual disability and motor impairments: Measurement invariance and group differences. *J. Intellect. Disabil. Res.* **2019**, *63*, 1413–1427. [CrossRef]
21. Shogren, K.A.; Wehmeyer, M.L.; Seo, H.; Thompson, J.R.; Schalock, R.L.; Hughes, C.; Little, T.D.; Palmer, S.B. Examining the reliability and validity of the Supports Intensity Scale-Children's Version in children with autism and intellectual disabilities. *Focus Autism Other Dev. Disabl.* **2017**, *32*, 293–304. [CrossRef]
22. Walker, V.L.; DeSpain, S.N.; Thompson, J.R.; Hughes, C. Assessment and planning in k-12 schools: A social-ecological approach. *Inclusion* **2014**, *2*, 125–139. [CrossRef]
23. Schalock, R.L.; van Loon, J.; Mostert, R. A systematic approach to enhancing the personal well-being of children and adolescents. *Int. J. Child. Youth Fam. Stud.* **2018**, *9*, 188–205. [CrossRef]
24. American Association on Intellectual and Developmental Disabilities. How organizations and systems use Supports Intensity Scales. Available online: https://www.aaidd.org/docs/default-source/sis-docs/howorganizationsusesis_webrev-final.pdf?sfvrsn=d4953021_0 (accessed on 15 April 2020).
25. Thompson, J.R.; Walker, V.L.; Snodgrass, M.R.; Nelson, J.A.; Carpenter, M.E.; Hagiwara, M.; Shogren, K.A. Planning supports for students with intellectual disability in general education classrooms. *Inclusion* **2020**, *8*, 27–42. [CrossRef]
26. Seo, H.; Shogren, K.A.; Little, T.D.; Thompson, J.R.; Wehmeyer, M.L. Construct validation of the Supports Intensity Scale–Children and Adult versions: An application of a pseudo multitrait-multimethod approach. *Am. J. Intellect. Dev. Disabil.* **2016**, *121*, 550–563. [CrossRef] [PubMed]
27. Verdugo, M.A.; Arias, V.B.; Guillén, V.M. Are type, frequency, and daily time equally valid estimators of support needs in children with intellectual disability? A multitrait-multimethod analysis of the Supports Intensity Scale for Children (SIS-C). *Assessment* **2019**, *26*, 1307–1319. [CrossRef]
28. Cronbach, L.J. Coefficient alpha and the internal structure of tests. *Psychometrika* **1951**, *16*, 297–334. [CrossRef]
29. Crocker, L.; Algina, J. *Introduction to Classical and Modern Test Theory*; Cengage Learning: Mason, OH, USA, 2008.
30. Embretson, S.E.; Hershberger, S.L. *The New Rules of Measurement*, 1st ed.; Erlbaum: Mahwah, NJ, USA, 1999.
31. Embretson, S.E.; Reise, S.P. *Item Response Theory for Psychologists*, 1st ed.; Erlbaum: Mahwah, NJ, USA, 2000.
32. Hambleton, R.K.; Swaminathan, H.; Rogers, H.J. *Fundamentals of Item Response Theory*, 1st ed.; Sage: Beverly Hills, CA, USA, 1991.
33. Samejima, F. A use of the information function in tailored testing. *Appl. Psychol. Meas.* **1977**, *1*, 233–247. [CrossRef]
34. Reise, S.P.; Waller, N.G. Item response theory and clinical measurement. *Annu. Rev. Clin. Psychol.* **2009**, *5*, 27–48. [CrossRef]
35. Hagiwara, M.; Shogren, K.A.; Shaw, L.A. Examining the impact of respondent-level factors on scores on the Supports Intensity Scale-Children's Version. *Am. J. Intellect. Dev. Disabil.* **2019**, *124*, 309–323. [CrossRef] [PubMed]
36. Tassé, M.J.; Craig, E.M. Critical issues in the cross-cultural assessment of adaptive behavior. In *Adaptive Behavior and Its Measurement: Implications for the Field of Mental Retardation*; Schalock, R.L., Ed.; American Association on Mental Retardation: Washington, DC, USA, 1999; pp. 161–184.
37. Muñiz, J.; Elosua, P.; Hambleton, R.K. Directrices para la traducción y adaptación de los tests: Segunda edición. *Psicothema* **2013**, *25*, 151–157. [CrossRef] [PubMed]
38. Samejima, F. Graded response models. In *Handbook of Item Response Theory*, 1st ed.; van der Linden, W.J., Ed.; Chapman and Hall/CRC: Boca Raton, FL, USA, 2016; Volume 1, pp. 123–136.
39. Timmerman, M.E.; Lorenzo-Seva, U. Dimensionality assessment of ordered polytomous items with parallel analysis. *Psychol. Methods* **2011**, *16*, 209–220. [CrossRef] [PubMed]
40. Ferrando, P.J.; Lorenzo-Seva, U. Assessing the quality and appropriateness of factor solutions and factor score estimates in exploratory item factor analysis. *Educ. Psychol. Meas.* **2018**, *78*, 762–780. [CrossRef]

41. Hancock, G.R.; Mueller, R.O. Rethinking construct reliability within latent variable systems. In *Structural Equation Modeling: Present and Future*; Cudek, R., duToit, S.H.C., Sorbom, D.F., Eds.; Scientific Software International: Lincolnwood, IL, USA, 2000; pp. 195–216.
42. Beauducel, A. Indeterminacy of factor scores in slightly misspecified confirmatory factor models. *J. Mod. Appl. Stat. Methods* **2011**, *10*, 583–598. [CrossRef]
43. Baker, F.B. *The Basics of Item Response Theory*, 2nd ed.; ERIC Clearinghouse on Assessment and Evaluation, University of Maryland: College Park, MD, USA, 2001.
44. Giné, C.; Adam, A.L.; Font, J.; Salvador-Bertran, F.; Baqués, N.; Oliveira, C.; Mumbardó, C.; Seo, H.; Shaw, L.A.; Shogren, K.A.; et al. Examining measurement invariance and differences in age cohorts on the Supports Intensity Scale-Children's Version-Catalan translation. *Am. J. Intellect. Dev. Disabil.* **2017**, *122*, 511–524. [CrossRef]
45. Shogren, K.A.; Seo, H.; Wehmeyer, M.L.; Palmer, S.B.; Thompson, J.R.; Hughes, C.; Little, T.D. Support needs of children with intellectual and developmental disabilities: Age-related implications for assessment. *Psychol. Sch.* **2015**, *52*, 874–891. [CrossRef]
46. Verdugo, M.A.; Arias, B.; Guillén, V.M.; Seo, H.; Shogren, K.A.; Shaw, L.A.; Thompson, J.R. Examining age-related differences in support needs on the Supports Intensity Scale-Children's Version-Spanish translation. *Int. J. Clin. Health Psychol.* **2016**, *16*, 306–314. [CrossRef]
47. Embretson, S.E.; McCollam, K.M.S. Psychometric approaches to understanding and measuring intelligence. In *Handbook of Intelligence*, 1st ed.; Sternberg, R.J., Ed.; Cambridge University Press: New York, NY, USA, 2000; pp. 423–444.
48. Wainer, H.; Dorans, N.J.; Eignor, D.; Flaugher, R.; Green, B.F.; Mislevy, R.J.; Steinberg, L.; Thissen, D. *Computerized Adaptive Testing: A Primer*, 2nd ed.; Lawrence Erlbaum Associates: Hillsdale, NJ, USA, 2001.
49. Amor, A.M.; Verdugo, M.A.; Calvo, M.I.; Navas, P.; Aguayo, V. Psychoeducational assessment of students with intellectual disability: Professional-action framework analysis. *Psicothema* **2018**, *30*, 39–45. [CrossRef]

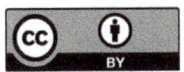

© 2020 by the authors. Licensee MDPI, Basel, Switzerland. This article is an open access article distributed under the terms and conditions of the Creative Commons Attribution (CC BY) license (http://creativecommons.org/licenses/by/4.0/).

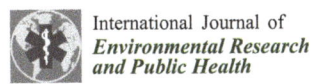

Review

State of the Art of Family Quality of Life in Early Care and Disability: A Systematic Review

Carmen Francisco Mora [1], Alba Ibáñez [2,3,*] and Anna Balcells-Balcells [1]

1. Faculty of Psychology, Education and Sports Sciences, Ramon Llull University, 08022 Barcelona, Spain; carmenrm@blanquerna.url.edu (C.F.M.); annabb0@blanquerna.url.edu (A.B.-B.)
2. Faculty of Education, University of Cantabria, 39005 Santander, Spain
3. Group in Health Economics and Management of Health Services, Instituto de Investigación Sanitaria Valdecilla (IDIVAL), 39011 Santander, Spain
* Correspondence: alba.ibanez@unican.es; Tel.: +34-(94)-2201165

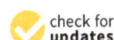

Received: 11 August 2020; Accepted: 27 September 2020; Published: 2 October 2020

Abstract: *Background*: In recent years, there has been a growing international interest in family quality of life The objective of this systematic review is to understand and analyze the conceptualization of the quality of life of families with children with disabilities between 0 and 6 years of age, the instruments for their measurement and the most relevant research results. *Method*: A bibliographic search was conducted in the Web of Science, Scopus and Eric databases of studies published in English and Spanish from 2000 to July 2019 focused on "family quality of life" or "quality of family life" in the disability field. A total of 63 studies were selected from a total of 1119 and analyzed for their theoretical and applied contributions to the field of early care. *Results*: The functional conceptualization of family quality of life predominates in this area, and a nascent and enriching holistic conceptualization is appreciated. There are three instruments that measure family quality of life in early care, although none of them is based on unified theory of FQoL; none of them focus exclusively on the age range 0–6 nor do they cover all disabilities. *Conclusions*: The need to deepen the dynamic interaction of family relationships and to understand the ethical requirement that the methods used to approach family quality of life respect the holistic nature of the research is noted.

Keywords: family quality of life; disability; early childhood intervention; conceptualization; measurement

1. Introduction

The field of early care (EC) is currently undergoing a significant conceptual change. The former clinical intervention model (expert model) is now being replaced by a social and transdisciplinary model (collaboration model) in which family and the environment are core dimensions [1,2]. Development studies have acknowledged the relevance of the social and cultural nature of human development since birth [3,4]. Yet, the role that the people surrounding the children and interacting with them from their birth and throughout their development process has been underestimated [5–9].

The focus now is on a positive understanding of disability and a knowledge "of the capacity for positive adaptation and of the strengths of families with children with disabilities" [10] (p. 2). Considering the positive impact that the families have in the development of kids with disabilities, the strategy now is to work with the families rather than working for the families [11], and to involve all the family members because what happens to any of the members has an impact on the rest of the family. Thus, it is important to take into consideration the individual needs of each of the family members as well as the needs of the family as a whole [12].

The new focus of EC on the family contributes to overcome some of the limitations that the ambulatory model had, especially regarding the time that the child can engage in learning opportunities and the type of learning opportunities that the family context offers [13]. The family involvement in turn fosters greater parental responsibility, improves family skills, and generates a higher level of satisfaction in the family [14]. Moreover, as Samuel et al., argue, "families that function well support societies and families with an effective quality of life are a social resource." [15] (p. 188). These are all solid reasons that support the adoption of this family model in EC, a model that has the family as a core dimension and whose ultimate goal is to promote a better quality of family life. In fact, Bhopti et al., stated that EC services should demonstrate "positive family outcomes annually" [12] (p. 192).

Family quality of life (FQoL), then, should be a relevant indicator of service quality [13]. The problem, however, is that there is no consensus in the definition of FQoL, nor it is easy to change the approach and purpose of some services [2]. One of the most accepted theorizations of the concept of FQoL argues that "family quality of life is a dynamic sense of well-being of the family, collectively and subjectively defined and informed by its members, in which individual and family-level needs interact" [16] (p. 262). This idea is reinforced by the unified theory developed by Zuna et al., according to which "[systemic factors] directly impact individual and family-level supports, services, and practices. Individual-member concepts (i.e., demographics, characteristics) are direct predictors of FQoL and interact with individual—and family-level support, services, and practices to predict FQoL. Singly or combined, the model predictors result in a FQoL outcome that produces new family strengths, needs, and priorities that re-enter the model as new input resulting in a continuous feedback loop throughout the life cycle" [16] (p. 269).

This integrative and multidimensional model does not make easy to assess FQoL. The current evaluation methods most recognized and used internationally are the International Family Quality of Life Project [17] and the Beach Center Family Quality of Life Scale [18]. Each one has a different operational definition of FQoL and each one identifies a different number of dimensions to focus on in the evaluation—nine in the former and five in the latter. At a national level, in Spain there is only one instrument to evaluate early care services—the Spanish Family Quality of Life Scale (FQoL-S) developed by Giné et al. [19]—which only covers until 18 years of age. The FQoL-S started including seven dimensions, but after a review of its psychometric properties in 2018, it was reduced to five dimensions. This scale was created and developed exclusively for population with intellectual disabilities. The limitations of this instrument do not allow us to know if the Spanish EC services are moving in the right direction. All of this limits us, while occupying our interest in how to know if our EC services are moving in a better direction.

The Spanish Federation of Associations of Early Care Professionals has already acknowledged that it is time to move towards a common early care model in Spain. They argued that early care must be recognized as a subjective right through a state law or regulation that includes all children from 0 to 6 years of age who have problems and developmental issues at some point in their development. This represents 10% of the child population of that age group, which means caring for 255,277 children in Spain in the Child Development and Early Care Centers (Centros de Desarrollo infantil y atención primaria, or CDIATs).

Our systematic review was based on all the factors mentioned above together with the fact that "the evolutionary and vital circumstances of children and their families are changing and are different from those that characterize early childhood" [2]. Our main goal was to provide answers to the following research questions:

(1) What has been the conceptualization of the quality of life of families with a child who has a disability or developmental concerns between 0 and 6 years?
(2) What instruments of FQoL directed to population with disability and that have adequate psychometric properties exist for the child stage (0–6 years)?
(3) What are the main findings of the existing studies on FQoL in the 0–6 years stage?

2. Method

The search focused on three databases, Web of Science, Scopus and Eric, and it was based on the following keywords: "Family Quality of Life" OR "Quality of Family Life" (in English) and "Calidad de Vida Familiar" (in Spanish). We decided to exclude the term 'disability' in our search in order to enrich our understanding on FQoL, to cover any type or diagnosis of disability and to improve our current measurements on disability related FQoL.

Our selection of the bibliographic materials was based on the following criteria:

(a) the empirical studies were based on studies with samples that included families of children with disabilities and/or developmental issues within the 0 to 6 years stage;
(b) the studies had been published after 1999, which is the year when the publications on FQL as a social construct and extension of the QoL of individuals with IDD started;
(c) the studies were written in English or Spanish, as these are the languages used in most of the publications on this topic and the languages mastered by the authors of this article;
(d) the studies were published in peer-review journals or as book chapters.

As for the exclusion criteria, we did not consider studies in which:

(a) disability was considered a disease, since that would have entailed to discard the systematic approach in favor of the rehabilitative medical model;
(b) FQoL was studied from an individual-based perspective (instead of the holistic model mentioned above which includes all the family members);
(c) FQoL was conceptualized from a rehabilitative medical perspective, since we are interested in disability from a psychosocial approach.

In order to ensure reliability, two independent researchers conducted the literature review and there was full agreement on their results. Besides, two separate searches were conducted in parallel: one focused on the scientific literature in English and another one focused on the scientific literature in Spanish.

3. Results

Our first bibliographic search retrieved a total of 1119 articles, 33 in Spanish and 1086 in English (see Table 1). From the 1119 articles, 493 were discarded as duplicate materials and seven more publications were incorporated from additional sources. The breakdown of these seven publications is as follows:

(1) four theoretical studies, which provide definitions of FQoL [16,20–22];
(2) the Family Quality of Life Survey (FQOLS-2006) [23] conducted by an international team of researchers;
(3) the study by García Grau et al. [24] published months after the searches were conducted;
(4) an empirical study [25] found as grey literature.

Table 1. Search procedures for English and Spanish publication.

Plataform	Results	Search	Languages
Scopus	563 9	"Family Quality of Life" OR "Quality of Family Life" "Calidad de Vida Familiar"	English Spanish
WOS	416 20	"Family Quality of Life" OR "Quality of Family Life" "Calidad de Vida Familiar"	English Spanish

Table 1. *Cont.*

Plataform	Results	Search	Languages
Eric	107	"Family Quality of Life" OR "Quality of Family Life"	English
	4	"Calidad de Vida Familiar"	Spanish
Total	1119		

The implementation of the inclusion and exclusion criteria reduced the total selection of articles to 663 records. Of these, 195 studies were removed after reading the titles and abstracts. After reading the full text of the remaining 438 records, 375 articles were also discarded. The reasons for their exclusion are included in the flowchart below (see Figure 1). Thus, the final number of articles in which our systematic review is based is 63, from which 60 are written in English and three in Spanish.

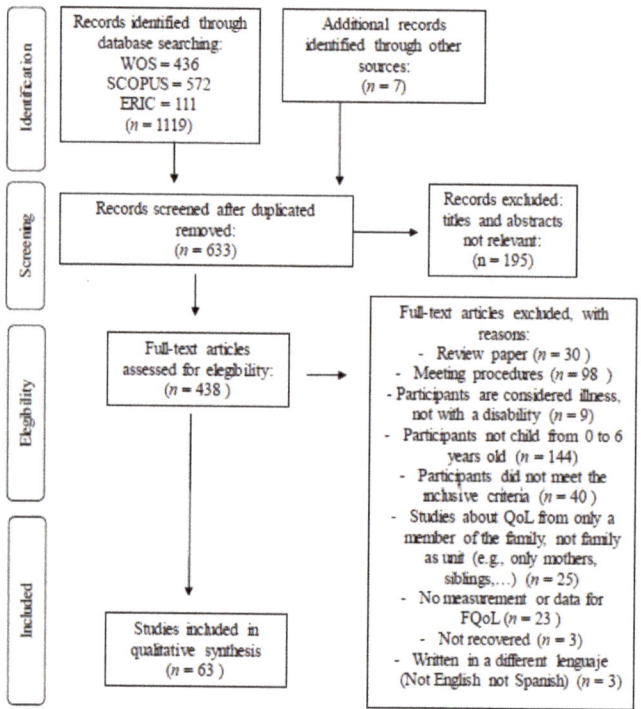

Figure 1. Flowchart of the selection process according to the recommendations of the Prisma statement. (Moher and Liberati [26]). Source: Own elaboration.

The selected articles were analyzed and classified according to the three research questions mentioned above.

3.1. The Conceptualization of FQoL in the 0 to 6 Year Stage

Considering the 63 articles reviewed, two ways of addressing the conceptualization of FQoL have been identified: (1) how it has been theoretically defined (Table 2) and (2) how it has been measured or operationalized (Table 3). Hu et al. [27] called this second approach "functional" because it identifies the areas or domains of family life that are measured through scales or other instruments. This Systematic Review (SR) follows Hu's functional approach.

Table 2. Theoretical conceptualization of FQoL.

Definitions of Family Quality of Life	Articles
Conditions where the family's needs are met, and family members enjoy their life together as a family and have the chance to do things which are important to them.	Turnbull et al. [22] Cited by Park et al. [28] (pp. 368)
It can be said that families experience a satisfactory quality of family life when: (a) they achieve what families around the world, and they in particular, strive to achieve; (b) they are satisfied with what families around the world, and they in particular, have achieved; (c) they feel empowered to live the lives they wish to live.	Brown and Brown [20] (pp. 32)
Family quality of life is a dynamic sense of well-being of the family, collectively and subjectively defined and informed by its members, in which individual and family-level needs interact.	Zuna et al. [16] (pp. 262)
Family quality of life is concerned with the degree to which individuals experience their own quality of life within the family context, as well as with how the family as a whole has opportunities to pursue its important possibilities and achieve its goals in the community and the society of which it is a part.	Brown and Brown [21] (pp. 2195)

Table 3. Conceptualization of FQoL across six researcher groups.

Beach Center FQoL scale (Hoffman et al. [18]) 5 Domains	FQoLsurvey-2006 International Project (Brown et al. [17]) 9 Domains	FQoL-S (Giné et al. [19]) 7 Domains	The Autism Family Experience Questionnaire (AFEQ) (Leadbiter et al. [29]) 4 Domains	ITP-Child Quality-of-Life Questionnaire (Barnard et al. [30]) 5 Domains	Feiqol-Family Early Intervention Quality of Life (Garcia-Grau et al. [24]) 3 Factors
1. Family Interaction 2. Parenting 3. Emotional Well-being 4. Physical-Well-being material 5. Disability Related Support	1. Health 2. Finances 3. Family Relationships 4. Informal Support 5. Service Support 6. Influence of values 7. Career path 8. Leisure and free time 9. Community	1. Emotional well-being 2. Family Interaction 3. Health 4. Final well-being 5. Organization and parenting skills 6. Accomodation of the family 7. Social Inclusion and Participation	1. Parents 2. Family 3. Child development 4. Child symptoms	1. Treatment side effect-related 2. Intervention related 3. Disease-related 4. Activity-related 5. Family-related	1. Family Relationships 2. Access to Information and Services 3. Child Functioning

3.1.1. Theoretical Conceptualization

Being aware of the different conceptualizations of FQoL is an important step in the field of disability because "it is difficult to advance in any field if a definition of the concept or phenomenon studied is not commonly shared and if there is uncertainty about what, in the first place, is supposed to be measured" [31] (p. 19). The existing definitions of FQoL are included in Table 2.

From a chronological point of view, the first definition was formulated in 2000 by Turnbull et al. [22] cited by Park et al. [28]. This definition includes the perceptions of family members, and for this reason some authors call it "subjective conceptualization" [32,33]. The influence of this conceptualization in the FQoL literature is relevant [34–37].

Four years later, in 2004, Brown and Brown [20] identified three components in FQoL. According to them, families experience quality of life when they (a) strive to achieve what they want; (b) are satisfied with what they have achieved; (c) feel empowered to lead the life they desire. Ten years later, these components were also included in another study by the same authors, which highlights how the FQoL construct "changes a little over time in response to our understanding of other related concepts, changing social values and norms and cultural and environmental conditions" [21] (pp. 2195).

In 2010, Zuna et al. [16] proposed a definition that highlights the dynamic meaning of the construct. This definition has been cited by 15 of the articles selected in this study [6,33,37–49].

3.1.2. Functional Conceptualization

From the operational or functional point of view, the FQoL is understood as "a global outcome of services" [50] (pp. 204). At first, the conceptualization of the FQoL was based on the one used in the field of the individual QoL, which led to the consideration of the FQoL as a multidimensional construct. Indeed, researchers of FQoL have focused on identifying the different domains that constitute the FQoL construct through the creation and validation of measurement instruments.

Table 3 shows the domains that constitute the instruments created to implement the FQoL construct, including the name and number of domains in each proposal. There are six functional conceptualizations so far. Although the number of domains in each of the proposals varies (from 9 domains by the FQOL Survey-2006 [17] to 3 of the FEIQoL [24]), the following domain names are repeated: family, supports and financial.

3.2. Instruments that Measure the FQoL in the 0 to 6 Years Stage

The results of the bibliographic search conducted for this review show that the majority of studies focused on the 0 to 6 years stage have used international FQoL scales, which were designed for all ages, such as the Beach Center FQoL Scale [18], the FQOL Survey-2006 [17] and FQoL-S [19]. Table 4 only includes the instruments designed to be applied in children between 0 and 6 years of age.

Table 4. FQoL instruments in the 0- to 6-year stage.

Instruments and Authors	Respond	Domains	Dimensions	Number of Items and Reliability
The Autism Family Experience Questionnaire (AFEQ) (Leadbiter et al. [29])	Parents	4 domains: (1) Parents; (2) Family; (3) Child development; (4) Child symptoms	Likert Scale of frequency 1 to 5 points (with "not applicable" option)	56 items
ITP-Child Quality-of-Life Questionnaire (Barnard et al. [30])	Parents	5 domains: (1) treatment side effect-related; (2) intervention related; (3) disease-related; (4) activity-related; and (5) family-related	Likert scale of frequency and importance 1 to 5 points	26 items
Family Early Intervention Quality of Life (FEIQoL) García Grau et al. [24] *		3 Factors: (1) Family Relationships; (2) Access to Information and Services; (3) Child Functioning	Likert Scale 1 to 5 points of "poor" to "excellent"	40 items

* The Family Early Intervention Quality of Life (FEIQoL) García Grau et al. [24] is the Spanish version of the original instrument developed by McWilliam and Casey 2013 (unpublished) [51].

There are three instruments designed to be applied in EC: (1) The Autism Family Experience Questionnaire (AFEQ) [29] for families with children with autism; (2) ITP-Child Quality-of-Life Questionnaire [30] for children with immune thrombopenic purpura; and (3) the adaptation of the Family Quality of Life (FaQoL) by McWilliam et Casey to the Spanish context (FEIQoL) [24] for children with all types of disabilities.

In the search for instruments to measure the FQoL and in addition to the instruments mentioned in Tables 3 and 4, we also identified 10 studies whose main objective is the development, adaptation and/or validation of the FQoL scales (see Table 5).

Table 5. Studies that adapt, develop or validate the FQoL scales.

Scales	Development, Validation or Adaptation Studies	Country
Beach Center FQoL Scale (Hoffman et al., 2006) [18]	Balcells-Balcells et al., 2011 [39]; Verdugo et al., 2005 [52] Chiu et al., 2017 [40]; Chiu et al., 2017 [53] Waschl et al., 2019 [54] Bello-Escamilla et al., 2017 [55]; Rivard et al., 2017 [56]	Spain Hong Kong Singapore Chile Canada
FQOL Survey-2006 (Brown et al., 2006) [17]	Perry e Isaacs 2015 [57]; Samuel et al., 2016 [15]; Samuel et al., 2018 [58]	USA

As we can see, these 10 studies refer to the most international FQoL scales.

3.3. Main Results on FQoL in the 0- to 6-Year Stage

In response to the third research question about the main finding of the studies on FQoL in the 0–6 years, the studies applied to this age group have been divided into two tables. The first table (Table 6) classifies 22 studies that describe, compare or relate QoL of families with young children with disabilities with other variables. The second table (Table 7) shows the studies that focus on the variables that predict FQoL.

Table 6. Descriptive, comparative or correlational studies.

Theme	Authors (Year) (Chronological Order)
Population	Córdoba et al., 2008 [59]; Neikrug et al., 2011 [60]; Clark et al., 2012 [61]; Rillotta et al., 2012 [35]; Giné et al., 2015 [62]; Mas et al., 2016 [6]; Schertz et al., 2016 [32]; García Grau et al., 2018 [44]; Rodrigues et al., 2018 [63].
Maternal Outcomes	McStay et al., 2014 [64,65].
Type of disability	Brown et al., 2006 [66]; Jackson et al., 2010 [48]; Schertz et al., 2016 [32]; Tait et al., 2016 [67]; Schlebusch et al., 2017 [37]; Tejada-Ortigosa et al., 2019 [68].
Ethnic perspective	Holloway et al., 2014 [69]; Algood and Davis, 2019 [70].
Attention to participants	Wang et al., 2006 [71]; Moyson and Roeyers, 2012 [72].
Supports	Steel et al., 2011 [73]; Escorcia-Mora et al., 2018 [25].

The breakdown of the results found in the studies included in Table 6 is as follows:

(a) Ten articles explicitly focus on describing the FQoL in the population of their respective countries. Spain [6,44,62] has three studies; Israel [32,60] has two, and Australia [36], Brasil [63], Colombia [59] and Malaysia [61] have one each.

(b) Two articles [64,65] relate FQoL to parental stress in families with children with autism.

(c) Six articles relate the FQoL to a specific type of disability. Brown et al. [66], for instance, compared the QoL of three types of families: families with a child with Down syndrome, families with a child with autism spectrum disorders, and families with none of their members having a disability. The other five articles focus on specific disabilities, namely deafness [48], intellectual disability [32,67], autism [37] and rare metabolic diseases [68].

(d) Two articles adopt an ethnic perspective. Algood et al. [70] address the issue of inequity in the care of African-American families compared to other ethnicities, while Holloway et al. [69] study QoL in California among Latino and non-Latino families.

(e) Two articles relate the FQoL to perspectives of some of the family members. Moyson and Roeyers [72] investigated the FQoL from the perspective of the siblings of the person with disabilities. Wang et al., determined "whether mothers and fathers similarly view the conceptual model of FQoL embodied in one measure" [71] (pp. 977). This study shows that there are no significant differences between the perceptions of fathers and mothers.

(f) Two studies investigate how families describe the supports and services they receive [24,71].

Following the proposal of Zuna et al. [8], the 21 studies analyzed in Table 7 identify the following components: (a) systemic concepts; (b) performance concepts; (c) individual-member concepts; and (d) family-unit concepts.

First, the systemic concept is integrated by three categories: (a1) systems; (a2) policies; and (a3) programs. Regarding the first two categories, no study has been identified. As for the third category ("programs"), Hielkema et al. [74] studied the effectiveness of "Coping with and Caring for infants with special needs (COPCA)", a family-focused program applied to 43 families with young children at high risk of cerebral palsy. The results related to the group that received COPCA show that the FQoL improved over time.

Second, the performance concepts focus on the following three categories: (b1) Services; (b2) Supports and (b3) Practices. Seven studies focus on services (b1), and all of them show that the services received by families with young children with disabilities favor FQoL [7,43,46,49,50,75,76]. Balcells-Balcells et al. [77] and Samuel et al. [75] identify an increase in parental satisfaction based on the information received by the services. Taub and Werner [49] found that both religious and secular families are satisfied with the support received from the spiritual community and the social services, respectively. Eight studies focus on supports (b2). The support of professionals to families has received significant attention, and it has become one of the strongest predictors of FQoL [58,78,79]. Emotional support is better considered than practical support from both services and other informal aids [35,41,73,76,80]. In fact, the study by Meral et al. [80] reveals that emotional support is the most important factor for the respondents. Svavarsdottir and Tryggvadottir [81], on the other hand, focus on the predictive nature of family support. Finally, considering the category of practices (b3), Davis and Gavidia Payne [79] recognize the value of the family-centered model as a safeguard for the needs of each family.

Third, the individual-member concepts integrates the following three categories: individual characteristics (c1), demographic aspects (c2) and beliefs (c3). In the individual characteristics category (c1), six articles were related to parental stress. The majority of them focus on studying how the support [33,79,81,82] and the information received [79,81] are predictive factors of the decrease in parental stress and, consequently, of the increase in FQoL [78]. Wang et al. [83] indicate that the efforts that parents with children with disabilities make in defending their kids generates considerable stress in them. Boehm et al. [84] investigate the relationship between the parents' religiosity and the improvement of the FQoL.

Table 7. Predictive studies of the FQoL.

Concepts of FQoL Theory (Zuna et al. [8])		Authors (Year) (Chronological Order)
Systemic concepts	Systems	No records have been identified
	Policies	No records have been identified
	Programs	Hielkema et al., 2019, [74]
Performance concepts	Services	Balcells-Balcells et al., 2019 [77]; Epley et al., 2011 [50]; Eskow et al., 2011 [43]; Kyzar et al., 2016 [46]; Samuel et al., 2012 [75]; Summers et al., 2007 [76]; Taub and Werner 2016 [49];
	Supports	Boehm et al., 2019 [84]; Cohen et al., 2014 [41]; Davis and Gavidia Payne, 2009 [79]; Hsiao et al., 2017 [78]; Kyzar et al., 2016 [46]; Kyzar et al., 2018 [85]; Meral et al., 2013 [80]; Samuel et al., 2011 [36]; Svavarsdottir and Tryggvadottir, 2019 [81]; Taub and Werner, 2016 [49]

Table 7. *Cont.*

Concepts of FQoL Theory (Zuna et al. [8])		Authors (Year) (Chronological Order)
	Practices	Davis and Gavidia Payne, 2009 [79]
Individual-member concepts	Individual characteristics	Boehm et al., 2019 [84]; Davis and Gavidia Payne, 2009, [79]; Hsiao et al., 2017 [78]; Hsiao 2018 [82]; Levinger et al., 2018 [86]; Meral et al., 2013 [80]; Vanderkerken et al., 2018 [33]; Wang et al., 2004 [83];
	Demographic aspects	Meral et al., 2013 [80]; Cohen et al., 2014 [41]; Hsiao 2018 [82]; Kyzar et al., 2018 [85]; Levinger et al., 2018 [86]; Vanderkerken et al., 2018 [33]; Boehm et al., 2019 [84]
	Beliefs	Svavarsdottir and Tryggvadottir, 2019 [81]
Family-unit concepts	Characteristics of the family	Boehm et al., 2019 [84]; Cohen et al., 2014 [41]; Davis and Gavidia Payne, 2009 [79]; Hsiao 2018 [82]; Hielkema et al., 2019 [74]; Kyzar et al., 2018; Schlebusch et al., 2016 [87]; Taub and Werner 2016 [49]; [85]; Wang et al., 2004 [83]
	Family dynamics	Schlebusch et al., 2016 [87]; Levinger et al., 2018; [86]; Vanderkerken et al., 2018 [33].

In the demographic aspects category (c2), nine articles consider as predictive variables for FQoL the following factors: the age of the child with a disability [41,80,83,85], the gender of the child [24,39,82], the type of disability [31,80,84], the degree of disability [80,81], the number of siblings [58,81], and the marital status of the parents [44].

Finally, in the category focused on beliefs, (c3), Svavarsdottir, and Tryggvadottir [81] conclude that the beliefs of the parents regarding the severe illness of the child significantly predicted the FQoL.

The last factor of the proposal by Zuna et al. [8] is the family-unit concepts, which integrates two categories: family unit (d1) and family dynamics (d2). In the section on the family unit (d1), 9 studies consider the predictive factors of FQoL. The results show that for the most part two-parent families enjoy better FQoL than single-parent families [62,82]; family income is predictive of better FQoL [79,82,87]; and belonging to one or another ethnic group [41,82], being part of a religious community [49] or having a spiritual faith [84] also determines the level of satisfaction of FQoL. Regarding family dynamics (d2), the study by Vanderkerken et al. [33] addresses the so-called homeostatic control and suggests asking the opinions of all family members about the FQoL.

4. Discussion

The discussion is developed in the order of the research questions stated at the outset of this review. Regarding the first question based on the FQoL conceptualization, there is an incipient holistic approach, but the functional conceptualization still prevails. We will analyze our findings in relation to two previous SRs focused on the conceptualization of the FQoL [88] and on the FQoL measurement tools, respectively. Both SRs found that the FQoL scales lack a theoretical framework and a definition of this construct. Most researchers who published their studies after these two SRs followed the functional conceptualization approach. For instance, in a theoretical study which integrated the perspectives of three authors from three different research teams—Schippers, Zuna and Brown—it was argued that "from the QoL conceptual development and research to date, we have a strong sense that it is usually a number of variables across a variety of life areas working in an interrelated fashion that are essential to improving QoL for individuals and families" [89] (pp. 151). Although these authors emphasize the interrelated dimension of the different variables considered, many studies that explicitly refer to the holistic theory developed by Zuna only identify the different domains of family life but do not integrate them in their studies.

Our SR has shown that the empirical studies arrive at different, and sometimes discordant, results. The discrepancies are based on how researchers have conceptualized FQoL, the number of the domains considered to evaluate FQoL, the methodology used (i.e., quantitative or mixed) and/or how many members of family have participated.

We agree with Boelsma et al. [90] on the need of taking into consideration the dynamic interaction between the individual and the family domains in the FQoL research. The fact that many studies refer to the holistic approach of FQoL by Zuna et al. [16] shows that this holistic understanding is becoming more and more solid in the conceptualization of the FQoL. What Zuna's definition adds to the rest of the existing definitions (see Table 2) is the dynamic character, referring to the sense of well-being and the collective dimension behind the definition and evaluation of the FQoL construct, since it is based on the interaction between individual and family needs [91], and among services, supports and practices.

The complexity underpinning this holistic approach does not reside in its multidimensionality but rather in its dynamic aspect. To study a dynamic reality entails understanding it from its capacity to face changes. Our understanding of this dynamic sense of family well-being follows Bhopti et al. [12] who emphasize how family well-being may change depending on significant events in the life of the family.

Considering the second research question, based on the FQoL assessment instruments, there are no scales developed specifically for the 0–6-year stage, nor do the developed scales address all disabilities and/or developmental concerns. The FQoL-S by Giné et al. [19] covers up to 18 years of age. The FEIQoL of García Grau et al. [24] focuses on the measurement of early care services [44] and puts emphasis on the factor "child functioning" [38]. These same authors [24] recognise not having conceptualized the EI as extensively as they did the other scales. This acknowledgment questions the solidity of the theoretical framework on which their conceptualization is based.

The FEIQoL scale takes into account both the dynamic sense of the FQoL and the fact that the dynamic sense can change in the different stages of the family life cycle. However, in the studies of these authors, the dynamic concepts mentioned by Zuna are not explicitly present in the FEIQoL, except for the notion of family routines.

Finally, regarding the third research question about the findings, this SR has found that research on FQoL has mainly focused on issues related to disability and chronic illnesses in children from 0 to 6 years of age, even though the FQoL is construct that can be applied to a wider typology of families (families with a child who has not been diagnosed).

Our analysis of the descriptive, comparative and correlational studies identified reveals that most of them focus on the individual concepts of the unified theory of FQoL by Zuna et al. [16]. Specifically, most of them focus on the characteristics of the individual, the characteristics of the child, and on demographic aspects.

Among the predictive studies of the FQoL, there is more interest in the studies related to supports and services, individual categories, and categories related to the family unit than in the studies that focus on systemic aspects and family dynamics. Considering the former, it is important to highlight that there are no conclusive results in relation to the variables indicated, in particular to the variables related to the age and the disability of the children [32,44,67]. There is only partial agreement in the studies that show how the FQoL of the families with children with disability in the first two years of age is less than the FQoL of the families with children with disability from three years of age on [44,62]. A wider agreement is reached among the studies that show that the greater the severity of the child's disability, the lower the degree of QoL in families [6,79,86,87]. We noticed that although quantitative studies predominate, there is an increase in others that incorporate qualitative [42,63,72] or mixed methodology [35,66,67,82]. We also identified the need of match the methods used with the ethical dimensions of the research.

Qualitative research studies are needed [42] if we want to evaluate family outcomes related to experiences "that can only be explained by considering the perceptions of the family members themselves, because ultimately it is these subjective perceptions that determine the individual's approach to life and how satisfied they are with life" [7] (pp. 17). In this regard, some researchers adapt their methodologies to the participants in their research. Van Heumen and Schippers [92], for instance, use the Photovoice methodology to allow the family members to speak about the images that are significant to them.

Finally, a few words on the ethical aspects of research in FQoL. As we know, one of the ethical requirements of research refers to the coherence between the objectives and intentions of the researchers and the results obtained. From the beginning, scholars doing research on FQoL identified a problem that presented both a practical and an ethical aspect. Poston et al., included in their study the opinions of various authors regarding the need to consider the perceptions of all family members. Yet, they soon identified a practical problem—despite trying to involve the other members, usually only the mother participated. From an ethical perspective, these authors consider this fact to be crucial to evaluate the realiability of the results [93]. In 2006, Wang et al., published a study in which they proposed to verify if both parents understood the QoL of their family in a similar way [71]. Both the fathers and the mothers responded in a similar way, which turned out to be promising for the use of the scales in the case that only one of the parents participated. This conclusion prompts some researchers to include only one of the parents in the research [6,8,10,50,63,69]. Although Vanderkerken et al., argued that the perceptions of fathers did not differ significantly from those of mothers in a study in which they had a broad representation of family members [33], it is still important to investigate the impact that the participation of one or more family members has in the FQoL.

There are numerous studies that explicitly address the limitations of not taking into account more than one of the parents, which shows that there is an ethical concern in this regard [35,39,42,43,45,46,53–55,60,75,82,84]. Gardiner and Iarocci [91] indicate that in the future, research on the FQoL should include the voices of the different members of the family. Hu et al., establish a connection between the holistic nature of the FQoL and the method used. To solve this problem, Brown et al., propose that one of the parents responds on behalf of the rest of the family [66], who would thus be represented by him or her [74,87,94]. However, as Giné et al., note, there is no way to ensure that this instruction of responding on behalf of the family has been followed by the family representative [58]. Feigin et al. [95] understand that the participation of brothers and sisters of the child with disabilities, in addition to the parents, is a requirement of the systemic nature of the family.

5. Implications

This SR clearly shows that the state of the art in the research of FQoL points to the ecological, systemic and inclusive vision of the family and, therefore, of the FQoL in the field of EC and disability. The inclusion of studies without the term "disabilities" as a keyword in this SR has contributed to including enriching studies on this topic and to cover any type or diagnosis of disability. This inclusive perspective is an invitation to all services and institutions to direct their attention to the dynamic interaction of personal and collective needs.

As this SR shows, there is a need to develop the emerging holistic conceptualization through mixed research and to be open to methodologies that overcome the limitations mentioned above. We also need to create instruments of measurement of the FQoL that are specific to this stage of life and family cycle from a systemic perspective.

6. Limitations

We were not able to get access to three studies found in the databases which were included in this review based on the title and/or the abstract [96–98].

7. Conclusions

Empirical studies of the QoL of families with a child with a disability or developmental concerns show a certain inertia of functional conceptualization. Yet, an incipient holistic conceptualization has also been noted. Among the selected articles, three instruments have been identified to measure the QoL of families with young children in the age range 0–6 years: (1) The Autism Family Experience

Questionnaire (AFEQ) [29]; (2) ITP-Child Quality-of-Life Questionnaire (Barnard et al. [30] and (3) Family Early Intervention Quality of Life (FEIQoL) [24]. These instruments however do not refer to all disabilities or do not have a holistic approach. Considering the main predictor variables studied here—the age of the child and the type of disability—there are no unanimous or conclusive results. After the investigation, the SR has become a State of the Art of the FQoL research, since it identifies the last contributions in conceptualization, and the epistemological and methodological deficiencies on the studies of FQoL. This SR identifies two key areas for future research: to deepen the understanding of the dynamic interactions of family relationships and to understand the ethical requirement of having the methods used to approach the FQoL respect the holistic nature of the research.

Author Contributions: Conceptualization, C.F.M. and A.B.-B.; methodology, C.F.M., A.I. and A.B.-B.; writing—original draft preparation, C.F.M. and A.I.; writing—review and editing, A.I., A.B.-B. and C.F.M. All authors have read and agreed to the published version of the manuscript.

Funding: This research received no external funding.

Conflicts of Interest: The authors declare no conflict of interest.

References

1. Escorcia, C.T.; García-Sánchez, F.; Sánchez-López, M.C.; Hernández-Pérez, E. Cuestionario de estilos de interacción entre padres y profesionales en atención temprana: Validez de contenido. *An. Psicol.* **2016**, *32*, 148–157.
2. Federación Estatal de Asociaciones de Profesionales de Atención Temprana (GAT). La Atención Temprana. La Visión de Los Profesionales. Available online: http://www.avap-cv.com/images/Documentos%20basicos/GAT-LA-VISI%C3%93N-DE-LOS-PROFESIONALES.pdf (accessed on 6 August 2020).
3. Bronfrenbrenner, U. *La Ecología del Desarrollo Humano*; Espasa: Barcelona, Spain, 1987.
4. Bruner, J.S. *La Educación, Puerta de la Cultura*; Visor: Madrid, Spain, 1997.
5. Guralnick, M.J. Why early intervention works. *Infants Young Child.* **2011**, *24*, 6–28. [CrossRef] [PubMed]
6. Mas, J.M.; Baques, N.; Balcells-Balcells, A.; Dalmau, M.; Gine, C.; Gracia, M.; Vilaseca, R. Family Quality of Life for families in early intervention in Spain. *J. Early Interv.* **2016**, *38*, 59–74. [CrossRef]
7. Rillotta, F.; Kirby, N.; Shearer, J.A. Comparison of two 'family quality of life' measures: An australian study. In *Enhancing the Quality of Life of People with Intellectual Disabilities: From Theory to Practice*; Kober, R., Ed.; Springer: Dordrecht, The Netherlands, 2010; pp. 305–348.
8. Zuna, N.I.; Turnbull, A.; Summers, J.A. Family Quality of Life: Moving from measurement to application. *J. Policy Pract. Intellect. Disabil.* **2009**, *6*, 25–31. [CrossRef]
9. Hadders-Algra, M.M.; Hielkema, A.G.B.; Hamer, E.G. Effect of early intervention in infants at very high risk of cerebral palsy: A systematic review. *Dev. Med. Child. Neurol.* **2017**, *59*, 246–258. [CrossRef]
10. Chiu, C.; Kyzar, K.; Zuna, N.; Turnbull, A.; Summers, J.A.; Aya Gómez, V. Family Quality of Life, Trends in family research related to family quality of life. In *The Oxford Handbook of Positive Psychology and Disability*; Wehmeyer, M.W., Ed.; Oxford University Press: New York, NY, USA, 2013; pp. 365–392.
11. Dunst, C.J.; Bruder, M.B. Valued outcomes of service coordination, early intervention, and natural environments. *Except. Child.* **2002**, *68*, 361–375. [CrossRef]
12. Bhopti, A.; Brown, T.; Lentin, P. Family Quality of Life: A Key Outcome in Early Childhood Intervention Services A Scoping Review. *J. Early Interv.* **2016**, *38*, 191–211. [CrossRef]
13. Jung, L.A.; Baird, S.M. Effects of service coordinator variables on individualized family service plans. *J. Early Interv.* **2003**, *25*, 206–218. [CrossRef]
14. Mahoney, G.; Perales, F. El papel de los padres de niños con síndrome de Down y otras discapacidades en la atención temprana. *Rev. Sínd. Down* **2012**, *29*, 46–54.
15. Samuel, P.S.; Pociask, F.D.; Dizazzo-Miller, R.; Carrellas, A.; LeRoy, B.W. Concurrent validity of the International Family Quality of Life Survey. *Occup. Ther. Health Care* **2016**, *30*, 187–201. [CrossRef]
16. Zuna, N.; Summers, J.A.; Turnbull, A.P.; Hu, X.; Xu, S. Theorizing about family quality of life. In *Enhancing the Quality of Life of People with Intellectual Disabilities: From Theory to Practice*; Kober, R., Ed.; Springer: Dordrecht, The Netherlands, 2010; Volume 41, pp. 241–278.

17. Brown, R.I.; Kyrkou, M.R.; Samuel, P.S. Family quality of life. In *Health Care for People with Intellectual and Developmental Disabilities across the Lifespan*; Rubin, I.L., Merrick, J., Greydanus, D.E., Patel, D.R., Eds.; Springer: Basel, Switzerland, 2016; pp. 2065–2082.
18. Hoffman, L.; Marquis, J.; Poston, D.; Summers, J.A.; Turnbull, A. Assessing Family Outcomes: Psychometric Evaluation of the Beach Center Family Quality of Life Scale. *J. Marriage Fam.* **2006**, *68*, 1069–1083. [CrossRef]
19. Giné, C.; Vilaseca, R.; Gràcia, M.; Mora, J.; Orcasitas, J.R.; Simón, C.; Torrecillas, A.M.; Beltran, F.S.; Dalmau, M.; Pro, M.T.; et al. Spanish Family Quality of Life Scales: Under and over 18 Years Old. *J. Intellect. Dev. Disabil.* **2013**, *38*, 141–148. [CrossRef] [PubMed]
20. Brown, I.; Brown, R.I. Concepts for Beginning Study in Family Quality of Life. In *Families and People with Mental Retardation and Quality of Life: International Perspectives*; American Association on Mental Retardation: Washington, DC, USA, 2004; pp. 25–49.
21. Brown, R.I.; Brown, I. Family Quality of Life. In *Encyclopedia of Quality of Life and Well-Being Research*; Michalos, A.C., Ed.; Springer: Dordrecht, The Netherlands, 2014. [CrossRef]
22. Turnbull, A.P.; Turnbull, H.R.; Poston, D.; Beegle, G.; BlueBanning, M.; Diehl, K.; Frankland, C.; Lord, L.; Marquis, J.; Park, J.; et al. *Enhancing Quality of Life of Families of Children and Youth with Disabilities in the United States. A Paper Presented at Family Quality of Life Symposium*; Seattle, W.A., Ed.; Beach Center on Families and Disability: Lawrence, KS, USA, 2000.
23. Brown, I.; Brown, R.I.; Baum, N.T.; Isaacs, N.J.; Myerscough, T.; Neikrug, S.; Wang, M. *Family Quality Life Survey: Main Caregivers of People with Intellectual or Development Disabilities*; Surrey Place Centre: Toronto, ON, Canada, 2006.
24. García-Grau, P.; McWilliam, R.A.; Martínez-Rico, G.; Morales-Murillo, C. Rasch analysis of the families in early intervention quality of life (FEIQoL) Scale. *Appl. Res. Qual. Life* **2019**, *14*, 1–17. [CrossRef]
25. Escorcia-Mora, C.T.; García-Sánchez, F.A.; Sánchez-López, M.C.; Orcajada, N.; Hernández-Pérez, E. Prácticas de intervención en la primera infancia en el sureste de España: Perspectiva de profesionales y familias. *An. Psicol.* **2018**, *34*, 500–509.
26. Moher, E.; Liberati, A. Revisiones Sistemáticas y Metaanálisis: La responsabilidad de Los Autores, Revisores, Editores y Patrocinadores. *Med. Clin.* **2010**, *135*, 505–506. [CrossRef]
27. Hu, X.; Summers, J.A.; Turnbull, A.; Zuna, N. The quantitative measurement of family quality of life: A review of available instruments. *J. Intellect. Disabil. Res.* **2011**, *55*, 1098–1114. [CrossRef]
28. Park, J.; Hoffman, L.; Marquis, J.; Turnbull, A.P.; Poston, D.; Mannan, H.; Wang, M.; Nelson, L.L. Toward assessing family outcomes of service delivery: Validation of a Family Quality of Life Survey. *J. Intellect. Disabil. Res.* **2003**, *47*, 367–384. [CrossRef]
29. Leadbiter, K.; Aldred, C.; McConachie, H.; Le Couteur, A.; Kapadia, D.; Charman, T.; Mcdonald, W.; Salomone, E.; Emsley, R.; Green, J. The Autism Family Experience Questionnaire (AFEQ): An ecologically-valid, parent-nominated measure of family experience, quality of life and prioritised outcomes for early intervention. *J. Autism Dev. Disord.* **2018**, 1042–1062. [CrossRef]
30. Barnard, D.; Woloski, M.; Feeny, D.; McCusker, P.; Wu, J.; David, M.; Bussel, J.; Lusher, J.; Wakefield, C.; Henriques, S.; et al. Development of disease-specific health-related quality-of-life instruments for children with immune thrombocytopenic purpura and their parents. *J. Pediatr. Hematol. Oncol.* **2003**, *25*, 56–62. [CrossRef]
31. Candel, D.; Dubois, D. Vers une définition de la « qualité de vie »? *Rev. Francoph. Psycho. Oncologie* **2005**, 18–22. [CrossRef]
32. Schertz, M.; Karni-Visel, Y.; Tamir, A.; Genizi, J.; Roth, D. Family Quality of Life among families with a child who has a severe neurodevelopmental disability: Impact of family and child socio-demographic factors. *Res. Dev. Disabil.* **2016**, *53–54*, 95–106. [CrossRef] [PubMed]
33. Vanderkerken, L.; Heyvaert, M.; Onghena, P.; Maes, B. Quality of Life in flemish families with a child with an intellectual disability: A multilevel study on opinions of family members and the impact of family member and family characteristics. *Appl. Res. Qual. Life* **2018**, *13*, 779–802. [CrossRef]
34. Ortiz-Quiroga, D.; Ariza-Araújo, Y.; Pachajoa, H. Family Quality of Life in Patients with Morquio Type IV-A Syndrome: The perspective of the colombian social context (South America). *Rehabilitación* **2018**, *52*, 230–237. [CrossRef]
35. Rillotta, F.; Kirby, N.; Shearer, J.; Nettelbeck, T. Family Quality of Life of Australian Families with a Member with an Intellectual/Developmental Disability. *J. Intellect. Disabil. Res.* **2012**, *56*, 71–86. [CrossRef]

36. Samuel, P.S.; Hobden, K.L.; LeRoy, B.W. Families of children with autism and developmental disabilities: A description of their community interaction. *Res. Soc. Science and Disabil.* **2011**, *6*, 49–83. [CrossRef]
37. Schlebusch, L.; Dada, S.; Samuels, A.E. Family Quality of Life of south african families raising children with autism spectrum disorder. *J. Autism Dev. Disord.* **2017**, *47*, 1966–1977. [CrossRef]
38. García-Grau, P.; McWilliam, R.A.; Martínez-Rico, G.; Grau-Sevilla, M.D. Factor structure and internal consistency of a spanish version of the family quality of life (FaQoL). *Appl. Res. Qual. Life* **2017**, *13*, 385–398. [CrossRef]
39. Balcells-Balcells, A.; Giné, C.; Guàrdia-Olmos, J.; Summers, J.A. Family Quality of Life: Adaptation to spanish population of several family support questionnaires. *J. Intellect. Disabil. Res.* **2011**, *55*, 1151–1163. [CrossRef]
40. Chiu, C.Y.; Seo, H.; Turnbull, A.P.; Summers, J.A. Confirmatory Factor Analysis of a family quality of life scale for taiwanese families of children with intellectual disability/developmental delay. *Intellect. Dev. Disabil.* **2017**, *55*, 57–71. [CrossRef]
41. Cohen, S.R.; Holloway, S.D.; Domínguez-Pareto, I.; Kuppermann, M. Receiving or believing in family Support? Contributors to the life quality of latino and non-latino families of children with intellectual disability. *J. Intellect. Disabil. Res.* **2014**, *58*, 333–345. [CrossRef]
42. Demchick, B.B.; Ehler, J.; Marramar, S.; Mills, A.; Nuneviller, A. Family quality of life when raising a child with pediatric autoimmune neuropsychiatric disorder associated with streptococcal infection (PANDAS). *J. Occup. Ther. Sch. Early Interv.* **2019**, *12*, 182–199. [CrossRef]
43. Eskow, K.; Pineles, L.; Summers, J.A. Exploring the effect of autism waiver services on family outcomes. *J. Policy Pract. Intellect. Disabil.* **2011**, *8*, 28–35. [CrossRef]
44. García-Grau, P.; McWilliam, R.A.; Martinez-Rico, G.; Morales-Murillo, C.P. Child, Family, and early intervention characteristics related to family quality of life in Spain. *J. Early Interv.* **2018**, *41*, 44–61. [CrossRef]
45. Hu, X.; Wang, M.; Fei, X. Family quality of life of chinese families of children with intellectual disabilities. *J. Intellect. Disabil. Res.* **2012**, *56*, 30–44. [CrossRef] [PubMed]
46. Kyzar, K.B.; Brady, S.E.; Summers, J.A.; Haines, S.J.; Turnbull, A.P. Services and supports, partnership, and Family Quality of Life: Focus on deaf-blindness. *Except. Child.* **2016**, *83*, 77–91. [CrossRef]
47. Parpa, E.; Katsantonis, N.; Tsilika, E.; Galanos, A.; Sassari, M.; Mystakidou, K. Psychometric properties of the family quality of life scale in greek families with intellectual disabilities. *J. Dev. Phys. Disabil.* **2016**, *28*, 393–405. [CrossRef]
48. Jackson, C.W.; Wegner, J.R.; Turnbull, A.P. Family Quality of Life following early identification of deafness. *Lang. Speech Hear. Serv. Sch.* **2010**, *41*, 194–205. [CrossRef]
49. Taub, T.; Werner, S. What support resources contribute to family quality of life among religious and secular Jewish families of children with developmental disability? *J. Intellect. Dev. Disabil.* **2016**, *41*, 348–359. [CrossRef]
50. Epley, P.H.; Summers, J.A.; Turnbull, A.P. Family Outcomes of early intervention: Families' perceptions of need, services, and outcomes. *J. Early Interv.* **2011**, *33*, 201–219. [CrossRef]
51. McWilliam, R.A.; Casey, A.M. Factor analysis of family quality of life (FaQoL). 2013; Unpublished manuscript.
52. Verdugo, M.A.; Cordoba, L.; Gomez, J. Spanish Adaptation and Validation of the Family Quality of Life Survey. *J. Intellect. Disabil. Res.* **2005**, *49*, 794–798. [CrossRef]
53. Chiu, S.-J.; Chen, P.-T.; Chou, Y.-T.; Chien, L.-Y. The mandarin chinese version of the Beach Centre Family Quality of Life Scale: Development and psychometric properties in taiwanese families of children with developmental delay. *J. Intellect. Disabil. Res.* **2017**, *61*, 373–384. [CrossRef] [PubMed]
54. Waschl, N.; Xie, H.; Chen, M.; Poon, K.K. Construct, Convergent, and Discriminant Validity of the Beach Center Family Quality of Life Scale for Singapore. *Infants Young Child.* **2019**, *32*, 201–214. [CrossRef]
55. Bello-Escamilla, N.; Rivadeneira, J.; Concha-Toro, M.; Soto-Caro, A.; Diaz-Martinez, X. Family Quality of Life Scale (FQLS): Validation and analysis in a chilean population. *Univ. Psychol.* **2017**, *16*, 20–29. [CrossRef]
56. Rivard, M.; Mercier, C.; Mestari, Z.; Terroux, A.; Mello, C.; Begin, J. Psychometric Properties of the Beach Center Family Quality of Life in french-speaking amilies with a preschool-aged child diagnosed with autism spectrum disorder. *J. Intellect. Dev. Disabil.* **2017**, *122*, 439–452. [CrossRef]
57. Perry, A.; Isaacs, B. Validity of the Family Quality of Life Survey-2006. *J. Appl. Res. Intellect. Disabil.* **2015**, *28*, 584–588. [CrossRef]
58. Samuel, P.S.; Tarraf, W.; Marsack, C. Family Quality of Life Survey (FQOLS-2006): Evaluation of internal consistency, construct, and criterion validity for socioeconomically disadvantaged families. *Phys. Occup. Ther. Pediatr.* **2018**, *38*, 46–63. [CrossRef]

59. Córdoba-Andrade, L.; Gómez-Benito, J.; Verdugo-Alonso, M.A. Family Quality of Life of people with disability: A comparative analyses. *Univ. Psychol.* **2008**, *7*, 369–383.
60. Neikrug, S.; Roth, D.; Judes, J. Lives of Quality in the face of challenge in Israel. *J. Intellect. Disabil. Res.* **2011**, *55*, 1176–1184. [CrossRef]
61. Clark, M.; Brown, R.; Karrapaya, R. An Initial look at the quality of life of malaysian families that include children with disabilities. *J. Intellect. Disabil. Res.* **2012**, *56*, 45–60. [CrossRef]
62. Giné, C.; Gràcia, M.; Vilaseca, R.; Salvador Beltran, F.; Balcells-Balcells, A.; Dalmau Montalà, M.; Adam-Alcocer, A.L.; Teresa Pro, M.; Simó-Pinatella, D.; Mas Mestre, J.M. Family Quality of Life for people with intellectual disabilities in Catalonia. *J. Policy Pract. Intellect. Disabil.* **2015**, *12*, 244–254. [CrossRef]
63. Rodrigues, S.A.; Fontanella, B.J.B.; de Avó, L.R.S.; Germano, C.M.R.; Melo, D.G. A Qualitative study about quality of life in brazilian families with children who have severe or profound intellectual disability. *J. Appl. Res. Intellect. Disabil.* **2019**, *32*, 413–426. [CrossRef] [PubMed]
64. McStay, R.L.; Trembath, D.; Dissanayake, C. Stress and Family Quality of Life in Parents of Children with Autism Spectrum Disorder: Parent Gender and the Double ABCX Model. *J. Autism Dev. Disord.* **2014**, *44*, 3101–3118. [CrossRef] [PubMed]
65. McStay, R.L.; Trembath, D.; Dissanayake, C. Maternal stress and Family Quality of Life in response to raising a child with autism: From preschool to adolescence. *Res. Dev. Disabil.* **2014**, *35*, 3119–3130. [CrossRef] [PubMed]
66. Brown, R.I.; MacAdam-Crisp, J.; Wang, M.; Iaroci, G. Family Quality of Life when there is a child with a developmental disability. *J. Policy Pract. Intellect. Disabil.* **2006**, *3*, 238–245. [CrossRef]
67. Tait, K.; Fung, F.; Hu, A.; Sweller, N.; Wang, W. Understanding Hong Kong chinese families' experiences of an autism/ASD diagnosis. *J. Autism Dev. Disord.* **2016**, *46*, 1164–1183. [CrossRef]
68. Tejada-Ortigosa, E.M.; Flores-Rojas, K.; Moreno-Quintana, L.; Muñoz-Villanueva, M.C.; Pérez-Navero, J.L.; Gil-Campos, M. Health and socio-educational needs of the families and children with rare metabolic diseases: Qualitative study in a tertiary hospital. *An. Pediatr.* **2019**, *90*, 42–50. [CrossRef]
69. Holloway, S.D.; Dominguez-Pareto, I.; Cohen, S.R.; Kuppermann, M. Whose job is it? Everyday routines and quality of life in latino and non-latino families of children with intellectual disabilities. *J. Ment. Health Res. Intellect. Disabil.* **2014**, *7*, 104–125. [CrossRef]
70. Algood, C.; Davis, A.M. Inequities in family quality of life for african-american families raising children with disabilities. *Soc. Work Public Health* **2019**, *34*, 102–112. [CrossRef]
71. Wang, M.; Summers, J.A.; Little, T.; Turnbull, A.; Poston, D.; Mannan, H. Perspectives of fathers and mothers of children in early intervention programmes in assessing Family Quality of Life. *J. Intellect. Disabil. Res.* **2006**, *50*, 977–988. [CrossRef]
72. Moyson, T.; Roeyers, H. The overall quality of my life as a sibling is all right, but of course, it could always be better'. Quality of Life of siblings of children with intellectual disability: The siblings' perspectives. *J. Intellect. Disabil. Res.* **2012**, *56*, 87–101. [CrossRef]
73. Steel, R.; Poppe, L.; Vandevelde, S.; Van Hove, G.; Claes, C. Family Quality of Life in 25 belgian families: Quantitative and qualitative exploration of social and professional support domains. *J. Intellect. Disabil. Res.* **2011**, *55*, 1123–1135. [CrossRef] [PubMed]
74. Hielkema, T.; Boxum, A.G.; Hamer, E.G.; La Bastide-Van Gemert, S.; Dirks, T.; Reinders-Messelink, H.A.; Maathuis, C.G.B.; Verheijden, J.; Geertzen, J.H.B.; Hadders-Algra, M. LEARN2MOVE 0–2 years, a randomized early intervention trial for infants at very high risk of cerebral palsy: Family outcome and infant's functional outcome. *Disabil. Rehabil.* **2019**, *41*, 1–9. [CrossRef] [PubMed]
75. Samuel, P.S.; Hobden, K.L.; Leroy, B.W.; Lacey, K.K. Analysing family service needs of typically underserved families in the USA. *J. Intellect. Disabil. Res.* **2012**, *56*, 111–128. [CrossRef] [PubMed]
76. Summers, J.A.; Marquis, J.; Mannan, H.; Turnbull, A.P.; Fleming, K.; Poston, D.J.; Wang, M.; Kupzyk, K. Relationship of perceived adequacy of services, family-professional partnerships, and Family Quality of Life in early childhood service programmes. *Int. J. Disabil. Dev. Educ.* **2007**, *54*, 319–338. [CrossRef]
77. Balcells-Balcells, A.; Gine, C.; Guardia-Olmos, J.; Summers, J.A.; Mas, J.M. Impact of supports and partnership on Family Quality of Life. *Res. Dev. Disabil.* **2019**, *85*, 50–60. [CrossRef]
78. Hsiao, Y.-J.; Higgins, K.; Pierce, T.; Whitby, P.J.S.; Tandy, R.D. Parental stress, family quality of life, and family-teacher partnerships: Families of children with autism spectrum disorder. *Res. Dev. Disabil.* **2017**, *70*, 152–162. [CrossRef] [PubMed]

79. Davis, K.; Gavidia-Payne, S. The impact of child, family, and professional support characteristics on the Quality of Life in families of young children with disabilities. *J. Intellect. Dev. Disabil.* **2009**, *34*, 153–162. [CrossRef]
80. Meral, B.F.; Cavkaytar, A.; Turnbull, A.P.; Wang, M. Family Quality of Life of turkish families who have children with intellectual disabilities and autism. *Res. Pract. Pers. Sev. Disabil.* **2013**, *38*, 233–246. [CrossRef]
81. Svavarsdottir, E.K.; Tryggvadottir, G.B. Predictors of Quality of Life for families of children and adolescents with severe physical illnesses who are receiving hospital-based care. *Scand. J. Caring Sci.* **2019**, *33*, 698–705. [CrossRef]
82. Hsiao, Y.-J. Autism Spectrum Disorders: Family demographics, parental stress, and Family Quality of Life. *J. Policy Pract. Intellect. Disabil.* **2018**, *15*, 70–79. [CrossRef]
83. Wang, M.; Turnbull, A.P.; Summers, J.A.; Little, T.D.; Poston, D.J.; Marman, H.; Turnbull, R. Severity of disability and income as predictors of parents' satisfaction with their family quality of life during early childhood years. *Res. Pract. Pers. Sev. Disabil.* **2004**, *29*, 82–94. [CrossRef]
84. Boehm, T.L.; Carter, E.W. Family Quality of Life and its correlates among parents of children and adults with intellectual disability. *Am. J. Intellect. Dev. Disabil.* **2019**, *124*, 99–115. [CrossRef] [PubMed]
85. Kyzar, K.; Brady, S.; Summers, J.A.; Turnbull, A. Family Quality of Life and partnership for families of students with deaf-blindness. *Remedial Spec. Educ.* **2018**, 1–13. [CrossRef]
86. Levinger, M.; Alhuzail, N.A. Bedouin hearing parents of children with hearing loss: Stress, coping, and Quality of Life. *Am. Ann. Deaf* **2018**, *163*, 328–355. [CrossRef] [PubMed]
87. Schlebusch, L.; Samuels, A.E.; Dada, S. South african families raising children with Autism Spectrum Disorders: Relationship between family routines, cognitive appraisal and Family Quality of Life. *J. Intellect. Disabil. Res.* **2016**, *60*, 412–423. [CrossRef] [PubMed]
88. Turnbull, A.P.; Summers, J.A.; Lee, S.-H.; Kyzar, K. Conceptualization and measurement of family outcomes associated with families of individuals with intellectual disabilities. *Ment. Retard. Dev. Disabil. Res. Rev.* **2007**, *13*, 346–356. [CrossRef] [PubMed]
89. Schippers, A.; Zuna, N.; Brown, I. A Proposed framework for an integrated process of improving quality of life. *J. Policy. Pract. Intellect Dis.* **2015**, *12*, 151–161. [CrossRef]
90. Boelsma, F.; Caubo-Damen, I.; Schippers, A.; Dane, M.; Abma, T.A. Rethinking FQoL: The dynamic interplay between individual and Family Quality of Life. *J. Policy Pract. Intellect. Disabil.* **2017**, *14*, 31–38. [CrossRef]
91. Gardiner, E.; Iarocci, G. Family Quality of Life and ASD: The role of child adaptive functioning and behavior problems. *Autism Res.* **2015**, *8*, 199–213. [CrossRef]
92. Van Heumen, L.; Schippers, A. Quality of Life for young adults with intellectual disability following individualised support: Individual and family responses. *J. Intellect. Dev. Disabil.* **2016**, *41*, 299–310. [CrossRef]
93. Roth, D.; Brown, I. Social and Cultural Considerations in Family Quality of Life: Jewish and Arab Israeli Families' Child-Raising Experiences. *J. Policy Pract. Intellect. Disabil.* **2017**, *14*, 68–77. [CrossRef]
94. Luijkx, J.; van der Putten, A.A.J.; Vlaskamp, C. "I love my sister, but sometimes I don't": A qualitative study into the experiences of siblings of a child with profound intellectual and multiple disabilities. *J. Intellect. Dev. Disabil.* **2016**, *41*, 279–288. [CrossRef]
95. Feigin, R.; Barnetz, Z.; Davidson-Arad, B. Quality of Life in family members coping with chronic illness in a relative: An exploratory study. *Fam. Syst. Health* **2008**, *25*, 267–281. [CrossRef]
96. Wang, M.; Mannan, H.; Poston, D.; Turnbull, A.P.; Summers, J.A. Parents' Perceptions of advocacy activities and their impact on Family Quality of Life. *Res. Pract. Pers. Sev. Disabil.* **2004**, *29*, 144–155. [CrossRef]
97. Liang, Z. The Quality of Family Life and lifestyle. In *The Chinese Family Today*; Xu, A., Defrain, J., Liu, W., Eds.; Routledge: Abingdon-on-Thames, UK, 2016; Volume 7, pp. 248–279. [CrossRef]
98. Vanderkerken, L.; Heyvaert, M.; Onghena, P.; Maes, B. Mother Quality of Life or Family Quality of Life? A survey on the Quality of Life in families with children with intellectual disabilities using home-based support in Flanders. *J. Intellect. Disabil. Res.* **2016**, *60*, 756.

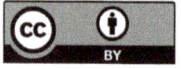

© 2020 by the authors. Licensee MDPI, Basel, Switzerland. This article is an open access article distributed under the terms and conditions of the Creative Commons Attribution (CC BY) license (http://creativecommons.org/licenses/by/4.0/).

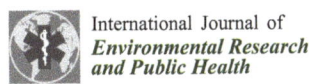

Article

The Spanish Family Quality of Life Scales under and over 18 Years Old: Psychometric Properties and Families' Perceptions

Anna Balcells-Balcells [1,*], Joana M. Mas [1], Natasha Baqués [1], Cecilia Simón [2] and Simón García-Ventura [1,3]

1. School of Psychology, Education and Sport Sciences Blanquerna, Ramon Llull University, 08022 Barcelona, Spain; JoanaMariaMM@blanquerna.url.edu (J.M.M.); natashaBA@blanquerna.url.edu (N.B.); simongv@blanquerna.url.edu (S.G.-V.)
2. School of Psychology, Autonomous University of Madrid, 28049 Madrid, Spain; cecilia.simon@uam.es
3. School of Psychology, Abat Oliba CEU University, 08022 Barcelona, Spain
* Correspondence: annabb0@blanquerna.url.edu

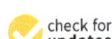

Received: 31 August 2020; Accepted: 22 October 2020; Published: 25 October 2020

Abstract: Background: Family quality of life (FQoL), just like individual quality of life, has become a priority outcome in the policies and services received by persons with intellectual and developmental disabilities (IDD) and their families. Conceptualizing, measuring, and theorizing FQoL has been the object of investigation in recent decades. The goal of this paper is to present a revision of the Spanish Family Quality of Life Scales, the CdVF-E < 18 and the CdVF-E > 18, and describe the FQoL of Spanish families with a member with IDD. Methods: The sample included a total of 548 families with a member under 18 years old and 657 families with a member over 18. Based on an Exploratory Factor Analysis (EFA) firstly and a Confirmatory Factor Analysis (CFA) secondly, the two scales' psychometric properties were explored. Results: The CdVF-ER < 18 and the CdVF-ER > 18 comprise 5 dimensions, containing 35 and 32 items, respectively, and they show good validity and reliability. The families obtained a high FQoL score, although some differences exist between the dimensions on which families with children under and over 18 score highest and lowest. Conclusion: The characteristics of the revised scales facilitate their use by professionals, administrations, and services.

Keywords: Family Quality of Life; intellectual and developmental disabilities; Family Quality of Life Scale; measure; Spanish Family Quality of Life Scales; CdVF-ER > 18; CdVF-ER < 18

---

1. Introduction

In the late 1970s and early 1980s, the concept of quality of life (QoL) emerged as a reference framework in the field studying individuals with intellectual and developmental disabilities (IDD) [1,2].

Increasing recognition that the QoL of the individual with IDD is closely related to their environment and, particularly, the role of the family in their life as a natural context of development [1,3–6] has established Family Quality of Life (FQoL) as an essential outcome for the services assisting these individuals [1,7–12]. In this sense, one of the most up-to-date FQoL definitions, and one of the most widely cited, is the one by Zuna et al. [13] (p.262), which highlights the relationship between the individual and the family in FQoL perception: "a dynamic sense of well-being of the family, collectively and subjectively defined and informed by its members, in which individual and family-level need to interact."

Indeed, in the last 20 years, FQoL has triggered researchers' interest in the field of IDD. Over these years, the studies conducted by researchers regarding FQoL have focused on: (1) conceptualizing FQoL; (2) developing measurement instruments and adapting them to different cultural contexts; and

(3) finding out about families' QoL to prepare a theory explaining the construct while identifying how FQoL behaves against specific predictors [14,15].

The early papers focused on conceptualizing FQoL, and they intended to discover what families understood as FQoL and identify its main components [16–19]. The studies in the second group are devoted to preparing measurement instruments to assess the construct. In many cases, these studies went hand in hand with the conceptualization studies where FQoL dimensions were identified [3,19,20].

The most internationally renowned instruments to measure FQoL according to Samuel et al. [21] are the Beach Center Family Quality of Life Scale (Beach Center FQoL) [22], originally developed in the USA, and the International Family Quality of Life Scale (FQOL-2006) [20,23], created by Australian, Canadian, Israeli, South Korean, and Taiwanese researchers. Both instruments were designed for families with members with IDD of all ages. They have been the object of investigation in many studies in order to optimize their tools [24–26], validate them in social and cultural contexts, e.g., Italy, Taiwan, China, Greece, Canada, Singapore, Spain [27–36], and studying their psychometric properties in more depth [20,37–39].

In parallel, other instruments have been developed to measure FQoL. Some of these are the Families in Early Intervention Quality of Life (FEIQoL) [40], initially prepared by McWilliam and Casey [41] and focusing on the stage of early intervention (children from 0–6 years old), the Spanish Family Quality of Life Scale for families with a child with IDD under 18 years old (CdVF-E < 18), and the Spanish Family Quality of Life Scale for families with a member with IDD over 18 years old (CdVF-E > 18) [42]. The last two are the object of study of this article.

Although all the scales above measure families' FQoL perception, here is how they differ: (a) sphere of application or the population they are intended for (whether culture, population, or ages of members with IDD); (b) characteristics of the instrument (closed-ended questions or a combination of open- and closed-ended questions); (c) the dimensions they assess (see Appendix A). As regards the latter aspect, it should be noted that each scale is made of different FQoL dimensions that allow researchers to measure the construct globally. Some of these dimensions are similar in different scales, although others are quite different [39,40].

Based on the different instruments, various studies focused on describing FQoL in specific populations from Spain, Colombia, Australia, or Brazil [40,43–46]. Other intended to describe what FQoL families perceived according to their individual and/or collective characteristics [24,47–50] or as a result of receiving certain supports or intervention practices [14,51–56].

These studies brought about the construct's theorization, i.e., defining an explicative theory that helped to holistically understand how FQoL factors and predictors are related. In this sense, Zuna et al. [13] made an explicative proposal in which they identified four factors that influence the families' FQoL: (a) the family unit; (b) the characteristics of the individuals who form the family; (c) performance; and (d) the system. The authors proposed middle-range theories that account for how these variables relate to one another to determine FQoL and urged researchers to validate these proposals through empirical research. They also requested an improvement in the existing instruments to measure FQoL, claiming that they are still not sensitive enough to perceive changes attributable to the factors comprised in their theoretical proposal Along the same lines, the Families Special Interest Research Group of the International Association for the Scientific Study of Intellectual and Developmental Disabilities [57] has repeatedly claimed that improving the FQoL instruments appears as one of the challenges of international research on FQoL. Either new proposals must be constructed, or the existing instruments must be refined to move forward, regarding the use of such instruments both in research and practice [13,15,22]. Consequently, just as happened with the individual QoL model, FQoL, understood as an outcome, has become a quality indicator of the policies, services, and programs received by individuals and families with IDD [22]. Likewise, it is also the framework to guide the planning of support and services for a better fit with families' actual needs. For administrations and services, using FQoL measurement instruments has in fact become an essential element to learn about the global situation of these families' lives.

The Spanish Family Quality of Life Scale for families with a child with IDD under 18 years old (CdVF-E < 18) and the Spanish Family Quality of Life Scale for families with a member with IDD over 18 years old (CdVF-E > 18), the two Spanish Family Quality of Life Scales (CdVF-E), were developed by the research group "Disability and Quality of Life: Educational Aspects" in 2013 [42]. These scales were the result, on the one hand, of the qualitative inquiry conducted to conceptualize FQoL in Spain and, on the other, a quantitative process that included trialing an early pilot version of the two scales as well as their final version in Spain.

There are two CdVF-E scales: one for children up to 18 years of age (CdVF-E < 18) and another for adults over 18 (CdVF-E > 18). The needs of individuals with IDD change substantially over time and, consequently, so do the needs of their families and the impact on their QoL perception. In Spain, the age of majority is 18. Reaching that age involves several changes; among them, the degree of disability and the family's financial compensation are revised. In addition, new choices open up: education, independent life, and employability. These choices vary according to each person's support needs and possibilities. In order to be more sensitive to such life changes and their possible impact on FQoL, the authors considered it advisable to have two different instruments [42].

The first psychometric approach conducted in Spain regarding the CdVF-E < 18 and the CdVF-E > 18 scales provided a one-dimensional measure. The items measured FQoL as a whole although they were constructed from seven conceptual areas: Emotional well-being, Family interaction, Health, Financial well-being, Organization and parental skills, Family accommodation, and Social inclusion and participation [44].

Since their creation, both scales have been subjected to adaptation and validation in other countries. In Costa Rica, Cordero [58] confirmed the multi-dimensionality of the CdVF-E < 18 in a 0–6-year-old population. More specifically, the author identified eight dimensions (Financial Well-being, Family Accommodation, Parental Abilities, Family Climate, Autonomy of the Member with Disability, Health, Formal Supports, and Informal Supports). However, Bitencourt [59] adapted and validated the CdVF-E > 18 scale in Brazil, and still found it to be one-dimensional.

Even though—as pointed out—numerous papers have in recent years have focused on the construction, validation, or study of tools to measure FQoL [14,20,22–39], authors agree on the need to continue to devote efforts to optimizing their internal structures and revising how they work in different populations in different contexts (socio-demographic, cultural, etc.) [25,29,31,39,40]. In this sense, after applying the CdVF-E < 18 and the CdVF-E > 18 scales for 5 years, we deemed it appropriate to revise them both and identify their internal structures for research [44,60] and intervention purposes in the Spanish context [61].

The purpose of that revision was twofold: on the one hand, to improve their efficiency by shortening them and thus improving the answer choices; and on the other, to study their psychometric properties according to reliability and validity criteria. More FQoL-sensitive instruments will provide better knowledge of the families' realities and, therefore, their needs will be better met.

Consequently, the goals of this article are: (a) to present the psychometric properties and final features of the new version of the scales named Spanish Family Quality of Life Scale for families with a child with IDD under 18 years old. Revised version in 2019 (CdVF-ER < 18) and Spanish Family Quality of Life Scale for families with a member with IDD over 18 years old. Revised version in 2019 (CdVF-ER > 18); and (b) to describe the FQoL perception of the families who participated in the study.

The ultimate objective is indeed to provide two tools to assess the FQoL of Spanish families that are more efficient and offer better psychometric guarantees, and which adapt to the period of life the families are undergoing. Therefore, the current paper should be understood as an extension of the measurement studies conducted in the field of FQoL thus far.

2. Materials and Methods

2.1. Type of Study

An instrumental type of study is presented for the first goal, classified among empirical studies as a quantitative methodology. The guidelines of the Standards for Educational and Psychological Testing [62] were observed in its preparation, since they compile different trustworthy procedures and strategies to guarantee a test's reliability and validity. The International Test Commission Guidelines [63] were also observed, which feature the general principles for the use of tests.

For the second goal, a descriptive study was conducted in order to present the participating families' FQoL perceptions.

2.2. Participants

A total of $N = 548$ families with one underage member with IDD participated in the study as well as $N = 657$ families with an adult member. They came from 13 Spanish Autonomous Communities. Table 1 shows the main characteristics of the individual who answered the scale and the member with IDD.

Table 1. Demographic characteristics of the family members who answer the scale and the person with intellectual and developmental disabilities (IDD).

	Families with One Member with IDD			
	Under 18 ($N = 548$)		Over 18 ($N = 657$)	
Characteristics	%	n	%	n
Sex of the person who answers				
Male	23	126	33.5	220
Female	75.9	416	65.1	428
Relation to the person with IDD				
Mother	83	455	47.9	315
Father	13.9	76	25.3	166
Sibling	0.2	1	23.3	153
Other	1.8	10	2.7	18
Age of the person who answers (year)				
Mean	41.52		56.91	
Age range	21–70		23–88	
Sex of the person with IDD				
Male	66.6	365	57.5	378
Female	31.9	175	4.3	265
Age range (years)				
0–6	33.6	184	-	-
7–12	39.8	218	-	-
13–18	24.8	136	-	-
19–40	-	-	69.6	457
41–60	-	-	25.4	167
>61	-	-	1.4	9
Degree of disability [1]				
Not recognized (15–33%)	5.7	31	0.5	3
Mild (33–64%)	42.7	234	10.5	69
Moderate (65–74%)	21	115	44.3	291
Severe (>75%)	20.1	110	42.9	282
In process	2	11	0.2	1
Not requested	6.2	34	-	-

Table 1. Cont.

Characteristics	Families with One Member with IDD			
	Under 18 (N = 548)		Over 18 (N = 657)	
	%	n	%	n
IDD-associated impairments				
Autism Spectrum Disorder (ASD)	42	211	6	28
Hearing impairment	2	10	7.5	35
Language disorder	15.9	80	13.5	63
Attention deficit disorder (ADHD)	9.6	48	4.1	19
Health	12	60	16.3	76
Conduct disorders	5.8	29	11.4	53
Visual impairment	6	30	13.5	63
Physical disability	17.1	86	21.7	101
Mental disorder	2	10	21.9	102
Other	26.1	131	-	-
Main service attended by the person with IDD				
School	55.8	306	4	26
Vocational training	3.3	18	28.9	190
Job	0.2	1	18.1	119
Daycare center	0.4	2	33.2	218
Leisure	0.4	2	0.8	5
Residence	0.5	3	9.4	62
Early intervention	24.5	134	-	-
Other	12.2	67	-	-

[1] The degrees of disability were defined according to the scales (%) provided by the Spanish Government.

The inclusion criteria for the participants were: (a) having a child with Intellectual or Developmental Disability diagnosed by the official social centers in each Autonomous Community and, (b) being a Spanish resident.

2.3. Instrument

The scales submitted for revision originated from the Spanish Family Quality of Life Scale, (CdVF-E) [42], both the version for families with an underage member with IDD (CdVF-E < 18), comprising 61 items, and the version for adults (CdVF-E > 18), comprising 67 items. Both were one-dimensional scales and featured seven areas interpreted as tendencies: Emotional well-being, Family interaction, Health, Financial well-being, Organization and parental skills, Family accommodation, and Social inclusion and participation. The answers were of the frequency type according to a 5-point Likert scale where 1 meant *never* and 5 *always*, plus one *it does not apply (NA)* choice. The scales' reliability was acceptable, with an internal consistency in agreement with a 0.96 Cronbach's alpha.

2.4. Procedure

Firstly, Plena Inclusión (Confederación Española de Organizaciones en favor de las Personas con Discapacidad Intelectual, one of the most important associations in Spain for persons with a disability and their families), through their different organizations, administered the CdVF-E scales [42] to the families. This process took place over 5 years in 13 Autonomous Communities of Spain. Regarding ethical safeguards, the participants were provided with information on the project as well as confidentiality safeguards. Secondly, the results were kept anonymously in a centralized computer database managed by Plena Inclusión. Prior to data storage, the families had to give their consent for their information to be added to the organization's computer file so they could be treated, analyzed, and published without prejudice to their rights, according to the applicable current law within the Ley Orgánica 15/1999, Protección de Datos de Carácter Personal de España (Spanish Personal

Data Protection Regulation). The ethical principles of the Spanish Psychological Association were also observed.

In total, information was gathered from 878 families of underage individuals with IDD and 2730 families with an adult member with IDD, all of them coming from the different organizations federated with Plena Inclusión. However, scales with over 20% of unanswered items were discarded from this study.

2.5. Dataset

Descriptive analyses of the items. The authors studied the descriptive statistics of each item to discover how each behaved. Additionally, they explored those that had answered *it does not apply* (NA) in 20% of the sample and considered them as lost data. As a result of those analyses, 11 items from the under-18 scale and 7 items from the adults scale were removed. Moreover, the answer *it does not apply* (NA) was discarded, given the families' tendency to choose this answer frequently.

Factor analyses. In this stage of the study, the authors explored the internal structure of both scales, and their reliability.

For this purpose, the samples were randomly divided into two datasets (under and over 18 years old). With one half of the sample, sample A, the authors conducted reliability and validity analyses by means of an Exploratory Factor Analysis (EFA), and assessed the results both empirically and theoretically. The extraction method used was the principal component analysis and the oblimim oblique rotation method. Later, in order to refine and empirically confirm the structure resulting from the EFA, a confirmatory factor analysis (CFA) was conducted with the other half of the sample, sample B, in both sets. The parameter estimation method used was Maximum Likelihood (ML) in the case of the under-18 scale, and Robust Maximum Likelihood (MLR) for the over-18 scale. To assess the global fit model, the authors calculated the Chi-square index (χ^2), associated likelihood p and the degrees of freedom (df), and the Root Mean Square Error of Approximation (RMSEA), in addition to the confidence intervals and the Standardized Root Mean Square Residual (SRMR). Regarding the incremental fit measures, they assessed the Normed Fit Index (NFI), the Non-Normed Fit Index (NNFI), or the Tucker Lewis Index (TLI), and the Comparative Fit Index (CFI). To increase each factor's consistency and explore alternative structures, Modification Indices (MI) were explored.

Study of reliability and normative scores. Lastly, the authors provided evidence of reliability through Cronbach's alpha coefficient, and calculated the central tendency and dispersion based on the mean, the standard deviation, the minimum, the maximum, and the percentiles, for the total and for each of the dimensions of both scales (CdVF-ER < 18 and CdVF-ER > 18).

Data analysis was conducted using the Statistical Package for the Social Sciences (SPSS) software, version 21.0 and MPlus software, version 7.4 [64].

3. Results

As a result of the scale refinement process through EFA, 15 items were removed from the under-18 scale (CdVF-ER < 18) and 28 items from the adults scale (CdVF-ER > 18). The EFA result for the CdVF-ER < 18 suggested a 5-factor solution that explained 50.83% of the variance and comprised 35 items. For the CdVF-ER > 18, a 5-factor solution was identified that explained 49.69% of the variance and comprised 34 items.

Below are the reliability and validity indices of the CdVF-ER < 18 and the CdVF-ER > 18 scales as well as their final characteristics after conducting the CFA, and the descriptive statistics of the population under study, in accordance with the two main goals of this study.

3.1. Reliability and Validity Indices and Final Characteristics of the Scales

Regarding the first objective of this study, presenting the psychometric properties identified in the new version of the scales, the validity indices for the CdVF-ER < 18 scale yielded highly acceptable results. As regards the absolute fit measurements, Chi-square Index (χ^2), and associated likelihood (959.989: $p < 0.001$), they indicated that the model proposed did not fit the data. However, to minimize the impact of the sample size, the magnitude was considered (χ^2/gl): at 1.79, this presented an acceptable value [65]. Regarding the RMSEA Index, the value was 0.052, which is indicative of a close fit [66], and the associated confidence intervals were (0.047–0.058). SRMR, with a value of 0.052, indicated an acceptable fit [67]. Concerning the incremental fit measurements, TLI was 0.934 and CFI 0.926, indicative of a good fit [68]. Table 2 shows the Goodness of fit indices for the final model of the CdVF-ER < 18 and the CdVF-ER > 18 scales.

Table 2. Goodness of fit indices for the final model of the CdVF-ER < 18 and CdVF-ER > 18 scales.

Goodness Indices	CdVF-ER < 18 Model	CdVF-ER > 18 Model
χ^2	959.989(537)	3117.430(496)
p	<0.001	<0.001
RMSEA	0.052	0.040
RMSEA (90%)	(0.047–0.058)	(0.034–0.046)
TLI	0.934	0.898
CFI	0.926	0.911
SRMR	0.052	0.051

X^2, Chi-square Index; RMSEA, Root Mean Square Error of Approximation; TLI, Tucker Lewis Index; CFI, Comparative Fit Index; SRMR, Standardized Root Mean Square Residual.

Regarding the latent variables, the Family resources dimension related significantly to the Family climate (0.445, $p = 0.000$), Financial well-being (0.4, $p = 0.002$), and Emotional stability (0.499, $p = 0.000$) dimensions. As for item reliability, standardized factor loadings yielded values between 0.120 (item 5) and 0.691 (item 3).

The reliability of the CdVF-ER < 18 scale, measured through Cronbach's alpha, was 0.91, and it ranged between 0.73 (Emotional stability and Family adaptation) and 0.86 (Family climate and Financial well-being) in each of the family dimensions. Table 3 presents these results.

Table 3. Cronbach's alpha of each dimension of the CdVF-ER < 18 scale.

Dimensions	Number of Items [1]	Cronbach's Alpha
Total	35	0.91
Family climate	12	0.86
Emotional stability	8	0.73
Financial well-being	8	0.86
Family adaptation	11	0.73
Family resources	9	0.79

[1] It should be noted that a number of items are repeated in different dimensions.

The final solution for the CdVF-ER < 18 scale comprises 5 FQoL dimensions and 35 items divided as follows: Family climate (12 items), Financial well-being (8 items), Emotional stability (8 items), Family adaptation (11 items), and Family resources (9 items).

As regards the CdVF-ER > 18 scale, the absolute fit measurement was 6.28 (x^2/gl), and the RMSEA index value was 0.040. The associated confidence intervals were 0.034 and 0.046 and the SRMR value was 0.051. Concerning the incremental fit measurements, TLI was 0.898 and CFI 0.911. Table 2 shows the Goodness-of-fit indices of the final model of both scales, the CdVF-ER < 18 and the CdVF-ER > 18.

All the latent variables yielded a significant relationship to one another ($p = 0.000$), where the most significant relationships were found between Family support for the person with IDD and Family climate (0.933), and between Family organization and Family climate (0.730).

On the other hand, the standardized loadings ranged between 0.115 (item 18) and 0.730 (item 22), while the limit of acceptable values is 0.30 according to some authors [69].

Regarding the reliability of the CdVF-ER > 18, Cronbach's alpha value for the total was 0.89 and the values for each area ranged between 0.81 for the Financial well-being area and 0.70 for Family support for the person with IDD. Table 4 presents Cronbach's alpha for the total and for each of the CdVF-ER > 18 scale's dimensions.

Table 4. Cronbach's alpha of the total and of each of the CdVF-ER > 18 scale's dimensions.

Dimensions	Number of Items [1]	Cronbach's Alpha
Total	32	0.89
Family climate	14	0.75
Autonomy of the person with intellectual and development disabilities (IDD)	12	0.79
Financial well-being	5	0.81
Family organization and functioning	11	0.77
Family support to the person with IDD	8	0.70

[1] It should be noted that a number of items are repeated in different dimensions.

The final solution for the CdVF-ER > 18 scale comprised 5 FQoL dimensions and 32 items divided as follows: Family climate (14 items), Autonomy of the person with IDD (12 items), Financial well-being (5 items), Family organization and functioning (11 items), and Family support to the person with IDD (8 items).

Given the existence of correlation between certain dimensions of both scales, some items load in more than one dimension at the same time [70]. An example of the items for both scales can be found in Appendix B.

3.2. Descriptive Statistics

With regard to the second objective, describing the FQoL perception of the families who participated in the study, Family quality of life perceived by the families with an underage child yielded a global mean of 3.99 ($SD = 0.49$). Regarding the FQoL dimensions, the highest score was Family adaptation ($M = 4.15$), followed by Family resources ($M = 4.15$). The lowest scores were obtained in the Financial well-being ($M = 3.73$) and Emotional stability dimensions ($M = 3.81$). Table 5 presents the scores obtained.

Table 5. Descriptive statistics of the total and each family quality of life dimension for the CdVF-ER < 18.

	M	Min	Max	SD
Family quality of life (FQoL) total	3.99	2.26	5.00	0.49
Family adaptation	4.25	2.18	5.00	0.48
Family resources	4.15	1.89	5.00	0.54
Family climate	4.08	2.17	5.00	0.58
Emotional stability	3.81	1.63	5.00	0.61
Financial well-being	3.73	1.13	5.00	0.73

M = Mean; Min = Minimum; Max = Maximum; SD = Standard Deviation.

As regards the family quality of life perceived by the families with an adult member, the global mean obtained was 4.03 (SD = 0.48). Concerning the FQoL dimensions, the highest score was Family organization and functioning (M = 4.15), followed by Financial well-being (M = 4.09). The lowest scores were obtained for Autonomy of the person with IDD (M = 3.75) and Family support to the person with IDD (M = 3.74). Table 6 presents the scores obtained.

Table 6. Descriptive statistics of the total and each family quality of life dimension for the CdVF-ER > 18.

	M	Min	Max	SD
FQoL Total	4.03	1.00	5.00	0.48
Family organization and functioning	4.15	1.00	5.00	0.54
Financial well-being	4.09	1.00	5.00	0.78
Family climate	4.08	1.00	5.00	0.48
Autonomy of the person with IDD	3.75	1.00	5.00	0.64
Family support to the person with IDD	3.74	1.00	5.00	0.72

M = Mean; Min = Minimum; Max = Maximum; SD = Standard Deviation.

4. Discussion

The present study pursued two goals: firstly, to show the psychometric properties and final features of the CdVF-ER < 18 and the CdVF-ER > 18 scales; and, secondly, to approach the way families perceive their FQoL.

As regards the first goal, similarly to the studies that have validated other FQoL scales, both for underage [22,25,27,32,34,36,39] and adult populations [31], the psychometric properties of the scales presented satisfactory reliability (with Cronbach's Alpha over 0.90) and validity indices. This guarantees that they can be used in the Spanish context for research and intervention purposes. With regard to the final features of the scales, like most existing scales that measure FQoL based on a series of dimensions, the present scales have shown they both consist of five dimensions, respectively, thus reflecting the multifactorial nature of FQoL [1,20,71]. On the one hand, the dimensions identified for the CdVF-ER < 18 were: Family climate, Financial well-being, Emotional stability, Family adaptation, and Family resources. On the other, the dimensions identified for the CdVF-ER > 18 were: Family climate, Autonomy of the person with IDD, Financial well-being, Family organization and functioning, and Family support to the person with IDD. Accordingly, two dimensions appeared in both scales: Family climate and Financial well-being.

The dimensions identified in both scales are not conceptually related in an accurate manner to the dimensions of the other existing FQoL scales, as is also the case among the scales developed thus far, and as proved by some authors [38,40]. Although some dimensions have similar names and assess very similar aspects, in other cases similar indicators are included in a different dimension or have been grouped into new dimensions. For this reason, trying to relate the dimensions of the CdVF-ER < 18 and the CdVF-ER > 18 scales to those of other scales is only carried out as an example of the coherence of some dimensions and indicators between scales, and can help explain each dimension's conceptual meaning.

To this effect, below are the descriptions of the dimensions found in both scales and their conceptual relationship with the dimensions of the rest of the FQoL scales presented in the introduction. Appendix A lists and defines the Beach Center FQoL dimensions [22] and the Family relationships of FQOL-2006 [20,23] and FEIQoL [40]. The first two scales concern families with a member with IDD of any age, whereas FEIQoL [40] focuses on families with children from 0–6 years old.

In this sense, the authors will first focus on the dimensions that the CdVF-ER < 18 and the CdVF-ER > 18 scales have in common, and then on the remaining ones.

Family climate refers to the quality of the relationship between the several members of the family (supporting and accepting each other as they are; having good communication; trusting each other; staying united and facing difficulties, etc.). This dimension agrees with Family interaction in the Beach Center FQoL [22], and Family relationships of FQOL-2006 [20,23] and FEIQoL [40], as can be seen in Appendix A. The Financial well-being dimension—related to the family's financial and material situation in facing the whole family's needs and the specific needs of the member with IDD—could be related to the Physical and Material Wellbeing dimensions of the Beach Center FQoL [22], or the Financial Wellbeing of FQOL-2006 [20,23].

As regards the other dimensions of the CdVF-ER < 18, we can observe that Emotional stability bears certain resemblance to Emotional wellbeing of the Beach Center FQoL [22], given that both are related to feelings of peace, quiet, personal projects, life as a couple, etc.

The rest of the CdVF-ER < 18 dimensions, such as Family resources and Family Adaptation, only share a few items with some of the dimensions of other FQoL scales and thus they cannot be likened, given that an important number of items of the scales presented in this paper have been grouped differently. However, we did find that Family resources–which focuses on both the family's emotional and service resources (formal supports) in facing their relative's needs—shares some resemblance with the Disability-related support dimension of the Beach Center FQoL [22], Support from other people and Support from disability-related services of the FQOL-2006 [23], and Access to Information and Services of FEIQoL [40]. For its part, Family Adaptation—understood as those aspects related to the family's acceptance and adaptation to their relative's disability, their needs and characteristics—resembles the Parenting dimension of the Beach Center FQoL [22].

The same applies to the rest of the CdVF-ER > 18 scale's dimensions. For example, Family organization and functioning—which concerns whether home chores and responsibilities are shared, as well as the care, attention, and education of the person with IDD—presents some items that also appear in the Parenting dimension of the Beach Center FQoL [22], among others. The dimension Family support to the person with IDD concerns the resources the family has to help their relative with IDD in solving daily life matters, managing their love and sex life, and planning their future. This dimension shares a few indicators with the following dimensions: Disability-related support of the Beach Center FQoL [22] and Support from other people and Support from disability-related services of the FQOL-2006 [20,23]. Lastly, yet another dimension identified in the CdVF-ER > 18 scale is Autonomy of the person with IDD. This dimension focuses on the perception families have regarding the autonomy of their relative with IDD according to their age; including their participation in community activities. Indicators of this dimension can be found in different dimensions of other scales, for instance, Community and civic involvement of the FQOL-2006 [20,23].

The second goal of the study was to describe the FQoL perception of the families who participated in the study. In agreement with other studies, the results showed a high global perception of FQoL for both types of families–under and over 18 years old—[14,44,60,72,73]. Similarly to other studies [60,72,74], families with an adult member show a higher FQoL perception than families with an underage member.

As regards FQoL perception, families with an underage member with IDD perceive they have better FQoL in relation to the Family adaptation and Family resources dimensions. On the other hand, the dimensions with the lowest scores are Financial well-being and Emotional stability.

Bearing in mind that Family adaptation encompasses items related to family accommodation, social inclusion and participation, and parental skills and organization, the results of the current study show that Spanish families perceive that they have adapted well to the needs of their relative's disability, and that they have integrated them well into their family dynamics. This agrees with other studies [73]. According to the authors, it makes sense that the families who scored high on this dimension also value the family's resources positively. This dimension includes not only the family's formal support, but also the capability they perceive they have in facing the challenges of their relative's development.

As regards more formal supports, the results presented here match those of other studies conducted in Spain [14,40] as well as in other countries [75].

As concerns the dimensions scored lowest by the families in this study, one of the dimensions that proves vulnerable for Spanish families is Financial well-being, in agreement with other studies [14,42,48,60,76]. More specifically, the families in this study indicate their lack of financial resources to face the future with confidence or to occasionally indulge themselves. However, the results obtained for Emotional stability—in light of other studies—are ambiguous. On the one hand, the results of this study agree with those of other studies conducted with other scales, like Balcells-Balcells et al. [14], Davis and Gavidia-Payne [51], or Summers et al. [54], where the Emotional well-being dimension was one of the least satisfactory for the families. On the other hand, the current results are not consistent with those obtained by some other studies conducted in Spain and with the scale's original version [42,44,60]. In the authors' opinion, the cause of this discrepancy lies in the fact that, in the current study, unlike in those previously mentioned, the FQoL measure used (CdVF-ER < 18) features statistically identified dimensions.

Concerning the families with an adult member with IDD, the dimensions with the highest scores are Family organization and functioning and Financial well-being, whereas the lowest scores go to Autonomy of the person with IDD and Family support to the person with IDD.

Similarly to the families with an underage child, these families perceive they have good Family organization and functioning, which implies that not only do they divide their house chores but also the functions and responsibilities related to their relative with IDD. This includes some aspects of emotional well-being. Unlike the families with an underage child with IDD, the families with adult children scored as high on the Financial well-being dimension. This would explain why the Family functioning dimension was high, among other reasons. The difference between the assessment of families with an underage and an adult member was also found in Giné et al. [60].

On the other hand, the dimensions with the lowest scores were Autonomy of the person with IDD and Family support to the person with IDD. In the authors' opinion, these results are explained by the fact that over 80% of the family members with IDD show a degree of disability between moderate and high, which involves important support needs. Likewise, the fact that the dimension Family support to the person with IDD obtains the lowest scores may be related to the degree of support the individuals need. It should be noted that this dimension enquires about aspects concerning the love and sex life of the person with IDD, and their plans for their future. These are complex subjects for the families and they frequently delegate them to professionals in the services their relative attends. In this sense, both Bertelli [77] and Jokinen and Brown [72] found that support-related dimensions were the least satisfactory for the families.

To sum up, the scales under revision in this article, the CdVF-ER < 18 and the CdVF-ER > 18, present good psychometric properties to measure the FQoL perception of families with an underage and an adult member. Moreover, the scales revised have certain strengths, which the authors would like to highlight. On the one hand, they allow researchers to measure the construct's multi-dimensionality based on 5 dimensions by scale; and on the other, they do so with shorter scales (with fewer items), and without the *it does not apply* choice, which facilitates the answering the scale for the families and applying and interpreting it for the professionals. Improved efficiency encourages administrations and services to use it more easily. The new format of the scales (fewer items and changes in the type of answer) make it easier to fill it out, thus reducing barriers when completing them: the time needed, and understanding the type of answer. Therefore, the revision of the scales met the two challenges that triggered this revision: the scale's multi-dimensionality and having more efficient scales that continue to provide relevant information to plan the necessary resources to improve the families' QoL. That had been, since the onset of the scales, an essential premise. In that way, they maintain the value of focusing on one specific evolution stage of the families (with underage or adult children) and consequently, they facilitate the planning of the most adequate support for each moment/situation in life.

Limitations

Most of the participants in this study were mothers. Wang et al. [78] proved there was no difference between fathers and mothers regarding FQoL perception. In consequence, most researchers sum up mothers' and fathers' perceptions globally, regardless of their role in the family [22,25,27,31,39]. Although some studies claim that fathers' perceptions do not differ significantly from those of mothers, Vanderkerken et al. [79] argue that it is still important to investigate the impact of the participation of one or more family members on the FQoL. There are no studies in Spain regarding the differences in the FQoL perceptions of fathers and mothers. It would be advisable to replicate this type of study to confirm this statement in the Spanish context.

This study presents another limitation, which is that the data was collected by the Plena Inclusión organization. Having the support of organizations to collect data is an advantage as concerns the number of participants the study has. But it also has some disadvantages, namely: (a) an important number of scales had over 20% unanswered items and, therefore, could not be used for the analyses; and (b) certain demographic information was not collected, for example, socio-economic level or place of residence. This information would have helped the authors interpret some aspects in more depth.

One relevant aspect that the current study also shares with most FQoL studies is the high scores the families give to the indicators that allow researchers to value the construct. Several colleagues like Chiu et al. [25] attribute this fact to the instruments being distributed by the children's assigned professionals. In any case, this is an aspect to bear in mind when analyzing the scores, both from the perspective of research and intervention. They should be complemented, especially in the latter case, with qualitative techniques such as interviews.

5. Conclusions and Implications for Research and Practices

The results obtained in this study as regards the psychometric properties and final features of the scales lead to the following conclusions:

- Since the first FQoL scales were created, the authors of the current paper have confirmed the reach of measuring FQoL, both for research (to improve knowledge) and intervention purposes (adjusting supports to the families' QoL).
- The results presented in this paper provide evidence that the CdVF-ER >18 and the CdVF-ER < 18 are both reliable and valid for measuring FQoL in Spain throughout the lifetime of the member with IDD. The CdVF-ER > 18 and the CdVF-ER < 18 scales have proved useful and easier to use than previous scales (in time and implementation). Furthermore, they are formed by several FQoL factors (5 dimensions each), which facilitates result interpretation and good validity and reliability.

As for the FQoL perception of the families who participated in this study, it can be argued that:

- Spanish families with a member with IDD have a high perception of their FQoL although families with an adult member show a higher FQoL perception than families with an underage member.
- Families with an underage member with IDD give a higher score to the Family adaptation and Family resources dimensions, whereas Financial well-being and Emotional stability obtained a lower score. For the families with an adult with IDD, Family organization and functioning and Financial well-being were the best-rated dimensions, better than Autonomy of the person with IDD and Family support to the person with IDD, which had with the lowest scores.

As far as research is concerned, it would be interesting to administer the scales to find out how they work on heterogeneous groups (ages, regions, family characteristics) and adapt them and validate them in other social and cultural contexts. This will allow researchers to explore whether the factors identified behave similarly in different places with different characteristics.

Using scales for research purposes would also allow investigators to shed light on certain FQoL-related questions and on the support the services provide, more specifically to assess the impact of the services and the efficacy of the programs on FQoL more efficiently, and to evaluate the role of quality in the relationships between the professionals and the families in FQoL, etc.

At the same time, the CdVF-ER > 18 and the CdVF-ER < 18 scales may have positive practical implications at different levels. Firstly, on a micro level, the information obtained from these scales—along with other data—will allow the professionals who work closely with the families to adapt their intervention better to each family's circumstances and needs. Secondly, at a program-service level, having data on how the families in the organization perceive their current FQoL will allow coordinators and directors to offer and/or design supports better adapted to their population. Finally, on a policy level, they should encourage policies that focus on fostering FQoL. Likewise, given that FQoL has also proved to be an important service outcome, the authors consider that the information provided by these scales should not only help design more adequate proposals, but also measure the impact of those proposals.

In short, being able to measure, and therefore, move forward in conceptualizing and discovering families' situations to provide more adequate support is not only going to help improve the general family context, but also each family member's situation. Schalock et al. [4], in their theoretical QoL proposal, defend the position that family-related aspects, such as FQoL, moderate the QoL of individuals with IDD. More specifically, the authors argue that the chances for the development of individuals with IDD are motivated by the family's characteristics. This justifies the services' current challenge: improving the QoL of individuals with IDD and also that of their families.

Author Contributions: Conceptualization, A.B.-B. and J.M.M.; Data curation, A.B.-B. and N.B.; Formal analysis, N.B. and S.G.-V.; Funding acquisition, J.M.M.; Investigation, A.B.-B. and J.M.M.; Methodology, N.B. and C.S.; Project administration, A.B.-B.; Supervision, J.M.M., N.B. and C.S.; Writing—original draft, A.B.-B. and J.M.M.; Writing—review & editing, A.B.-B., J.M.M., C.S. and S.G.-V. All authors have read and agree to the published version of the manuscript.

Funding: This research was funded by Plena Inclusión (Confederación Española de Organizaciones en favor de las Personas con Discapacidad Intelectual). And the APC was funded by School of Psychology, Education and Sport Sciences Blanquerna, Ramon Llull University.

Acknowledgments: The authors thank Plena Inclusión (Confederación Española de Organizaciones en favor de las Personas con Discapacidad Intelectual) in helping us gather the information from families and the families that have participated in this study for dedicating their time to it and sharing their knowledge with us.

Conflicts of Interest: The authors declare no conflict of interest.

Appendix A

Table A1. Dimensions of the Beach Center FQoL [22], FQOL-2006 [20,23], and FEIQoL [39] and their definitions.

Beach Center FQoL [22]	- Family interaction: relationships among family members. - Parenting: activities that adult family members do to help children grow and develop. - Emotional well-being: the aspects of family life that address the emotional needs of family members. - Physical/material well-being: the aspects of family life that address the physical needs of family members. - Support for the family member with a disability: informal and formal support to benefit the family member with a disability.
FQOL-2006 [20,23]	- Health of family: sometimes one or more members of a family have health problems and these problems affect the other members of the family. - Financial well-being: coping financially. Individual members of the family earn different amounts of money and have different financial needs. - Family relationships: general atmosphere or feeling that is usually present in the family. - Support from others: families sometimes get practical and emotional support from a variety of other people, such as relatives, friends, neighbors and others. - Support from disability services: support received from disability-related services to the member with IDD or the family as a whole. - Influence of values: the influence of personal, spiritual, religious, and cultural values on the family. - Careers and preparing for careers: this regards the adult's work life or the child's life in learning. - Leisure and Community involvement: the family's leisure and recreation activities.
FEIQoL [39]	- Family Relationships: this regards the families' perceptions of communication within the family, parenting, relationships with extended family, and participation in social activities. - Access to Information and Services: this focuses on the families' knowledge of child development, managing challenging behaviors, specific demands of their child, and their access to resources in their community. - Child Functioning: this regards the families' perceptions of the child's engagement, independence, and social relationships in daily routines. - Overall Life Situation: this regards the families' perceptions of the fulfillment of family needs in areas such as family health status, family economy, and employment.

Appendix B

Table A2. Dimensions, number and examples of the CdVF-ER < 18 and the CdVF-ER > 18 scales' items.

Scale	Dimension	Number of Items	Item Example
CdVF-ER < 18	Family climate	12	All my family members show love and affection towards each other.
	Emotional stability	8	All our family members carry out our life projects (personal and professional).
	Financial well-being	8	My family can cover the cost of basic needs (food, clothing, etc.).
	Family adaptation	11	My family adapts to the needs of the relative with IDD.
	Family resources	9	My family feels well treated by the health professionals.
CdVF-ER >18	Family climate	14	All my family members show love and affection towards each other.
	Autonomy of the person with IDD	12	The relative with IDD can manage physically autonomously.
	Financial well-being	5	My family can cover the cost of basic needs (food, clothing, etc.).
	Family organization and functioning	11	In my family we share the chores and responsibilities related to the relative with IDD in a balanced way.
	Family support to the person with IDD	8	My family searches for existing resources and support to improve their quality of life.

References

1. Brown, I.; Brown, R. Concepts for beginning study in family quality of life. In *Families and People with Mental Retardation and Quality of Life: International Perspectives*; Turnbull, A.P., Brown, I., Turnbull, H.R., Eds.; American Association on Mental Retardation: Washington, DC, USA, 2004; pp. 25–47.
2. Schalock, R.L.; Gardner, J.F.; Bradley, V.J. *Quality of Life for People with Intellectual and Other Developmental Disabilities: Applications Across Individuals, Organizations, Communities, and Systems*; American Association on Intellectual and Developmental Disabilities: Washington, DC, USA, 2007.
3. Park, J.; Hoffman, L.; Marquis, J.; Turnbull, A.P.; Poston, D.; Mannan, H.; Wang, M.; Nelson, L.L. Toward assessing family outcomes of service delivery: Validation of a family quality of life survey. *J. Intellect. Disabil. Res.* **2003**, *47*, 367–384. [CrossRef] [PubMed]
4. Schalock, R.L.; Verdugo, M.A.; Gomez, L.E.; Reinders, H.S. Moving us toward a theory of individual quality of life. *Am. J. Intellect. Dev. Disabil.* **2016**, *121*, 1–12. [CrossRef] [PubMed]
5. Summers, J.A.; Poston, D.J.; Turnbull, A.P.; Marquis, J.; Hoffman, L.; Mannan, H.; Wang, M. Conceptualizing and measuring family quality of life. *J. Intellect. Disabil. Res.* **2005**, *49*, 777–783. [CrossRef] [PubMed]
6. Turnbull, A.P. La calidad de vida de la familia como resultado de los servicios: El nuevo paradigma. In *Investigación, Innovación y Cambio*, Verdugo, M.A., Jordán de Urríes, F.B., Eds.; Amarú: Salamanca, Spain, 2003; pp. 61–82.
7. Schalock, R.L.; Verdugo, M.A. *Calidad De Vida. Manual Para Profesionales De La Educación, Salud y Servicios Sociales*; Alianza: Madrid, Spain, 2003.
8. Bailey, D.B.; Bruder, M.B.; Hebbeler, K.; Carta, J.; Defosset, M.; Greenwood, C.; Kahn, L.; Mallik, S.; Markowitz, J.; Spiker, D.; et al. Recommended outcomes for families of young children with disabilities. *J. Early Interv.* **2006**, *28*, 227–251. [CrossRef]
9. Mannan, H.; Summers, J.A.; Turnbull, A.P.; Poston, D.J. A review of outcome measures in early childhood programs. *J. Policy Pract. Intellect. Disabil.* **2006**, *3*, 219–228. [CrossRef]
10. Schalock, R.L. Moving from individual to family quality of life as a research topic. In *Families and People with Mental Retardation and Quality of Life: International Perspectives*; Turnbull, A.P., Brown, I., Turnbull, H.R., Eds.; American Association on Mental Retardation: Washington, DC, USA, 2004; pp. 11–24.
11. Turnbull, A.P.; Summers, J.A.; Lee, S.H.; Kyzar, K. Conceptualization and measurement of family outcomes associated with families of individuals with intellectual disabilities. *Ment. Retard. Dev. Disabil. Res. Rev.* **2007**, *13*, 346–356. [CrossRef]
12. Turnbull, A.P.; Turnbull, R.; Poston, D.; Beegle, G.; Blue-Banning, M.; Diehl, K.; Frankland, C.; Mische Lawson, L.; Lord, L.; Marquis, J.; et al. Enhancing quality of life of families of children and youth with developmental disabilities in the United States. In *Families and People with Mental Retardation and Quality of Life: International Perspectives*; Turnbull, A.P., Brown, I., Turnbull, H.R., Eds.; American Association on Mental Retardation: Washington, DC, USA, 2004; pp. 51–100.
13. Zuna, N.; Summers, J.A.; Turnbull, A.P.; Hu, X.; Xu, S. Theorizing about family quality of life. In *Enhancing the Quality of Life of People with Intellectual Disabilities: From Theory to Practice*; Kober, R., Ed.; Springer: Dordrecht, The Netherlands, 2010; pp. 241–278.
14. Balcells-Balcells, A.; Giné, C.; Guàrdia-Olmos, J.; Summers, J.A.; Mas, J.M. Impact of supports and partnership on family quality of life. *Res. Dev. Disabil.* **2019**, *85*, 50–60. [CrossRef]
15. Hu, X.; Summers, J.A.; Turnbull, A.; Zuna, N. The quantitative measurement of family quality of life: A review of available instruments. *J. Intellect. Disabil. Res.* **2011**, *55*, 1098–1114. [CrossRef]
16. Aldersey, H.M.; Francis, G.L.; Haines, S.J.; Chiu, C.Y. Family quality of life in the Democratic Republic of the Congo. *J. Policy Pract. Intellect. Disabil.* **2017**, *14*, 78–86. [CrossRef]
17. Aznar, A.S.; Castañón, D.G. Quality of life from the point of view of Latin American families: A participative research study. *J. Intellect. Disabil. Res.* **2005**, *49*, 784–788. [CrossRef]
18. Gràcia, M.; Vilaseca, R.; Balcells, A.; Simó, D.; Salvador, F. Family quality of life-scale (FQOL-S) (younger and older than 18 years old). *J. Appl. Res. Intellect. Disabil.* **2010**, *23*, 505. [CrossRef]
19. Poston, D.; Turnbull, A.; Park, J.; Mannan, H.; Marquis, J.; Wang, M. Family quality of life: A qualitative inquiry. *Ment. Retard.* **2003**, *41*, 313–328. [CrossRef]

20. Isaacs, B.J.; Brown, I.; Brown, R.I.; Baum, N.; Myerscough, T.; Neikrug, S.; Roth, D.; Shearer, J.; Wang, M. The international family quality of life project: Goals and description of a survey tool. *J. Policy Pract. Intellect. Disabil.* **2007**, *4*, 177–185. [CrossRef]
21. Samuel, P.S.; Rillotta, F.; Brown, I. The development of family quality of life concepts and measures. *J. Intellect. Disabil. Res.* **2012**, *56*, 1–16. [CrossRef]
22. Hoffman, L.; Marquis, J.; Poston, D.; Summers, J.A.; Turnbull, A. Assessing family outcomes: Psychometric evaluation of the Beach Center Family Quality of Life Scale. *J. Marriage Fam.* **2006**, *68*, 1069–1083. [CrossRef]
23. Brown, I.; Brown, R.I.; Baum, N.T.; Isaacs, B.J.; Myerscough, T.; Neikrug, S.; Roth, D.; Shearer, J.; Wang, M. *Family Quality of Life Survey: Main Caregivers of People with Intellectual or Developmental Disabilities*; Survey Place Centre: Toronto, ON, Canada, 2006.
24. Balcells-Balcells, A.; Giné, C.; Guàrdia-Olmos, J.; Summers, J.A. Proposal of indexes to evaluate Family Quality of Life, Partnership, and Family support needs. *Revista Iberoamericana de Psicología y Salud* **2016**, *7*, 31–40. [CrossRef]
25. Chiu, C.Y.; Seo, H.; Turnbull, A.P.; Summers, J.A. Confirmatory factor analysis of a family quality of life scale for Taiwanese families of children with intellectual disability/developmental delay. *Intellect. Dev. Disabil.* **2017**, *55*, 57–71. [CrossRef]
26. Zuna, N.I.; Seiling, J.P.; Summers, J.A.; Turnbull, A.P. Confirmatory factor analysis of a family quality of life scale for families of kindergarden children without disabilities. *J. Early Interv.* **2009**, *31*, 111–125. [CrossRef]
27. Balcells-Balcells, A.; Giné, C.; Guàrdia-Olmos, J.; Summers, J.A. Family quality of life: Adaptation to Spanish population of several family support questionnaires. *J. Intellect. Disabil. Res.* **2011**, *55*, 1151–1163. [CrossRef]
28. Bello-Escamilla, N.; Rivadeneira, J.; Concha Toro, M.; Soto, A.; Díaz Martínez, X. Escala de Calidad de Vida Familiar: Validación y análisis en población chilena. *Univ. Psychol.* **2017**, *16*, 1–10. [CrossRef]
29. Chiu, S.J.; Chen, P.T.; Chou, Y.T.; Chien, L.Y. The Mandarin Chinese version of the Beach Centre Family Quality of Life Scale: Development and psychometric properties in Taiwanese families of children with developmental delay. *J. Intellect. Disabil. Res.* **2017**, *61*, 373–384. [CrossRef] [PubMed]
30. Hu, X.; Wang, M.; Fei, X. Family quality of life of Chinese families of children with intellectual disabilities. *J. Intellect. Disabil. Res.* **2012**, *56*, 30–44. [CrossRef] [PubMed]
31. Parpa, E.; Katsantonis, N.; Tsilika, E.; Galanos, A.; Mystakidou, K. Psychometric properties of the family quality of life scale in greek families with intellectual disabilities. *J. Dev. Phys. Disabil.* **2016**, *28*, 393–405. [CrossRef]
32. Rivard, M.; Mercier, C.; Mestari, Z.; Terroux, A.; Mello, C.; Bégin, J. Psychometric Properties of the Beach Center Family Quality of Life in French-speaking families with a preschool-aged child diagnosed with autism spectrum disorder. *Am. J. Intellect. Dev. Disabil.* **2017**, *122*, 439–452. [CrossRef]
33. Sainz, M.; Verdugo, M.A.; Delgado, J. Adaptación de la escala de calidad de vida familiar al contexto español. In *Cómo Mejorar la Calidad De Vida de las Personas Con Discapacidad. Instrumentos y Estrategias de Evaluación*; Verdugo, M.A., Ed.; Amarú: Salamanca, Spain, 2006; pp. 300–323.
34. Verdugo, M.A.; Córdoba, L.; Gómez, J. Spanish adaptation and validation of the Family Quality of Life Survey. *J. Intellect. Disabil. Res.* **2005**, *49*, 794–798. [CrossRef]
35. Verdugo, M.A.; Rodríguez, A.; Sáinz, F. *Escala de Calidad de Vida Familiar*; Universidad de Salamanca, INICO: Salamanca, Spain, 2012.
36. Waschl, N.; Xie, H.; Chen, M.; Poon, K.K. Construct, Convergent, and Discriminant Validity of the Beach Center Family Quality of Life Scale for Singapore. *Infants Young Child.* **2019**, *32*, 201–214. [CrossRef]
37. Perry, A.; Isaacs, B. Validity of the family quality of life survey-2006. *J. Appl. Res. Intellect. Disabil.* **2015**, *28*, 584–588. [CrossRef]
38. Samuel, P.S.; Pociask, F.D.; DiZazzo-Miller, R.; Carrellas, A.; LeRoy, B.W. Concurrent validity of the international family quality of life survey. *Occup. Ther. Health Care* **2016**, *30*, 187–201. [CrossRef]
39. Samuel, P.S.; Tarraf, W.; Marsack, C. Family quality of life survey (FQOLs-2006): Evaluation of internal consistency, construct, and criterion validity for socioeconomically disadvantaged families. *Phys. Occup. Ther. Pediatr.* **2018**, *38*, 46–63. [CrossRef]
40. García-Grau, P.; McWilliam, R.A.; Martínez-Rico, G.; Grau-Sevilla, M.D. Factor structure and internal consistency of a Spanish version of the family quality of life (FaQoL). *Appl. Res. Qual. Life.* **2018**, *13*, 385–398. [CrossRef]

41. McWilliam, R.A.; Casey, A.M. *Factor Analysis of Family Quality of Life (FaQoL)*; Unpublished Manuscript: Nashville, TN, USA, 2013.
42. Giné, C.; Vilaseca, R.; Gràcia, M.; Mora, J.; Orcasitas, J.R.; Simón, C.; Torrecillas, A.M.; Beltran, F.S.; Dalmau, M.; Pro, M.T.; et al. Spanish family quality of life scales: Under and over 18 years old. *J. Intellect. Dev. Disabil.* **2013**, *38*, 141–148. [CrossRef] [PubMed]
43. Córdoba, L.; Gómez, J.; Verdugo, M.A. Calidad de vida familiar en personas con discapacidad: Un análisis comparativo. *Univ. Psychol.* **2008**, *7*, 369–383.
44. Mas, J.M.; Baqués, N.; Balcells-Balcells, A.; Dalmau, M.; Giné, C.; Gràcia, M.; Vilaseca, R. Family quality of life for families in early intervention in Spain. *J. Early Interv.* **2016**, *38*, 59–74. [CrossRef]
45. Rillotta, F.; Kirby, N.; Shearer, J.; Nettelbeck, T. Family quality of life of Australian families with a member with an intellectual/developmental disability. *J. Intellect. Disabil. Res.* **2012**, *56*, 71–86. [CrossRef] [PubMed]
46. Rodrigues, S.A.; Fontanella, B.J.; de Avó, L.R.; Germano, C.M.; Melo, D.G. A qualitative study about quality of life in Brazilian families with children who have severe or profound intellectual disability. *J. Appl. Res. Intellect. Disabil.* **2019**, *32*, 413–426. [CrossRef]
47. Boehm, T.L.; Carter, E.W. Family quality of life and its correlates among parents of children and adults with intellectual disability. *Am. J. Intellect. Dev. Disabil.* **2019**, *124*, 99–115. [CrossRef]
48. Meral, B.F.; Cavkaytar, A.; Turnbull, A.P.; Wang, M. Family quality of life of Turkish families who have children with intellectual disabilities and autism. *Res. Pract. Pers. Sev. Disabl.* **2013**, *38*, 233–246. [CrossRef]
49. Mori, Y.; Downs, J.; Wong, K.; Anderson, B.; Epstein, A.; Leonard, H. Impacts of caring for a child with the CDKL5 disorder on parental wellbeing and family quality of life. *Orphanet. J. Rare. Dis.* **2017**, *12*, 16:1–16:15. [CrossRef]
50. Wang, M.; Turnbull, A.P.; Summers, J.A.; Little, T.D.; Poston, D.J.; Mannan, H.; Turnbull, R. Severity of disability and income as predictors of parents' satisfaction with their family quality of life during early childhood years. *Res. Pract. Pers. Sev. Disabl.* **2004**, *29*, 82–94. [CrossRef]
51. Davis, K.; Gavidia-Payne, S. The impact of child, family, and professional support characteristics on the quality of life in families of young children with disabilities. *J. Intellect. Dev. Disabil.* **2009**, *34*, 153–162. [CrossRef]
52. Hielkema, T.; Boxum, A.G.; Hamer, E.G.; La Bastide-Van Gemert, S.; Dirks, T.; Reinders-Messelink, H.A.; Maathuis, G.B.; Verheijden, J.; Geertzen, J.H.B.; Hadders-Algra, M. LEARN2MOVE 0–2 years, a randomized early intervention trial for infants at very high risk of cerebral palsy: Family outcome and infant's functional outcome. *Disabil. Rehabil.* **2019**. [CrossRef] [PubMed]
53. Hsiao, Y.J. Autism spectrum disorders: Family demographics, parental stress, and family quality of life. *J. Policy Pract. Intellect. Disabil.* **2018**, *15*, 70–79. [CrossRef]
54. Summers, J.A.; Marquis, J.; Mannan, H.; Turnbull, A.P.; Fleming, K.; Poston, D.J.; Wang, M.; Kupzyk, K. Relationship of perceived adequacy of services, family–professional partnerships, and family quality of life in early childhood service programmes. *Int. J. Disabil. Dev. Ed.* **2007**, *54*, 319–338. [CrossRef]
55. Vanderkerken, L.; Heyvaert, M.; Onghena, P.; Maes, B. The Relation Between Family Quality of Life and the Family-Centered Approach in Families With Children With an Intellectual Disability. *J. Policy Pract. Intellect. Disabil.* **2019**, *16*, 296–311. [CrossRef]
56. Zeng, S.; Hu, X.; Zhao, H.; Stone-MacDonald, A.K. Examining the relationships of parental stress, family support and family quality of life: A structural equation modeling approach. *Res. Dev. Disabil.* **2020**, *96*, 103523. [CrossRef] [PubMed]
57. Families Special Interest Research Group of IASSIDD. Families supporting a child with intellectual or developmental disabilities: The current state of knowledge. *J. Appl. Res. Intellect. Disabil.* **2014**, *27*, 420–430. [CrossRef] [PubMed]
58. Cordero, B. *Calidad de Vida y Necesidades de Apoyo de las Familias de Personas con Discapacidad en Edades Tempranas en Costa Rica*. Ph.D. Thesis, Universitat Ramon Llull, Barcelona, Spain, 2019.
59. Bitencourt, D.S.; Gracia, M.G.; Beltran, F.S. Family quality of life: Content validity of a tool for families of adults with intellectual disabilities in Brazil. *Eurasia Proc. Educ. Soc. Sci.* **2015**, *3*, 57–65.
60. Giné, C.; Gràcia, M.; Vilaseca, R.; Salvador Beltran, F.; Balcells-Balcells, A.; Dalmau Montala, M.; Adam-Alcocer, A.L.; Pro, M.T.; Simó-Pinatella, D.; Mas, J.M. Family Quality of Life for People With Intellectual Disabilities in Catalonia. *J. Policy Pract. Intellect. Disabil.* **2015**, *12*, 244–254. [CrossRef]

61. Gràcia, M.; Simón, C.; Salvador-Beltran, F.; Adam Alcocer, A.L.; Mas, J.M.; Giné, C.; Dalmau, M. The transition process from center-based programmes to family-centered practices in Spain: A multiple case study. *Early Child Dev. Care* **2019**. [CrossRef]
62. American Educational Research Association; American Psychological Association; National Council on Measurement in Education. *The Standards for Educational and Psychological Testing*; American Educational Research Association: Washington, DC, USA, 2014.
63. International Test Commission. International Guidelines for Test Use. *Int. J. Test.* **2001**, *1*, 93–114. [CrossRef]
64. Muthén, L.K.; Muthén, B.O. *Mplus User's Guide*, 7th ed.; Muthén & Muthén: Los Angeles, CA, USA, 2015.
65. Wheaton, B.; Muthen, B.; Alwin, D.F.; Summers, G.F. Assessing reliability and stability in panel models. *Sociol. Methodol.* **1977**, *8*, 84–136. [CrossRef]
66. Browne, M.W.; Cudeck, R. Alternative ways of assessing model fit. *Sociol. Methods Res.* **1992**, *21*, 230–258. [CrossRef]
67. Thompson, B. *Exploratory and Confirmatory Factor Analysis: Understanding Concepts and Applications*; American Psychological Association: Washington, DC, USA, 2004.
68. Hu, L.T.; Bentler, P.M. Cutoff criteria for fit indexes in covariance structure analysis: Conventional criteria versus new alternatives. *Struct. Equ. Modeling* **1999**, *6*, 1–55. [CrossRef]
69. Kim, J.O.; Mueller, C.W. *Factor Analysis: Statistical Methods and Practical Issues*; Sage Publications: Beberly Hills, CA, USA, 1978.
70. Lohelin, J.C.; Beaujean, A. *Latent Variable Models: An Introduction to Factor, Path, and Structural Equation Analysis*; Routledge: New York, NY, USA, 2017.
71. Wang, M.; Brown, R. Family quality of life: A framework for policy and social service provisions to support families of children with disabilities. *J. Fam. Soc. Work* **2009**, *12*, 144–167. [CrossRef]
72. Jokinen, N.S.; Brown, R.I. Family quality of life and older-aged families of adults with an intellectual disability. In *Enhancing the Quality of Life of People with Intellectual Disabilities: From Theory to Practice*; Kober, R., Ed.; Springer: Dordrecht, The Netherlands, 2010; pp. 377–398.
73. Mas, J.M.; Giné, C.; McWilliam, R.A. The adaptation process of families with children with intellectual disabilities in Catalonia. *Infants Young Child.* **2016**, *29*, 335–351. [CrossRef]
74. Brown, R.I.; Hong, K.; Shearer, J.; Wang, M.; Wang, S.Y. Family quality of life in several countries: Results and discussion of satisfaction in families where there is a child with a disability. In *Enhancing the Quality of Life of People with Intellectual Disabilities: From Theory to Practice*; Kober, R., Ed.; Springer: Dordrecht, The Netherlands, 2010; pp. 377–398.
75. Valverde, B.B.D.R.; Jurdi, A.P.S. Analysis of the Relationship Between Early Intervention and Family Quality of Life. *Revista Brasileira de Educação Especial* **2020**, *26*, 171–186. [CrossRef]
76. Clark, M.; Brown, R.; Karrapaya, R. An initial look at the quality of life of Malaysian families that include children with disabilities. *J. Intellect. Disabil. Res.* **2012**, *56*, 45–60. [CrossRef]
77. Bertelli, M.; Bianco, A.; Rossi, M.; Scuticchio, D.; Brown, I. Relationship between individual quality of life and family quality of life for people with intellectual disability living in Italy. *J. Intellect. Disabil. Res.* **2011**, *55*, 1136–1150. [CrossRef]
78. Wang, M.; Summers, J.A.; Little, T.; Turnbull, A.; Poston, D.; Mannan, H. Perspectives of fathers and mothers of children in early intervention programmes in assessing family quality of life. *J. Intellect. Disabil. Res.* **2006**, *50*, 977–988. [CrossRef]
79. Vanderkerken, L.; Heyvaert, M.; Onghena, P.; Maes, B. Mother Quality of Life or Family Quality of Life? A survey on the Quality of Life in families with children with intellectual disabilities using home-based support in Flanders. *J. Intellect. Disabil. Res.* **2016**, *60*, 756.

Publisher's Note: MDPI stays neutral with regard to jurisdictional claims in published maps and institutional affiliations.

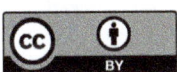

© 2020 by the authors. Licensee MDPI, Basel, Switzerland. This article is an open access article distributed under the terms and conditions of the Creative Commons Attribution (CC BY) license (http://creativecommons.org/licenses/by/4.0/).

MDPI
St. Alban-Anlage 66
4052 Basel
Switzerland
Tel. +41 61 683 77 34
Fax +41 61 302 89 18
www.mdpi.com

International Journal of Environmental Research and Public Health Editorial Office
E-mail: ijerph@mdpi.com
www.mdpi.com/journal/ijerph

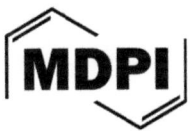

www.ingramcontent.com/pod-product-compliance
Lightning Source LLC
LaVergne TN
LVHW070709100526
838202LV00013B/1058